MASTERS OF HEALTH

Masters of Health

RACIAL SCIENCE AND SLAVERY
IN U.S. MEDICAL SCHOOLS

CHRISTOPHER D. E. WILLOUGHBY

THE UNIVERSITY OF NORTH CAROLINA PRESS

Chapel Hill

Designed by Richard Hendel
Set in Utopia by codeMantra
Manufactured in the United States of America

Cover illustration: Samuel Morton's facial goniometer.
Photo courtesy of the Huntington Library, San Marino, Calif.

Library of Congress Cataloging-in-Publication Data
Names: Willoughby, Christopher D. E., author.
Title: Masters of health : racial science and slavery in
U.S. medical schools / Christopher D. E. Willoughby.
Other titles: Racial science and slavery in U.S. medical schools
Description: Chapel Hill : The University of North Carolina Press,
[2022] | Includes bibliographical references and index.
Identifiers: LCCN 2022020606 | ISBN 9781469671840 (cloth ; alk. paper) |
ISBN 9781469672120 (paperback) | ISBN 9781469671857 (ebook)
Subjects: LCSH: Medicine—Study and teaching—United States—
History. | Scientific racism—United States—History. | Discrimination
in medical education—United States—History. | Medical colleges—
United States—History. | Medical education—Political aspects. |
Monogenism and polygenism. | Slavery—United States—History. |
African Americans—Social conditions—History.
Classification: LCC R745 .W54 2022 | DDC 610.76—dc23/eng/20220625
LC record available at https://lccn.loc.gov/2022020606

A version of chapter 7 originally appeared as "'His Native,
Hot Country': Racial Science and Environment in Antebellum
American Medical Thought," *Journal of the History of Medicine and
Allied Sciences* 72, no. 3 (July 2017): 328–51. Reprinted with permission.

For Urmi and my parents

CONTENTS

FIGURES

ABBREVIATIONS

MCSC
Medical College of South Carolina

MDUP
Medical Department of the University of Pennsylvania

UVA
University of Virginia

MASTERS OF HEALTH

INTRODUCTION

In fact, from having been trained & drilled to certain duties;
[the enslaved person's] body has become a mere machine
subservient to his master's will.
—Joseph Hinson Mellichamp, "On the Causes of Insanity in the
    United States," M.D. thesis, Medical College of South Carolina, 1852

On July 1, 1857, Samuel Forwood, an enslaver from south Alabama, wrote a letter to his son, Dr. William Stump Forwood, about an article the younger Forwood had written in that May's *Medical and Surgical Reporter*. Three years prior, William had graduated from the Medical Department of the University of Pennsylvania (MDUP). He was one of the hundreds of southern students who traveled to Philadelphia for medical education each year in the decades leading up to the Civil War. Like other young and ambitious physicians, William Stump Forwood contributed essays to medical journals both to add legitimacy to his new practice and to build a reputation in the nation's rapidly expanding medical profession. This particular article was entitled "The Negro—a Distinct Species." Over the course of the essay, he argued that Black people were a distinct species as defined by their supposed anatomies, heavily citing Joseph Leidy, his former anatomy professor at MDUP.

As the letter revealed, William's slaveholder father found the piece offensive. Samuel was a very religious man, and like many antebellum Christians, he thought polygenesis—the theory that each race was created separately—blasphemous. Though he supported free intellectual inquiry into the subject, Samuel nonetheless believed that it amounted to "a conflict with sacred history to occupy such a ground." Despite being a southern enslaver, Samuel Forwood balked at the idea of permanent divisions of humanity dating back to God's creation.[1]

The letter went on to report that Samuel Forwood had shared the issue of the *Medical and Surgical Reporter* with two local doctors. One ardently agreed with William, and the other was currently reading the article with interest. While this was no poll of the national medical profession, it was telling. Both doctors were intimately familiar with the theory, and at least one subscribed to it. Moreover, throughout that year and the next in the *Medical and Surgical Reporter*, physicians continued to debate polygenesis. While the belief was not universally held, the journal reflected the degree to which study of racial difference and human origins had gained significant traction among medical professionals in the decade before the Civil War.[2]

Even when physicians disagreed with polygenesis as a causal explanation for racial difference, they nevertheless tended to agree that essential racial differences existed, even if time or climate might erase them. In his June 1857 refutation of Forwood and polygenesis, for example, Senex agreed with many of Forwood's descriptions of Black people's bodies. He just disputed the primordial nature of these differences. He even concluded, "Whilst I deny that the negro is of another species from the European, I readily admit his inferiority." He went on to explain, "God permits the enslaving of the Africans, though this does not justify the conduct of their captors." "I am no 'northern abolitionist,'" he asserted.[3] In short, what separated Forwood and Senex most clearly was not whether they supported slavery or believed in essentialist racial differences. Rather, they disagreed over whether white supremacy was the product of distinct biblical creations that justified species differentiation. Both agreed that racial differences were real and embodied.

This anecdote captures much of the central argument of this book. First, it reveals how racial slavery created a market for the production of racial medicine. Doctors like William Stump Forwood used their racial expertise to navigate the southern political and economic landscape, and claims to racial knowledge made them appealing experts for enslavers. It was also no coincidence that William attended the University of Pennsylvania to study medicine. Northern schools sought to attract southern students like Forwood through their racial pedagogy, and this choice had a corollary effect of creating a national medical discourse about race. Second, *Masters of Health* argues that racial thinking underwrote the professionalization of medicine in the United States. In short, as medicine created socially and culturally powerful institutions of education, physicians also embraced racist ideas about the nature of humanity and health. These ideas were critical to creating a national medical culture. This unified medical culture created durable professional bonds in an era of national division over slavery, culminating in the outbreak of civil war in 1861. Thus, in the 1850s, even when some southern-nationalist doctors criticized northern schools as abolitionist, other southern doctors like Forwood could point to northern schools' racial curricula to defend their own training and their alma maters. In a time of division, then, racial science allowed doctors to stay remarkably unified.

Likewise, this book also argues that the theory of polygenesis was central to the creation of racial medicine and racial thinking more broadly in the United States. Though historians have documented this debate over creation and human origins, they often focus on the apparent fracture among scientists about the origins of racial difference. This tendency, though, has masked the level of agreement that prevailed among early national and antebellum physicians when it came to applying polygenesis to notions of embodied difference. Polygenists' most critical legacy, I argue, did not relate to the origins of racial difference. In this regard, their theory was closer to the blip on the radar as described by historians of racial science. In this narrative, polygenesis came into ascendancy in the middle of the nineteenth century only to be quickly rendered archaic by Charles Darwin's theory of natural selection. However, polygenists' most important and lasting contribution to science, medicine, and racism was how they depicted racial differences as enduring and embodied. Since the founding of the first U.S. medical school, MDUP, in 1765, medical faculty had been discussing race with their students as a part of their pedagogy. By the antebellum era, medical school pedagogies reproduced many of polygenists' concepts of racial bodily difference, even as physicians were not required to believe in polygenists' revisions to biblical creation. In this sense, this book reveals that by the end of the antebellum era, many of polygenists' central ideas were widely held and largely unchallenged within the medical profession. This belief did not disappear in the wake of the Darwinian revolution but continued to haunt medicine.

As well as being sites of production of racial theories, U.S. medical schools were also important nodes of their dissemination. After completing their education, physicians entered countless towns, cities, and rural areas in the South, the Midwest, and the West. Like Samuel Forwood's neighbors, local physicians were often the leading, if not only, trained scientists in their communities. Thus, their opinions carried considerable weight. Many of these doctors were not doctrinal polygenists, even as they practiced a version of medicine shaped by the theory. As with Senex and Forwood, whether or not doctors disagreed about racial origins, most believed that blackness was accompanied by embodied essential traits that affected Black people's health outcomes.

When William Stump Forwood wrote "The Negro—a Distinct Species" in 1857, Abraham Lincoln's election as president remained years away. Even so, the ongoing regional civil war known as "Bleeding Kansas," endemic white fears of enslaved rebellion, and decades of political fracture shaped the urgency of Forwood's and others' writings. The sectional conflict over slavery had been gestating since the revolution, yet despite this political conflict that had been simmering for decades, Forwood and many other white southern males attended medical schools in the North until secession made it nearly impossible. These schools were not bastions of abolitionism, and they hoped to attract southern students. They came into being during the tumultuous century of debates over slavery from the 1760s to 1860, and built slavery and racial thinking into the foundations of the nation's medical education.

Once they graduated, physicians acted as the foot soldiers for racial science and medicine, and they were a part of an emergent managerial class in American life. Faculty at colonial North American and later U.S. medical schools taught that race had a profound impact on medical practice. In his 1798 printed syllabus, MDUP professor, abolitionist, and signer of the Declaration of Independence Benjamin Rush included a section for students to take notes on the "peculiar diseases of negroes." In his lectures in 1809-10, MDUP professor Benjamin Smith Barton told his students that humanity comprised five races or varieties: "Caucasian," "Mongolians," "Etheopica," "Americana," and "Malaical—or those inhabiting the islands of the South Seas." In the 1858 edition of his textbook *A Treatise on the Practice of Medicine*, MDUP professor George B. Wood told his student readers that Black patients were less affected by miasmatic fevers. Wood also asserted that they required less quinine than whites in cases of intermittent fever.[4] Faculty at other institutions made similar claims. Some even directly supported slavery in their writings and teachings. These professors' prescriptions represented just a small sample of the racial pedagogy developed and disseminated in the first century of U.S. medical schools.

By the end of the antebellum period, American medical students in the North and South were taught the prevailing scientific theories about the origins of racial difference: polygenesis and monogenesis. In contrast to polygenists, monogenists asserted that races shared a common point of origin but had been changed into their current forms by climate and other external forces. With a few exceptions, though, white antebellum scientists on neither side of the debate supported any plan approximating racial equality. In contrast, by the end of the antebellum period, most monogenists shared polygenists' belief that Black people's bodies had essential differences. This represented a shift from earlier racial theorists who thought doctors might be able to turn Black people white or maybe that Black people would naturally turn white in a temperate climate. Even this hope for equality through whitening assumed the superiority of a white culture and skin color.

In the first century of medical schools in the United States, professors and their students created a structural relationship between medical education and the dissemination of racial science. This story began in colonial

North America when William Shippen Jr. dissected a Black man during a series of public medical lectures in 1762 in Philadelphia.[5] Building on these initial lectures, three years later, Shippen and John Morgan founded the first medical school at the College of Philadelphia (referred to afterward as the Medical Department of the University of Pennsylvania, or MDUP). This early period also coincided with a growing white interest in abolishing slavery in some British North American colonies, as well as the Atlantic slave trade itself. Medical schools in the United States, then, gestated alongside political debates about the future of slavery, culminating with the Civil War.

Giving racial essentialism a greater veneer of legitimacy, faculty provided students opportunities to gain direct experience in manipulating and analyzing Black people's bodies. Polygenesis came into prominence at the height of "empirical" medicine in the Atlantic World. Polygenist physicians such as MDUP anatomy professor Joseph Leidy were a part of the movement that discarded eighteenth-century models of disease causation in favor of clinical observation, pathological anatomy, and environmental determinism.[6]

Clinical and anatomical medicine directly emphasized experience. Through empirical approaches, professors taught students to think of diseases as caused by different afflictions local to specific parts of the body. Simultaneously, they depicted people of African descent's bodies as defined by small, local anatomical distinctions dispersed across the organs and skeletal structure. The apparent racial issues inherent to the sectional political conflict certainly caused racial science to come to the forefront of American medicine. Yet empirical medicine's focus on anatomy and observation-based evidence most clearly shaped the texture of the language and arguments undergirding polygenesis.

By the middle of the nineteenth century, anatomical and epidemiological notions of racial difference worked symbiotically to depict people of African descent as a distinct species that required unique treatments. In his racial science research notes, for example, William Stump Forwood enunciated many of the definitive medical and social concepts that had been incorporated into medical education during the first half of the nineteenth century. Forwood's headings in his notes include "Climate, effects of," "Negro's Diseases," and "Longevity of the Negro." Forwood claimed that people of African descent were suited for hard labor in hot climates and constitutionally protected from southern scourges like malaria and yellow fever. As well as justifying slavery, physicians attempted to frame the biological limitations and policy of European and U.S. imperial projects. As a result, medical professionals fashioned themselves as authorities and health regulators over the flow of peoples and goods that made up the Atlantic World and burgeoning global economy.[7]

Discussion of disease susceptibility and the environment only represented one part of the equation for naturalizing Black people as inferior. Forwood's notes also reflect the influence of anatomical thinking in medical education. Similar to other physician-polygenists, Forwood focused his readings on subjects such as "Approach of Negro to Animals," "Negro Brain + Physiognomy," "Anatomical Peculiarities," "Antiquity of the Types," "Intellect in Africa," and the "Negro's Incapacity for Civilization."[8] Antebellum medical professors shaped their racial pedagogies around similar topics, and Forwood actively reproduced them. Through environmental medicine, racial scientists and physicians shaped the geographic and social limits of Black people. Using anatomy, they framed the differences of people of African descent through an imagined and racially specific physical structure.

Medical faculties' embrace of biologically determinist race constructs occurred simultaneously with growth in the number of medical schools in the United States. These developments were symbiotic, with physicians obtaining further social power through their perceived ability to define racial difference just as schools grew numerically. The proliferation of medical schools also allowed physicians to lay claim to being a geographically diverse profession with a shared ideology and set of practices. In the eighteenth century and before, when medical education was primarily based in apprenticing, claims to shared knowledge were harder to sustain. As a result, in the late antebellum era, a whole generation of physicians emerged that were trained to see racial groups as defined by imagined anatomical and physiological differences. When he was a student at MDUP in the early 1850s, Forwood was part of a graduating class that likely comprised more than 300 students.[9] At MDUP, they learned about racial determinants of disease contraction, supposedly distinctive anatomies of each racial group, and even aspects of controlling enslaved patients' behavior, also known as plantation management. Prefiguring the so-called search for the missing link in popular culture and post-Darwinian biology, polygenists had already begun to frame the bodies of African descendants as an intermediary between apes and white humanity.

Masters of Health argues that institutional medical education served to create a much larger medical profession with claims to expertise in defining racial difference. Likewise, educators in these institutions worked to develop a broad consensus among physicians on the indefinite and embodied nature of racial differences. When discussing polygenesis and monogenesis, previous scholars often depicted these causal explanations for racial differences as diametrically opposed. In some ways, they were. Of course, people who believed that Black and white people descended from a shared ancestry differed intellectually from those who did not. Likewise, monogenists' belief in the possibility of bodily changes that created racial differences implied that this process could theoretically be reversed. Yet by the middle of the nineteenth century, few white American monogenists still claimed that race could be changed quickly. Instead, they argued that Black people needed tutelage from whites on plantations or in segregated societies, and that the embodied differences that separated Black and white people would persist indefinitely. In some respects, late antebellum monogenists and polygenists disagreed about the causes of racial differences. Still, most shared a commitment to a belief that racial differences were embodied and likely to persist for the foreseeable future.

Similarly, in telling the history of slavery and racial science in medical education, it is essential to consider how these ideas were being applied to support burgeoning empire and global capitalism in the United States. Racial science and medicine emerged out of systems of enslavement and colonialism, but as these ideas became embedded in medical thought and education, they were able to mature and persist after slavery's abolition. Thus, this book helps explain why racial thinking rooted in the history of slavery has been so difficult to expunge from contemporary medical practice.

Even before slavery was abolished, medical racial theories were connected to and being applied to other social and political issues, ensuring that these ideas' utility would outlive the slave system. Collections of racial skulls held in medical school museums were built through the networks and violence of global empires and capitalism as well as Atlantic slavery. Likewise, many elite antebellum medical professors traveled abroad, and they constructed concepts of race and health in the tropics. These theories represented some of the earliest enunciations of what would become tropical medicine. Professors' observations on health in the tropics combined with globally sourced racial skull collections encouraged students to compare peoples globally. At Harvard for example, students could study skulls from Hawaii, Senegal, and India. This meant that polygenists influenced more than domestic racial politics and social structures. They also shaped white Americans' international outlook just as the United States was beginning to expand its influence around the world.

Thus, *Masters of Health* embraces a transnational framework for understanding the history of U.S. medicine, while also arguing for an expansion of medical history's purview. The book follows medical students, faculty, and institutional forces where their minds, bodies, and professional networks wandered. In some chapters, this means engaging with students' political beliefs about slavery, imperialism, and the genocide of non-white races outside the United States. This is political, intellectual history, but the venue, an M.D. thesis, is inherently medical. Chapter 5, as an example, makes forays into the history of the Opium Wars in China, British colonization of southern Africa, and one of the largest slave revolts in Brazilian history, the Muslim uprising. These conflicts directly contributed to the death and disruption of the lives of people whose skulls were held in Harvard's medical school.

Stories of these conflicts and the ways that they turned people into cadavers and remains on display at Harvard's Warren Anatomical Museum are not sad appendices in the history of medical education. They represent the hidden foundation of exploitation that exists beneath much of the history of medicine and medical education in the United States. Like slavery, capitalism and imperialism helped wed the world together, and medicine and medical schools did not exist outside that world. Instead, medical faculty exploited it for knowledge production, opportunities for transatlantic travel, and professional prestige. This book contends that stories of medical politics and victims of museum collectors hold a central place in medical history. Properly understanding that history requires centering the ideas, people, and places that were discussed in medical schools but are not neatly captured in histories of individual medical theories or epidemics.[10]

In his classic 1960 study *The Leopard's Spots: Scientific Attitudes toward Race in America, 1815–59*, historian William Stanton argues that polygenists, despite their racism, advanced a secular approach to science that opened the door for Charles Darwin's theory of evolution.[11] While there is some merit to this argument, racial anatomy continued to be taught in medical schools long after Darwinian evolution became widely accepted, just with a different causal mechanism. The notion that race could be defined bodily and medically endured for many future generations because early theorists of essentialist racial medicine had succeeded in creating an intellectual home for these ideas: the medical school.

The history of racial thinking in medical schools challenges previous depictions of U.S. racial science and medicine as a distinctively southern set of phenomena. In this frame, scholars depict polygenists as primarily focused on using science to shore up support for a southern slave system threatened by abolitionism in the late eighteenth- and nineteenth-century Atlantic World. Since 1971, when George Fredrickson first published *The Black Image in the White Mind: The Debate over Afro-American Character and Destiny, 1817–1914*, political historians who study polygenesis have often focused on its influence over the proslavery movement. Fredrickson and more recent political historians discussing polygenesis emphasize the ideology's support for the southern slave system, and how it laid an intellectual groundwork for Jim Crow segregation. In this framework, racial scientists themselves often appear as craven secessionist plotters with little commitment to the validity of their theories.[12]

Likewise, when scholars discuss polygenesis's popularity in the North, they focus on just that, its popular appeal. Fredrickson's readers likely would not assume that polygenesis had a significant foothold in Ivy League medical schools, which remain some of the leading higher education institutions in the United States. This should not be taken to mean that polygenesis did not have popular appeal, or that it was not used to garner support for slavery and segregation. Fredrickson is right.[13] Understanding polygenesis's most enduring legacy, though, requires situating its proponents alongside a different set of contemporary ideas and an alternative audience from those discussed in political histories. Instead, we must examine medical theory, faculty, and students. Through this framing, key racial theorists appear in a different light, and a new and perhaps more important class of trained racial essentialists emerges—the average American physician. This approach also helps explain why essentialist racial thinking has been so difficult to extricate from medical practice and training in the more than a century and a half after emancipation. Simply put, early medical faculty built racial essentializing into the foundations of these institutions in the North and the South.

Analyzing both the medical and political context, *Masters of Health* contends that polygenesis and essentialist racial medicine evolved through the shifting tides of racial and medical theory in the United States and abroad. Historians of science have long recognized that polygenesis's appeal resided in the theory's ability to speak the language of both nineteenth-century racism and science. Scholars such as Terence Keel, Nancy Stepan, and Melissa Stein have emphasized how, for much of the eighteenth and nineteenth centuries, science and politics were not seen as in conflict. In short, there was nothing incongruous or unethical about overtly shaping political and social ideologies through science and medicine or vice versa. In fact, consciously or unconsciously, these were the forces that routinely shaped polygenist thought. This dynamic is why scholars avoid terms such as "pseudoscience" to describe antiquated racial science. Polygenists would certainly be considered pseudoscientists today. In the nineteenth century, however, they were on the cutting edge, claiming that their opponents opposed secular science and lacked an empirical understanding of race.

Understanding polygenesis and racial medicine as having been considered good science in their historical context undermines the use of scientific authority to support spurious racial theories in the present.[14] Polygenists rose to prominence during a period of great flux in medicine and science generally. Inspired by religion, eighteenth-century theories of human health and human origins no longer seemed to explain the world that scientifically literate whites saw unfolding around them.[15] Polygenesis's prominence among antebellum doctors, rather than being an aberration, explains how seemingly dedicated scientists and physicians in the present continue to treat race as a biological category.[16] Historians of science, though, largely focus on elite theorists, leaving underexamined how average readers understood polygenesis. Analysis of medical students' reception of racial theories makes plain another route for the dispersal of essentialist racial constructs. Scattering after graduation, doctors who had studied racial science as a part of their medical education made their homes in communities across the United States.

In addition to scholarship on antebellum racial science, this monograph also builds on decades of scholarship about the health and health-care practices of enslaved people. Previous historians of medicine and slavery in the Atlantic World have emphasized how physicians served a vital support role in many slave societies. Writing in the 1970s and 1980s about the South and the British Caribbean, Todd Savitt and Richard Sheridan revealed some of the profound biomedical effects of enslavement. Their works depict slavery as causing myriad health risks in addition to its brutal regimes of corporal punishment.[17] Nearly twenty years ago, pathbreaking scholar Sharla Fett argued that issues like epidemic disease only told one part of the history of medicine and health on Atlantic plantations. Instead, she reframed plantation medicine as contests of power between enslaver, physician, and patient. Fett's analysis emphasizes how white physicians could use medicine to heal or punish, and enslaved people employed their own healing practices to survive and resist bondage.[18] Building on Fett, Savitt, and Sheridan's work, *Masters of Health* examines the training and ideologies physicians brought to practice on plantations.

Other recent scholarship on the history of medicine and slavery has examined the role of African diasporic healers in the medical marketplace of the early modern Americas. Black healers, thinkers, and spiritual leaders analyzed and described the natural world. Like white thinkers, naturalists, and physicians, African diasporic commenters worked to create authoritative knowledge of health and nature in the Americas. They cataloged the plants of the Americas to create new healing techniques. In the diverse early Americas, African-descended healers influenced the cosmologies of white medics, Native healers, and vice versa.[19] These varied marketplaces of early modern medicine and healing provide an important context for this study. Constructing medical schools and valorizing formal training represented an effort to separate allopathic physicians from the array of healers selling their services in the eighteenth century. In fact, it was the most effective way to define physicians' legitimacy and denigrate other healing traditions in the United States.

Furthering this theme, scholars have shown that medical practice on enslaved people in the nineteenth century spurred the professionalization and institutionalization of southern medicine. Rana A. Hogarth's study of medical practice on enslaved people in Jamaica and South Carolina explains how physicians in turn-of-the-nineteenth-century slave societies relied on institutions such as hospitals and local medical schools to increase their power and market share. Likewise, Deirdre Cooper Owens emphasizes how pathbreaking gynecological surgeons such as J. Marion Sims created the new field of gynecology through a brutal trial-and-error approach toward enslaved women's bodies. These practitioners tested surgical cures for gynecological ailments commonly found on plantations and caused by hard labor and malnutrition. Stephen C. Kenny also has analyzed the relationship between slavery and medical institution building, uncovering how medical museums in the South were literally constructed from the remains of enslaved people. Finally, Civil War historian Jim Downs has probed how Union army medics approached practice on formerly enslaved people fleeing plantations. Downs finds that Union medics both exploited and neglected these self-liberated refugees. Hogarth, Cooper Owens, Kenny, and Downs draw out how physicians in slave societies understood institutionalization and professionalization as routes to garner more power and profit. Yet except for Downs's work on the Civil War and Reconstruction, none of these studies closely analyze the national appeal of the institutionalization of racial medicine.[20]

Masters of Health, though, is not a history of plantation health or politics or primarily a work of southern history, even as it contributes to each of these fields. Instead, it considers the history of slavery and medicine through the lens of institutional racism and the transnational nature of U.S. politics, medicine, and intellectual culture. In this sense, the book builds on recent trends in the history of slavery that connect slavery and its nineteenth-century proponents to both national and transnational forces of capitalism and institutional development. For well more than a decade, many universities have inquired into their historical entanglements in slave economies. Likewise, scholars like Walter Johnson and Daina Ramey Berry have analyzed the diverse ways that enslavers calculated the value of enslaved people's bodies in markets of exchange. Moreover, in *Ebony & Ivy: Race, Slavery, and the Troubled History of America's Universities*, Craig Steven Wilder reveals how Black people's enslavement, Native American genocide, and land expropriation were foundational to the rise of colonial North American universities. Other scholars ranging from Eric Williams and Sidney Mintz to Sven Beckert have revealed how the commodities enslaved people produced shaped capitalist economic development outside of the Americas and vice versa. These analyses illustrate that U.S. slavery was far from just a local or regional concern.[21]

This book embraces a similar framing. It argues that the acceleration of global commerce, the rise of U.S. universities, and the practice of closely analyzing non-white bodies were foundational to the construction of this new medical education system. Moreover, these factors were the context for the emergence of a medical profession with claims to expert knowledge on the meaning of blackness. Medical schools trained students to analyze Black people's bodies. These schools often were affiliated with the universities that Wilder discusses. Finally, the institutions benefited from and made exchanges across the networks of trade in goods and ideas that comprised nineteenth-century commercial capitalism.

Studying the history of medical education and slavery is also a route to demystifying racial thinking and unveiling its fundamentally flawed nature. Building on works by Troy Duster, Dorothy Roberts, Michael Yudell, and Harriett Washington, exposing early racial thinking's illogic reveals long-standing similarity between the ways in which antiquated and contemporary racial science became accepted by the medical community. Racial science and medicine act as forms of what scholars Karen Fields and Barbara Fields describe as "racecraft." Racecraft, they explain, represents a set of phenomena akin to witchcraft, where illogical fantasies like race become so deeply held that they take on the appearance of reality for adherents. As they assert, "Racecraft originates not in nature but human action and imagination; it can exist in no other way. The action and imagining are collective yet individual, day-to-day yet historical, and consequential even though nested in mundane routine." In many ways, racecraft is the subject of this book. Racecraft is the trappings that make the false biological concept of race seem real to its adherents. It naturalizes race, which becomes the justification for treating groups unequally based on perceptions of ancestry, or racism.[22] Thus, as well as seeking to understand historically specific questions about how the slave system and early racial science influenced the development of U.S. medical education, the following chapters provide some insights into why race continues to be reproduced by medical practitioners today.

While *Masters of Health* relies on the published and archival records of well-known physicians and scientists, it differs from previous studies of racial science by focusing on medical students as avatars for the average American physician. Analysis of over 4,000 dissertations written from 1807 to 1861 by students at the Medical College of South Carolina in Charleston (MCSC), Transylvania University in Lexington, Kentucky, the University of Nashville in Tennessee, and the University of Pennsylvania in Philadelphia makes it clear that racial science garnered a wide professional audience. Theses act as a sort of mirror for understanding medical pedagogy. In his 1860 "An Essay on Thesis," MDUP student L. B. Hayley described most theses as "nothing more than an incompletely disguised compilation."[23] As a result, theses provide insight into the education students received from their professors and textbooks. Aspiring physicians often restated or even plagiarized what they learned with little or no analytical additions. The pedagogical aim of these theses was to show how much students had learned about a specific topic during their medical education. As a result, the works reflect medical pedagogy, as opposed to original scholarship. Theses—combined with lecture notes, museum records, and the manuscript records of medical faculty at Columbia University, Harvard University, and the University of Virginia (UVA), among many other institutions—reveal how race became an established and relatively standardized part of medical education in the North and the South.

Just as with any medical topic, not every or even most students discussed race in their thesis. Approximately 10 percent of the students assessed included race in their theses, or a little more than 400 students. Within this subset, most students did not focus on race; rather, they brought it up organically as a part of discussing a separate medical topic. Even fewer students overtly defended or critiqued slavery. In passages on race from theses on topics ranging from lactation to tuberculosis, racial thinking manifests as a part of the patchwork of the medical curriculum, not the central focus. Like most twenty-first-century physicians' incidental forays into racial thinking, most early American medical students discussed race for overtly medical rather than political reasons.

Through these sources, *Masters of Health* revises our understanding of the legitimacy and influence of polygenesis in early U.S. medicine, as well as the destructive career of racial thinking in medical practice that endures into the present. Most clearly, this work argues that racial science instead of a niche field was a foundational part of the fabric of U.S. medical training, a part that was spread through the mundane operations of institutional medical education.

There are significant gaps in this story. Most notably, in the broader literature on early modern racial science through the nineteenth century, white scientists in the Americas and Atlantic World were perhaps as interested in categorizing Native Americans as they were in classifying people of African descent. In simply considering leading U.S. polygenist Samuel Morton's titles for his key texts Crania Americana; *or, a Comparative View of the Skulls of Various Aboriginal Nations* and Crania Aegyptiaca; *or, Observations on Egyptian Ethnography*, it becomes clear that racial scientists were not just interested in describing the bodies of Black people. Yet medical students and professors simply did not discuss Native Americans nearly as much as they did people of African descent, even as American racial scientists often examined both groups thoroughly. Where faculty talked about Native Americans readily was in the most transparent introduction of racial science into medical education: collections of and conversations about skulls and their measurement. Medical museums, much like natural history museums, collected the crania of all racial groups, but racial analysis based in medical practice was mostly reserved for people of African descent. Likewise, doctors confined discussions of Native Americans' bodies mostly to their skulls, where medical faculty posited a whole host of anatomical differences between white people's and Black people's bodies. In short, medical faculty discussed Native Americans within the traditional confines of racial science, but they did not create a larger set of medical practices meant to racialize Native American groups as they did for people of African descent.

Medical faculty and students discussed Native Americans much less for two key reasons. First, unlike in the case of enslaved people, where the paying customer was actually the enslaver, there was little financial incentive to construct a broad pedagogy on American Indian health care and anatomy (beyond skull measurements). Likewise, arguments about Black inferiority were meant to impress white enslaver consumers, not enslaved people themselves. While some physicians would practice on Native Americans on reservations or from remote forts, these practitioners were much smaller in number than the army of doctors that worked on plantations. These factors, combined with the successful displacement and genocide of many tribes east of the Mississippi River, simply made practice on Native Americans financially unimportant.

Second, Native Americans' laboring bodies were not valued by whites. In contrast, African descendants' bodily health needed to be preserved to maintain the prosperity of elite whites. In the case of Native Americans, whites viewed their continued existence as an impediment to forming a prosperous white nation. Native Americans' health and continued possession of lands east of the Mississippi actually prevented further development of land for cotton production and slave labor. Thus, just as James Fenimore Cooper was authoring *The Last of the Mohicans* and predicting the ultimate, if tragic, extinction of Native Americans, white Americans more broadly encouraged their disappearance through active displacement and genocide. In short, if doctors felt both financially and racially incentivized to preserve the bodies of people of African descent, the opposite was true of their feelings toward Native Americans. This active white desire for American Indian displacement and death helps explain why racially distinctive medical practices were mostly constructed for the bodies of African descendants.

Masters of Health is divided into three parts. Part 1 examines the emergence and coalescing of two worlds: medical education and racial science. These chapters argue that medical students participated in the development of a novel racial pedagogy built on the slave system, the rise of polygenesis, the expansion of medical schools, and the growing influence of numerical and clinical methodologies. Where part 1 is interested in large-scale structural and intellectual shifts, part 2 considers how this new medical education was experienced. Through examination of routine dissection, an anatomical pedagogy based in tactile and visual learning, and rare cases of experimentation on Black people's bodies, part 2 reveals how practical experience was essential to learning medicine and racial science. Finally, part 3 considers how these ideas were applied to social and political questions outside of the medical school. Particularly, these three chapters look at how physicians applied racial medicine to questions of domestic, Atlantic, and international racial politics.

Part 1 studies the rise of medical schools, polygenesis, and empirical medicine in light of growing debates about the future of slavery. Building the foundation of the book, chapter 1 unpacks the parallel evolutions of U.S. medical schools and the debate over racial origins from 1765 up to the Civil War. Racial-theorist medical faculty including Josiah Nott, Charles Caldwell, James Lawrence Cabell, and Samuel Morton produced essentialist racial science just as medical schools grew in the number of institutions and degrees granted. Chapter 2 argues that medical schools' racial pedagogies were built on knowledge produced on plantations and in the most elite sites of medical education in the first half of the nineteenth century: the Parisian clinics. Polygenists' methods—collecting, measuring, and aggregating thousands of sets of human remains—were rooted in the method of Parisian clinics and southern slave markets. Part 1 reveals how in just a century, U.S. medical education evolved from primarily local apprenticeships to dozens of medical schools producing graduates with claims to racial expertise.

Part 2 studies the training that made medics think and feel like "masters."[24] It examines how students were trained to see blackness, emphasizing the experiential and tactile nature of medical education. Chapter 3 unpacks the animalization and commodification of Black people's bodies through dissection and experimentation in medical schools. When dissecting and experimenting, students turned racial science into a series of actions that aped enslavers' control and commodification of Black people's bodies. Through hands-on experience, students learned to subordinate Black people in medical practice. Developing further the hands-on nature of this pedagogy, chapter 4 relates the quotidian operations of racial science in anatomical instruction. Racial anatomical pedagogy developed over the course of the first half of the nineteenth century, as can be seen in textbooks, lectures, and the anatomical museum. In short, medical faculty developed a coherent, multilayered racial anatomical pedagogy, where students could apply their learning from textbooks and lectures to dissection and the curated material culture of the museum.

This history would not be complete without reckoning with how these theories were applied to practice, the politics of slavery, and nascent U.S. imperialism, the foci of part 3. In chapter 5, I address the geopolitical origins of medical schools' skull collections, analyzing the routes of acquisition for stolen human remains from imperial conflicts from around the world. Likewise, this chapter tells the life stories—albeit fragmented ones—of two men in the African diaspora whose skulls were collected. Their histories reveal in intimate detail how medical schools benefited from racial violence. Chapter 6 tells the story of Harvard professor and physician Jeffries Wyman, and how living in and traveling to slave societies shaped his ideas about race, anatomy, and climate. His story reveals how many physicians routinely practiced and reproduced racial ideologies during their careers, whether they were from New Orleans or Boston, as in Wyman's case. Chapter 7 moves beyond anatomy, expounding on concepts of environmental health. Physicians claimed that Black people were either created or adapted for plantation labor in the tropics, underscoring the practical and political effects of racial medicine. Moreover, while the peak of European nations' imperial presence in the global tropics and the "scramble for Africa" remained a few decades away, American physicians were already articulating a racial framework that would be applicable to not only the politics of slavery but also global capitalism and imperialism.

The book ends with an epilogue emphasizing that *Masters of Health* represents the early chapters of a longer, ongoing history of how racial thinking has plagued medicine. Thus, the epilogue begins just after the Civil War, with northern and southern medical professors rekindling their professional networks. In fact, they picked up right where they had left off, exchanging favors, local gossip, and anecdotes meant to prove racial difference. In short, the history related in the following pages represents only the beginning of a much longer history of the braiding together of medicine and racism in the United States.

PART 1

FOUNDATIONS
FOR A RACIALIZED
CURRICULUM

1

RACIAL SCIENCE AND MEDICAL SCHOOLS IN EARLY AMERICA

In the summer of 1796, Henry Moss arrived in Philadelphia and quickly became a sensation with the local white population and MDUP's faculty. Moss was a Black man, but in 1792, spots of white skin had begun to appear all over his body. Recognizing the marketability of such a condition in a society weighing the future of slavery, he began to present himself as a curiosity in his home state of Virginia. Prior to this, Moss had worked as a farmer and soldier, having obtained 100 acres of land for serving in the Continental Army. In Virginia, Moss profited from many who paid to gawk at his appearance. Elite whites like the French aristocrat the duc de La Rochefoucald-Liancourt and Joseph Holt gave written testimony as to the validity of his story. This attention made Moss a popular medical attraction in 1796 in Philadelphia.[1]

Almost as soon as they heard of Moss's condition, MDUP faculty members such as Benjamin Rush, Benjamin Smith Barton, and student Charles Caldwell began conducting experiments on and examinations of his body in exchange for money, room, and board. In these examinations, the faculty hoped to understand race better and to discover whether it was permanent or transitory. Barton found Moss's transformation perplexing because his skin had changed, but his physiognomy appeared the same. The instructor began his description of Moss's body with the statement "Moss has the negro physiognomy, or aspect." Working from a century of natural historians' previous discussions of race, Barton compared Moss to an already established Black physiognomy. He continued, "[Moss] has the *frons brevis*, or short forehead; the *nasus quasatus*, and the *tibiæ incurvæ*, so common among the blacks. He has, likewise, the heavy eye of the blacks, and their crisped hair, or wool, upon his head."[2] Barton then noted that the change in complexion had not altered "the peculiar odour of the perspiration of the blacks."[3] This commentary highlights how physicians already had begun to tie blackness to a broad range of phenotypical features beyond just skin color.[4] Confronted with Moss's white skin but supposedly Black body type, medical educators such as Barton could not decide how to classify him—a puzzle that would continue to confront physicians.

Like Barton, Caldwell and Rush also found Moss intriguing, but instead of simply examining the man, they initiated several painful experiments. Rush blistered Moss's skin, testing his theory that blackness could be erased or cured, as the professor saw it. While Caldwell also raised blisters, he had Moss engage in intense exercise to see whether he might sweat off his remaining darkness.[5] These experiments highlighted medical educators' growing interest in researching blackness just as racial science remained in its adolescence. In many ways, Rush's, Caldwell's, and Barton's writings on Moss encapsulated the changing nature of American medicine in the late colonial and early national periods.

During these years, medical schools became sites for the production and dissemination of scientific ideas about race and blackness in particular. Aspects of this story are not especially novel, even if the total picture stands apart from previous histories of medical education or racial science. Historians of medicine have long pointed to this period as one of significant institutional growth in U.S. medicine. They also depict it as a time when medical practitioners increasingly sought out a more formal education to complement apprenticing.[6] Likewise, other scholars have argued that historians need to study racial science in its scientific context, as well as in light of debates over the abolition of slavery.[7] More recently, historians have argued that slavery was foundational to the growth and success of universities in early America.[8] These works have been instrumental to crafting this depiction of how racial science and slavery shaped U.S. medical education since its inception.[9]

Medical schools, medical journals, and a desire to use medicine to understand and define racial difference were essential elements for creating a national medical profession. As this chapter shows, these schools created a profession and a medical identity based on white male fraternity that transcended regional boundaries and was truly national. Barton and Rush were Philadelphians, but Caldwell, their student, had grown up in North Carolina. Medical schools in the North and eventually the South provided venues for white male youths to come together to learn their profession, to make friends and professional connections, and to handle and study Black people's bodies. Journals contributed to this medical culture by keeping physicians in this intellectual fraternity after graduating from school.[10] And, finally, medical professionals' continued interest in studying racial difference and teaching medical white supremacy allowed for northern schools to attract southern students. Long after northern states had begun to abolish slavery, southern students continued to travel to MDUP and other northern institutions, knowing that a belief in inherent racial difference was shared by physicians nationally.[11] All of these institutional and ideological changes started in the eighteenth century, but they culminated in the United States in the late antebellum period. In short, this chapter lays out much of the foundation on which the medical profession's culture of racism was based, including the growing importance of both medical schools and racial science to creating an influential national medical profession.

THE RISE OF RACIAL THINKING IN ATLANTIC MEDICINE

While this book tracks the rise of racial thinking in U.S. medical schools, it would be inaccurate to think that either racial science or racial medicine originated in the medical school, or solely in the United States or even colonial British North America.[12] While debate among historians persists over the origins of the race concept, anti-Black ideologies among Europeans have some roots at least in the medieval period. These anti-Black ideas, however, existed alongside folklore about powerful Black African rulers with expansive states. During the centuries of European exploration prior to the settlement of British North America, travelers wrote accounts of various parts of Africa, the Americas, and Asia that depicted these places and their inhabitants as exotic and different. Likewise, European states in the northern Mediterranean had been in contact with North African Muslim societies that had long enslaved sub-Saharan Africans. These slave-trading societies also trafficked in anti-Black ideologies.[13]

Building on this foundation, in North America in the seventeenth century, British colonials began to consider whether racial differences were cultural or embodied and inheritable. At this time, all but a few Europeans held beliefs about racial difference rooted in the Christian narrative of human creation, where all humans derived from a single pair, Adam and Eve. Even though most seventeenth-century Europeans might have considered Africans and their descendants in the Americas culturally inferior non-Christians, they upheld the essential unity of humanity. Early commenters on race described cultural practices and religious differences that corresponded to a group's skin color. When seventeenth-century authors discussed embodied differences between racial groups outside of skin color, they did so mostly in the context of body modification, though, like the Islamic practice of circumcision or the musculature of Native Americans.[14] In other words, these authors understood race—even physical attributes excepting skin color—as something largely cultural, not essential.

While most Europeans accepted monogenesis in the sixteenth and seventeenth centuries, there were outliers and controversies around polygenesis in this period. The discovery of entirely new continents and peoples in the Americas, in particular, caused serious questions among some European elites about the origins of these new people and their relation to biblical history. In 1550 during a papal junta in Valladolid, Spain, for example, controversy erupted over whether American Indians were a separate species. Spanish scholar Juan Ginés de Sepúlveda supported polygenesis in this case, claiming Native Americans were "fundamentally bestial and fitted only for slavery," explains historian David Livingstone. Bartolomé de Las Casas, the bishop of Chiapas and former vicar of Guatemala, disagreed. The question was not solved in 1550, and occasional controversies such as this occurred over the following two centuries.[15]

These early colonial discussions of difference also revealed how racial medicine in many ways predated racial science. Most whites' descriptions of physical differences in the seventeenth century were largely superficial and not yet used to create racial categories rooted in inherited physical attributes. In contrast, the racial scientists of the eighteenth century would focus on classifying human bodies into races based on inherited morphology or anatomy. This would be the real genesis of what would be called racial science in the nineteenth century, with its focus on bodily classification. In the seventeenth century, though, some medical thinkers did consider inherited and embodied approaches to race and health, or racial medicine, even if they applied this frame unevenly. These more impressionistic discussions of the people and illnesses of the Atlantic World's colonial periphery predated the more systematic attempts to understand racial difference by mostly Continental philosophers and natural historians during the Enlightenment. Prior to the late eighteenth century, then, producers of racial medicine and racial science remained largely separate, even if they were intellectually related.[16]

In the seventeenth century, some British colonists interpreted epidemic illnesses through burgeoning concepts of racial difference. Or, rather, interpretations of epidemics served as an early basis for thinking about different groups in North America, racially. During the sixteenth and seventeenth centuries, a combination of European warfare, enslavement, and illness caused the deaths of thousands of Native Americans in British North America and millions more across the continents. Literate colonials, perhaps to assuage collective guilt, emphasized disease as the primary cause of Native deaths, not their own militarism. As Native American deaths outpaced the still-high mortality of whites, British colonists argued that bodily weakness made Native Americans unsuited to the diseases of the American climate. Not simply desiring to protect public health, though, colonists believed this dynamic made Native Americans poor enslaved workers. In contrast, historian Joyce Chaplin explains, "European assessments of Africans had already emphasized that they were capable of hard labor, nearly insensitive to pain and physical want, and could be transplanted into any hot climate." Thus, ideas of Native Americans' susceptibility to illness led whites to push for greater importation of enslaved Africans, even as the African slave trade already had deep roots in the Atlantic World.[17]

British colonists and physicians further shaped nascent racial medicine in the eighteenth century, just as they increased the importation of enslaved Africans. Proponents of racial medicine in the Anglo-Atlantic World focused their attention on the idea that Black Africans and their Creole descendants had inherited resistance to some of the worst illnesses in American plantation societies. This belief should not be taken at face value, though, as historians have amply shown that the extreme mortality of the African slave trade and plantation labor proved the opposite.[18] Historian Suman Seth has argued that racial medicine came into existence when physicians saw race as a cause rather than an effect of health patterns. In many eighteenth-century theories, physicians argued that environmental and climatic forces shaped differential health outcomes among racial groups. The facts of high mortality in the slave trade and on tropical American plantations seemed to prove that Black Africans were not any better suited to this climate than anyone else. A minority of commenters began to argue that race shaped peoples' relationships to diseases and climates rather than the corollary.[19]

During this period, primarily colonial authors produced a slow trickle of texts that discussed both illness and race. Building on more impressionistic accounts from the seventeenth century, a few physicians in the Americas argued that Black people and Native Americans possessed an inherent promiscuity that made them prone to venereal disease. This combination of racial typology and seeming health patterns was the definitive feature of racial medicine in the first half of the eighteenth century. Yet for the most part, these physicians showed little interest in whether white and Black people shared a common origin.[20]

In the eighteenth century, racial science emerged through a significant shift in racial classification and thought. Beginning with Carolus Linnaeus, naturalists began a project of classifying the entire plant and animal kingdoms into massive taxonomies. While Linnaeus classified people of African descent, Europeans, Asians, and Native Americans as members of one species, he did give each group its own taxonomic description as a subgroup within that unified species. Linnaeus, though, saw the human form as remarkably malleable, able to be shaped by the environment and sexual intercourse between races that created fertile progeny. Thus, for different reasons, he was a precursor to both Benjamin Rush, who believed racial difference could be erased, and Charles Caldwell, who wrote a monograph in 1830 arguing that Black people could be classified as a distinct species.[21]

Furthering this theme of malleable bodies in eighteenth-century Atlantic naturalism, Georges-Louis Leclerc, the French naturalist better known as the Comte de Buffon, posited that exposure to wind darkened human skin, claiming to witness this occurrence among the inhabitants of Peru. In many ways, Buffon's theories were analogous to those of his contemporaries, who posited that ill-health was caused by either over- or understimulation of the human body by environmental factors.[22] Eighteenth-century naturalists / racial theorists such as Buffon and Linnaeus set the theoretical questions that would be explored by antebellum monogenists. What was the degree of difference between the varieties of the human species? Were these differences alterable by time, environment, and interracial coupling? If so, what would this timeline look like, and what did it bode for the immediate social future of enslaved African descendants and other groups like Native Americans?

During this period, polygenists also emerged as a significant minority voice in Atlantic science.[23] In contrast to the changing complexion of monogenists' arguments from the eighteenth to the nineteenth century, the core basis of polygenesis remained largely the same—namely, that bodies did not change, and type was permanent. In his 1776 monograph *Six Sketches on the History of Man*, Scottish philosopher Henry Home, Lord Kames, argued for the permanence of each racial type. At their core, Home and other eighteenth-century polygenists such as David Hume, Voltaire, and Thomas Jefferson, to an extent, separated themselves from contemporary monogenists including Linnaeus and Buffon due to their confidence in the immutable forms of human bodies.[24] For example in *Notes on the State of Virginia*, Jefferson explained that he suspected that African descendants, whether by different development or natural creation, were intellectually inferior. He believed that education could lessen but not erase African descendants' supposed ingrained deficiency in intellect. Jefferson further depicted Black people in physiological and anatomical terms. Among other stereotypes, he claimed that Black people both smelled bad due to possessing more skin glands and needed less sleep, and that orangutans were attracted to Black women.[25]

The transatlantic backgrounds of these writers also highlight the ways in which debates about racial science were not inherently defined by geography or a person's direct relationship to slavery. Where Linnaeus and Buffon saw elements such as wind, climate, and diet constantly shaping the human form, Home argued that bodily types were permanent. Home concluded that instead of the environment shaping bodies into races, the races had been built for specific environments. He explained, "The African negroes, though living in the hottest known country, are yet stout and vigorous, and the most healthy people in the universe."[26] Home, however, differentiated himself from many of his progeny in one regard: he felt uncertain whether African descendants had no potential for civilization or intellectual equality.[27] Thus, by the second half of the eighteenth century, racial science had emerged as a relatively coherent field of inquiry with two central questions: Were human races permanently separated? And did these races share a common origin?

Thus, as the eighteenth century came to a close, scientific and medical approaches to understanding racial difference had emerged and were growing in influence in the Atlantic World. However, for the most part, these two approaches to race remained largely separate. Unsurprisingly, physicians were much more focused on questions of health and disease transmission. Doctors portrayed Black people as hypersexual, and thus, their supposed instincts were the cause of perceived high rates of venereal disease among African descendants. During this period, some physicians also began to argue that people of African descent had an inherited protection to yellow fever, a position that is not supported by twenty-first-century science. Even so, these racial medical theories and theorists remained relatively small in number, even as physicians increasingly subscribed to some anecdotal ideas about disease susceptibility and resistance among Native Americans and people of African descent.[28]

Likewise, Enlightenment thinkers and naturalists began to focus their attention on how to classify racial difference. Most thinkers promoted the notion that all human races were the same species and shared the same point of origin. A minority of naturalists and philosophers, however, began to argue the opposite—that each race was created separately and was a different species. Polygenesis thus was a minority opinion throughout the Enlightenment, but the belief had gained multiple influential adherents. In the first half of the nineteenth century, though, polygenesis and essentialist racial medicine would grow in influence, and medical schools would develop into an important site for the distribution of these ideas.

THE EMERGENCE OF MEDICAL SCHOOLS IN
THE UNITED STATES, 1765–1861

At the same time as scientists around the Atlantic World were beginning to use natural history to define race, physicians were founding medical schools in North America.[29] Doctors started only two schools during the colonial period, MDUP in 1765 and the New York College of Physicians and Surgeons at King's College (Columbia University) in New York City in 1767. Physicians established Harvard's medical school in 1783, just as war with Britain ended. In these early years, schools did not need to be too competitive, although Benjamin Rush held some apprehension about the necessity of two medical schools and the future of MDUP with King's College nearby.[30]

While these new institutions shaped much of the future of medical education in the United States, most physicians during this period, and many still during the antebellum era, learned the medical trade exclusively through apprenticing with a practicing physician. Pupils apprenticed for three years with their preceptor (usually their local physician). The system created a highly localized medical culture where physicians were largely isolated from other practitioners. As a result, apprenticeships presented significant roadblocks to creating a unified medical profession in early America. The quality of apprentices' education relied almost solely on the competence and theoretical approach of their preceptors. Through apprenticing, physicians could rarely build a reputation beyond their local communities, thus inhibiting their mobility and the potential for a larger medical profession. In contrast, medical schools provided doctors with nationally recognized credentials and networks.[31] Medical schools played an essential role in changing physicians from a diffuse set of practitioners into members of a much more unified profession with common ideas, experiences, and professional networks.

As early as the 1760s, with the founding of MDUP and the New York College of Physicians and Surgeons, physicians had established many of the basic components of a medical school education in the United States. With the hiring of Benjamin Rush and three other professors in 1769, MDUP had gone from offering just two courses of lectures by William Shippen Jr. and John Morgan—another MDUP faculty member who studied race—to having six professors teaching seven different courses.[32] In order to receive their degree, students took two courses of lectures on Anatomy, Surgery, and Midwifery; Chemistry; Materia Medica (early pharmacology); Theory and Practice of Medicine; Clinical Lectures at the Pennsylvania Hospital; Natural and Experimental Philosophy; and Botany.[33] Graduation requirements in the eighteenth century were fairly simple and would largely remain the same well into the next century. To graduate, students were required to attend two courses of lectures lasting sixteen to twenty weeks, pass an oral exam, write a thesis, and apprentice for three years.[34]

By the time of the American Revolution, much of the general structure of the curriculum for medical students had been set for the next century, including the types of courses they took and the way in which the faculty assessed them for graduation. These changes to the structure of medical education also coincided with increased debates over the abolition of the slave trade and slavery in northern states. Pennsylvania passed a gradual abolition law in 1780, and other states followed suit in the ensuing decades.[35] However, abolition in the North did not end white racial anxiety in any region of the United States. Quite the opposite, political and social anxiety over race and slavery increased.[36] Likewise, during these early abolition debates, some physicians began to argue that anatomical racial difference justified slavery and discrimination.[37] As time went on, medical professionals in the North and South amplified their interest in and research on racial difference.

Medical schools also created institutional and structural methods to exclude Black people from the medical profession. Despite Rush's support for abolition, free people of African descent were mostly not admitted into MDUP, one more indication that abolishing slavery was not tied to a belief in racial equality. Not until after the Civil War would Black people be able to establish their own medical schools, and with only a few exceptions, medical schools during this period did not admit African-descended students. Moreover, no schools admitted Black pupils in large numbers. As a result, before the Civil War, very few African descendants were able to practice medicine.[38] Professors did not even seriously consider admitting Black students into these schools until the end of the antebellum period. By excluding African descendants and women, physicians made early medical schools a white male–dominated space. By creating a place for white youths to study Black people's bodies in private, professors further attached medical identity to whiteness.

By the end of the eighteenth century, the number of medical schools had expanded to a total of four, but graduating classes remained small. During this period, U.S. medical schools only granted 221 degrees. Institutions graduated few students due to small class sizes and the fact that many pupils took lectures in an à la carte fashion to complement their apprenticeships.[39] While the structures had emerged that would eventually become dominant in U.S. medical education, eighteenth-century American physicians still largely defined medical training through apprenticing. In this context, a unified approach to medical practice was impossible, much less the dissemination of racial theories across the medical profession.

The first two decades of the nineteenth century represented a crucial moment for U.S. medical schools. While growth was slow during the colonial era, the rate of expansion grew precipitously during this twenty-year period and afterward. By 1820, the number of medical schools had increased to thirteen. These new institutions were largely located in the Northeast, with ten of the thirteen founded in that region and none in the Deep South. The number of students also increased. From 1810 to 1819 alone, U.S. medical schools granted degrees to over 1,000 students, over four times the number that had graduated during the entire eighteenth century.[40]

Medical schools continued to expand rapidly throughout the antebellum era. Growth occurred in three interrelated measures: the number of students, the number of schools, and the geographical distribution of the schools. First, from 1820 to 1839, nearly 10,000 students graduated from medical schools compared to the fewer than 2,000 who received degrees in the first two decades of the century. That number reached a total of nearly 30,000 students for the last two decades of the antebellum era alone. Second, by 1860, forty-seven medical schools were granting degrees in the United States. Finally, establishments became distributed more evenly across the country. In 1860, only sixteen of the forty-seven schools in operation were in the Northeast. The rest were spread across the West and the South.[41] Likewise, many of the graduates went on to rural practice in the South and West, where competition for business was not as fierce as in urban centers.[42] While these institutions could hardly be compared to the medical schools of the twentieth and twenty-first centuries, their proliferation was a dramatic and consequential change. The lone country doctor became much less isolated from his profession. He was more likely to have graduated from a medical school. In addition, he could subscribe to medical journals, and a medical school was likely within a few days' ride of his home. Even if the country doctor was physically isolated, through their training, medical school graduates maintained a shared set of ideas and experiences with other practitioners.

Even though medical schools represented the most successful institutional means to legitimize the medical profession during this period, physicians also sought other tools to bolster their status in the United States. At the end of the eighteenth century, state legislatures across the country began to enact laws that required practicing physicians to obtain licenses through state and local medical societies. While these laws were largely ineffective in preventing alternative healers from practicing, they did help define a legitimate white medical identity. Moreover, they publicly set apart allopathic physicians from alternative healers whose ranks regularly included Native Americans, people of African descent, and lower-class whites.[43] As they were with medical schools, free Black people were largely left out of medical licensing until after the Civil War.[44] In January 1831, for example, the Medical Society of South Carolina rescinded the license of John W. Schmidt Jr., the son of a local elite physician in Charleston. The society members formed a special committee as soon as they heard rumors that Schmidt might be "of mixed blood." During the next meeting, they voted to invalidate the young doctor's license.[45] While these institutional shifts served the goal of legitimizing the medical profession, reformers also created an exclusively white medical identity through changes in education and licensing that began in the late eighteenth century.

Unlike licensing, medical schools were an effective tool for homogenizing the profession. During the eighteenth century and first half of the nineteenth century, MDUP and other established schools in the Northeast resided at the center of this increasingly unified field, influencing educational institutions across the country. Beginning in the 1820s, medical schools began to emerge in the Deep South and Old West. MDUP graduates and racial theorists such as Charles Caldwell, Daniel Drake, Samuel Henry Dickson, and Josiah Nott played influential roles in the development of regional medical schools and the distribution of medical and scientific theories about blackness. By training physicians from all around the country, MDUP greatly influenced U.S. medical pedagogy in the first half of the nineteenth century. In the 1850s, one newspaper described Philadelphia as the "Medical Metropolis of the United States." They continue, "She is far ahead of her sister cities in the number of her medical colleges, the number of her students, and the learning and skill of her professors, and not far, if any behind even Paris and Edinburgh in the patronage accorded her schools."[46]

Despite the growing importance of regional schools, especially in prominent cities such as Charleston, Louisville, New Orleans, and Richmond, northern establishments continued to have little trouble attracting southern students. In Philadelphia's leading schools, the proportional enrollments of southern pupils reached an all-time high at the end of the antebellum era. From 1850 to 1859, southerners constituted a majority of graduates at both MDUP and Jefferson Medical College in Philadelphia. At MDUP in the 1850s, the proportion of southern students was a little more than 50 percent. This figure represented a slight decline. In prior decades, southern students had usually made up more than 60 percent of the graduates. In the early decades of the antebellum era, southern students made up less than 50 percent of the students at Jefferson Medical College. However, throughout the 1850s, they represented a majority of students.[47] In 1853, for example, David Pusey, a medical student from Kentucky, wrote in his diary, "All practicing physicians should spend one winter in [Philadelphia]—To better prepare himself to relieve suffering humanity."[48] During this period, an impressive population of physicians emerged who were inculcated with medical and scientific ideas about African descendants' bodies as taught in the nation's medical schools and widely discussed in professional journals.

Through practice in rural and urban spaces, doctors interacted with patients in their local communities across class and racial boundaries.[49] The seeds of this large and diffuse profession were planted during the eighteenth century. Physicians' early interest in explaining race helped keep them unified long after regional divisions had defined U.S. politics.

As the number of schools in the antebellum period grew, physicians also established numerous medical journals. Before the Civil War, physicians founded hundreds of periodicals, even though most only lasted a few issues. Often connected to medical schools, these publications were usually small, with between 400 and 700 subscribers. They printed original research, book reviews, and news about the local medical community.[50] By producing journals, physicians worked to solidify the professional identity created by medical schools. As with educational institutions, journals first emerged in the Northeast, but as the antebellum era progressed, they spread across the rest of the country. Before the Civil War, for example, physicians published five medical journals in the city of Charleston alone and ten in the state of Louisiana.[51] Medical periodicals even fomented an international medical community, regularly reprinting articles from European journals.[52]

Ambitious young physicians such as 1854 MDUP graduate and racial scientist William Stump Forwood published in and subscribed to journals across regional and national boundaries. In the late 1850s and 1860s, Forwood subscribed to a total of fourteen different medical periodicals, including London's the *Lancet*, the *British & Foreign Medico-Chirurgical Review*, the *Medical and Surgical Reporter* (Pennsylvania), and the *Virginia and Maryland Medical and Surgical Journal*, among others.[53]

Medical periodicals not only grew in number, but they also acted as a forum to debate the medical and biological meanings of race. While full-scale debates over ethnology in medical journals did not occur until the antebellum era, many U.S. periodicals had been publishing articles on race since their earliest issues, like Benjamin Smith Barton's account of Henry Moss.[54] Through discussion of race, these journals further solidified the bonds between northern and southern physicians.

Through medical schools and journals, physicians increasingly had a well of shared experiences in handling people of African descent's bodies. Similarly, medical schools in the eighteenth century had established a pattern of exploiting the persons of enslaved and free Black people and lower-class whites.[55] From the inception of U.S. medical schools, physicians shaped their professional identity and their elite status through their perceived proprietary rights over the bodies of enslaved people, free African descendants, and working-class whites.

While the new schools were initially concentrated in the Northeast, by the end of the period, they were spread more evenly across the United States. Likewise, the number of graduates grew from a few hundred in the entire eighteenth century to more than a thousand annually during the two decades preceding the Civil War. Moreover, medical schools, like other early efforts at professionalizing medicine, were designed to exclude non-whites from becoming physicians. Thus, as well as emerging alongside racial science, these institutions actively sought to tie medical practice to whiteness. These white-dominated spaces would become a critical site for the production and mass dissemination of theories depicting African descendants as naturally inferior and suited for hard labor in the U.S. South and, more broadly, the tropics.

HETERODOX NO MORE: THE RISE OF
POLYGENISTS IN THE ANTEBELLUM ERA

At the beginning of the nineteenth century, physicians were beginning to see the fruits of their labor toward creating a national medical profession with a perceived expertise on race. In 1808 in New York City, a court case, *The Commissioners of the Alms-House vs. Alexander Whistelo*, required some of the city's leading physicians to act as racial experts. The doctors needed to decide whether the father of Lucy Williams's daughter was Black. Two years earlier, Williams, a free mixed-race woman, had been raped by two men— once by Whistelo, a Black man who worked for Dr. David Hosack and once by an unnamed white man with a gun, who interrupted Whistelo. Extreme sexual violence was all too common against Black women in early America, and Whistelo's lawyers never disputed that he committed the act, although they insinuated that Williams was secretly consenting. In the published court proceedings, no mentions were made of separate trials for the sexual violence against Williams, nor did they discuss any attempt to track down the white perpetrator. Instead in 1808, the New York Alms-House sued Whistelo to take responsibility for Williams's child. Hosack, Whistelo's employer, was a prominent physician in the city, and he later worked at Rutgers University's and Geneva College's medical schools. Since the case featured the almshouse and Hosack, many of New York's most prominent doctors mounted the witness stand to decide the race of the father.[56]

The case illustrates the increased power of medical professors in defining race in the early national period. The almshouse's star witness was Samuel L. Mitchell, a professor at the New York College of Physicians and Surgeons. In fact, outside of Lucy Williams, nearly all of the witnesses in the trial were doctors, and it was they who decided the race of the child's father. After the initial proceedings left the jurors divided, the mayor and various other city officials became Williams's jurors. Once Williams testified that she believed Whistelo was the father, twelve physicians testified that the unnamed white man was the father. Lucy Williams's daughter, they all explained, had a lighter complexion than her mother. In fact, the only doctor who seemed to believe Lucy Williams was Mitchell, the eminent professor.[57]

Mitchell's testimony captured the ongoing conflict over whether bodies could rapidly change, and whether racial differences were permanent. Make no mistake, questions of embodied change like Henry Moss's were key to doctors deciding whether white and Black people were the same species. Mitchell rested his belief that Whistelo was the father on Lucy Williams's testimony and a conviction that blackness could emerge or be erased rapidly. Relying on a history of the West Indies, Mitchell began by outlining the idea that Williams's child was by racial definition either a "quadroon"—the progeny of a white and "mulatto"—or a "sambo"—the progeny of a Black person and a "mulatto." Having defined his terms, Mitchell explained that there were various medical causes for a child to resemble a "quadroon" even if he or she was a "sambo." Social and environmental factors could affect Williams's daughter's appearance during gestation or even afterward, he asserted. Here, the doctor relied on the research of other medical faculty like Benjamin Rush and Benjamin Smith Barton. He explained that in the case of Henry Moss, "who was born of black parents," he actually "began to grow white."[58]

The cross-examiner then asked Mitchell whether changes like these could occur in the womb because of the mother's imagination. Mitchell affirmed the idea. He claimed that in New York, a woman had birthed a child with no arms and "distorted feet" after seeing the feet of a slaughtered cow. Likewise, Mitchell recited the case of a poem about a Scotsman who spilled ink on his wife's feet, after which she gave birth to a Black child. The physician concluded, "If such cases as the last are true (and there is strong authority for it) then the mere change of color or complexion is not difficult to believe." In the end, the mayor and the other jurors sided with the twelve other doctors, and Lucy Williams appeared to be left to raise her daughter alone.[59] As well as providing a disturbing window into elites' callous response to sexual violence against Black women at the turn of the nineteenth century, the case also illustrated the growing authority of the medical profession to define race in early America.

New York's city government expected physicians to be knowledgeable about the latest developments in racial thinking as a part of their trade. Thus, practitioners like Mitchell were seen as racial experts because they had studied medicine. Mitchell and the other physicians' beliefs about racial difference did not appear to be based in personal experience. Instead, their knowledge reflected debates over racial formation that had occurred during the Enlightenment. Moreover, the social power that doctors possessed over defining race would only grow as medical schools multiplied. While philosophers and naturalists were more likely to define race in the eighteenth century, in the nineteenth century, physicians began to produce racial science as well as racial medicine at a rapid rate. Testimony like Mitchell's and Hosack's represented early examples of medical professionals' growing responsibility to characterize difference. Moreover, this period marked the accelerated erosion of the divide between racial medicine and racial science. In their classes, professors increasingly made racial science speak to the needs of the medical profession. Therefore, it should be no surprise that antebellum medical faculty dominated the debate between polygenists and monogenists.

Even as physicians emerged as race experts in the early national period, they remained divided over racial difference's permanent or transitory nature. For example, when Benjamin Rush experimented on Henry Moss, he hoped to prove that blackness could be erased or "cured." In fact, Rush saw blackness as a literal illness, arguing that it was a form of leprosy. This contention was both racial medicine and racial science, as it pertained to perceptions of health and racial classification. Rush believed that it was physicians' duty to study and eradicate this disease of blackness. As a result, he taught his students at MDUP about Moss's case, and about his belief that Black people could be turned white through medical intervention. Rush even said that phenotypical stereotypes of blackness, such as "a big lip, flat nose & offensive smell," were symptoms of the illness.[60]

While Rush was yet to find a total cure for the condition, he did believe that he had found partial measures to alleviate this leprosy or blackness. He explained, "[When African descendants'] diet & manner of life is changed for the better, the color becomes much lighter; the juice of unripe peaches, friction & bloodletting are said to change their skin of a lighter color." Like other eighteenth-century naturalists, Rush believed real physical differences existed between African descendants and white people, but he also asserted that they were reversible.[61] Rush, however, represented the last vestiges of Enlightenment monogenism. He still envisioned a white United States. He also argued that interracial coupling should be prevented until a cure for communicable blackness was discovered. Even during the last decades of Rush's life and tenure on the medical faculty at MDUP, other professors began to teach that embodied racial differences would endure either permanently or indefinitely.

With the belief that racial distinctions were either permanent or not easily erased came an emphasis on anatomical differences. Beyond just skin color, late eighteenth-century physicians–racial scientists invented additional methods for defining difference. In particular, they studied human skulls to construct notions of inherited intelligence and race. In the 1770s, the Dutch anatomist Petrus Camper developed a technique for measuring the facial angle of human skulls, which he classified by race. He did not go so far as to call African descendants inferior, but when he arranged his skulls on his shelf, the Black skull sat next to the orangutan's. In fact, at Harvard in 1805, Professor Benjamin Waterhouse taught students Camper's method even as he admitted some skepticism about its validity. Waterhouse particularly feared that this approach could be used to further justify subjugating people of African descent.[62]

In 1799, the English surgeon Charles White wrote a detailed case for the anatomical inferiority of Black people, one of the first studies of its kind. His arguments closely resembled those made famous by late antebellum physicians and polygenists such as Samuel G. Morton and Josiah Nott. Notably, White contended that African descendants had a smaller cranial capacity.[63] He then concluded, "In whatever respect the African differs from the European, the particularity brings him nearer to the ape."[64] By 1799, White had set out many of the core arguments of polygenists. Similarly, he had helped to establish the type of expertise a physician could bring to the question of race in social relations.

While many American physicians did not adopt polygenesis as the causal mechanism of racial difference until later, in the first decades of the nineteenth century, medical professors increasingly focused on enduring anatomical differences when discussing race. In many ways, this new line of pedagogy opened medical schools up to polygenesis. Fifteen years after Rush's 1798 lectures on blackness, New York College of Physicians and Surgeons anatomy professor John Augustine Smith gave a lecture to his students that affirmed much of Charles White's analysis. At the same time, Smith claimed to still be committed to monogenesis. He informed his pupils that Black and white people were members of the same species who had enduring differences. Like some other faculty in this period, Smith tended to argue for monogenesis and permanent distinctions. He described African descendants' bodies as radically different from whites', so much so that the disparities could not have been caused recently or exclusively by the environment. Moreover, Smith explained that African descendants were a type somewhere between apes and whites, even though they shared the taxonomic classification as the same species.[65] While Rush certainly fetishized whiteness, and he presented an all-white future for the United States, Smith argued that the condition of Black people was likely permanent and could not be affected by improving social or environmental conditions. Smith and others like him made any attempt at broad social improvement seem futile, even significantly racist projects like Rush's that were intended to aid Black people.

Rush's and Smith's differing approaches to monogenesis displayed the fissures emerging among the theory's proponents in the first half of the nine-teenth century. Smith's lecture underscored how in many ways the origins debate was an ancillary part of a larger set of questions about the present and future of racial differences. While Smith claimed to believe in a common human origin, his depiction of African descendants' bodies more closely resembled polygenists'. Similarly, he was not searching for a cure for black-ness because he did not see it as transitory. Instead, Smith, like some late antebellum monogenists, argued that racial change at least took millennia. Thus, many monogenists only provided a nominal alternative to the perma-nent racial social systems that polygenesis would seem to endorse anatom-ically. Instead, like polygenists, many antebellum monogenists argued that racial differences would persist indefinitely, and that whites were intellec-tually superior to other races.

Simultaneous to increased discussion of permanent racial difference in antebellum medical schools was a rise in pro-polygenesis publications by medical faculty. In the 1830s up to the U.S. Civil War, Samuel Morton (Penn-sylvania Medical College), Josiah Nott (University of Louisiana [now Tulane University] and the Medical College of Alabama [now the medical school at the University of Alabama at Birmingham]), Samuel Henry Dickson (MCSC [now the Medical University of South Carolina], the New York University Medical College, and the Jefferson Medical College), and Jeffries Wyman (Hampden-Sydney College and Harvard University) produced books, pamphlets, and articles in support of polygenesis. In 1830, though, Charles Caldwell (the University of Pennsylvania, Transylvania University, and the University of Louisville) wrote the first monograph in favor of polygenesis by an American author. In 1830, Caldwell had held the position of professor of theory and practice for ten years at the Medical Department of Transylvania University, where he taught future racial scientist and polygenist Samuel Cartwright. In his monograph, Caldwell began by brushing aside the Bible as a source of natural history. This disregard for the Bible, rather than the racism of polygenesis, made the theory controversial among many white Americans.[66]

Like Charles White's work and later monographs in support of polygen-esis, Caldwell employed a variety of arguments for claiming that white and

Black people were different species. His key arguments hinged on anatomy and reproduction. Caldwell, like later authors and professors, argued that Black people were anatomically distinct, and he assembled long lists of anecdotal observations of embodied differences to supposedly prove his point.[67] Echoing Thomas Jefferson and eighteenth-century Jamaican planter and polygenist writer Edward Long, Caldwell also claimed that apes were particularly attracted to African women. This represented a reply to monogenists who argued that instances of sexual attraction between racial groups made them the same species. Myths about apes being attracted to and copulating with African women were meant to counteract this notion.[68] In many respects, these early exchanges reflected the dominant controversies in racial science. For antebellum scientists, embodied differences played out in significant ways behaviorally in terms of sexual attraction and propensity for education. These debates centered on the definition of species, whether mutual sexual attraction connoted a shared species status, and the degree to which species were defined by successful procreation between races.

Despite the seemingly preposterous nature of some of Caldwell's arguments, polygenists gained significant concessions from monogenists during the antebellum period. Prominent monogenists came to argue that each race had significant anatomical differences. Some, like Smith, even argued that racial differences would continue to exist for the foreseeable future. In the antebellum era, two men represented the vanguard of the Anglo American monogenesis movement: the English physician, anthropologist, and abolitionist James Cowles Prichard and the South Carolina naturalist and proslavery advocate the Reverend John Bachman. Similar to Johann Friedrich Blumenbach's 1775 thesis on race at the University of Göttingen, the first version of James Cowles Prichard's influential monogenist text *The Natural History of Man* was his 1808 doctoral thesis at the Medical Department of the University of Edinburgh. In writing his medical thesis on race, Prichard underscored the position of the medical school as a site for producing racial science in the Atlantic World. Moreover, he believed science could be used as a tool to prove and elucidate a biblical natural history.[69] Like many other proponents of monogenesis, Prichard saw polygenesis and its attendant materialist outlook as an attack on Christianity.

Pritchard opposed slavery, and he believed that Black and white people were morally and intellectually equal, but he also thought that the races possessed significant bodily differences. He argued that each race represented "permanent varieties" whose racial "peculiarities in question are not coeval with the tribe, but sprang up in it since the commencement of its existence, and constituted a deviation from its original character."[70] For

Prichard and many other antebellum monogenists, the forms of the human species appeared as though on a spectrum with a center. Even as Prichard argued for the unity of the human species, he conceded that at least slight anatomical differences existed between the human races, including length of the forearm, shape of the leg bones, degree of facial angle, and shape of the foot. He used two main arguments to counter the notion that these disparities constituted a need to divide humanity into different species. First, individuals' bodies within each racial group varied more than the aggregated differences between each race. Second, these racial distinctions were slight enough to be the product of a process akin to the domestication of animals, with social and physical environment producing racial difference.[71]

Prichard's arguments held significant weight for Anglo-Atlantic science and politics. In contrast to many proslavery monogenists writing at the time, Prichard saw the unity of the human species as a key argument for a humanist racial politics that opposed slavery. In his European travel memoirs from 1841, MDUP's professor of surgery William Gibson recalled attending a lecture in England given by Prichard, his "old acquaintance and fellow student" from their days studying medicine in Edinburgh. Prichard devoted the talk to the protection of the "aborigines." As the discussion grew more heated, he called on Gibson "loudly by name" to discuss race relations in the United States. Gibson explained, "I was obliged, reluctantly, to mount the rostrum and make a speech, and had the satisfaction of receiving, for my pains, especially from Mr. Thomson, a straggling fire—about Indian and African persecution in the United States—which I returned, with interest, but not without bringing a hornet's nest about my ears from all quarters."[72]

Gibson's story demonstrates the political implications of these scientific theories for Atlantic politics and slavery, in particular. As an American physician, Gibson was required to take a side in this Atlantic debate, and he firmly defended slavery. For many elite doctors, the medical profession consisted of a set of transnational personal and professional relationships, where traveling American physicians could be called on to make witness to the U.S. racial experience. It is also worth noting that, while Prichard disliked Gibson's proslavery politics, there is no evidence that this dislike altered his affection for his old classmate or vice versa.

In contrast to Prichard, the Reverend John Bachman of Charleston, South Carolina, the other influential antebellum proponent of monogenesis, was ardently proslavery and believed that it would take millennia for African descendants to become equal with whites, if that was ever possible. Bachman argued that Black and white people were the same species, but each human race was adapted to a specific climate and position. Ever a proslavery advocate, Bachman even gave the opening prayer at the signing of the South Carolina Ordinance of Secession.[73]

While John Bachman was best known for his work on avian species with the famous naturalist and painter John James Audubon, he also produced several articles on monogenesis and one significant monograph in the 1850s, *The Doctrine of the Unity of the Human Race Examined on the Principles of Science*. In many ways, Bachman shared Prichard's ideas about the causes of racial difference. Humans were susceptible to influences akin to domestication. While anatomical differences existed between each race, they were slight. Bachman believed the unity of the human species was proved by the fact that Black and white people produced fertile offspring. Prichard also made this argument. As proof, Bachman cited mixed-race families in Charleston and New York going back at least five generations.[74] For him, the ability for two animals to interbreed successfully meant that they were the same species.

Despite being a monogenist, Bachman believed physical racial traits were passed from parent to child, and these traits were innate or at least could not be erased simply through education. Giving examples relating to lambs, sheep, dogs, and other domesticated animals, he contended, "Domestication during successive generations produces an influence on the dispositions of the progeny." Human offspring's inheritance of domesticated traits allowed Bachman simultaneously to uphold a loose interpretation of biblical creation while deploying science to support the indefinite subjugation of people of African descent.[75] Bachman's work pointed to a significant shift in racial science in the nineteenth-century United States. While the English physician Prichard saw monogenesis as a significant argument against slavery, many U.S. monogenists saw no such conflict. White Americans' defenses of monogenesis did not necessarily represent a liberating force for enslaved people. Sometimes these arguments were merely a different route to naturalizing racial difference and, by extension, the social system attached to slavery.

While Charles Caldwell represented an important early call for polygenesis from a U.S. scientific author, Samuel G. Morton would be the most important figure in shaping the arguments of the American School of Ethnology. Born in 1799 in Philadelphia, Morton earned his first medical degree at MDUP in 1820 and his second from the University of Edinburgh in 1823 before returning to Philadelphia to practice. Morton and other physicians' transatlantic educational backgrounds illustrate how these ideas gestated in a larger Atlantic World and not just in the proslavery South. Throughout his career, Morton remained active in the Philadelphia academic community, teaching anatomy at the Pennsylvania Medical College from 1839 to 1843 and working at the Academy of Natural Sciences while maintaining a medical practice.[76]

Even though physicians such as Samuel Henry Dickson commended Morton for his medical texts, he garnered much more fame for his work on the comparative measures of human crania, which he ultimately used to argue that each human race was a distinct species.[77] For example, in 1840, Morton's work on skulls and race was the talk of the Phrenological Association's meeting in Glasgow, underscoring the persistence of this debate in Atlantic science.[78] And through correspondence and exchange with friends and admirers around the world, Morton gathered in Philadelphia one of the largest collections of human crania, dubbed by contemporaries the "American Golgotha."[79] He even entertained doctors at home and at the "Golgotha" when they passed through Philadelphia. For instance, in the mid-1840s, when Jeffries Wyman returned home to Boston during breaks from teaching at Hampden-Sydney College in Richmond, Virginia, he regularly visited Morton for company and to see his skull collection. Afterward, Wyman's sister followed, analyzing Morton's skulls for herself. Finally, illustrating the connections between monogenists and polygenists, Morton's first monograph on craniometry, Crania Americana; or, a Comparative View of the Skulls of Various Aboriginal Nations, was dedicated to James Cowles Prichard.[80]

Morton's methods of collecting and measuring human skulls were foundational for antebellum polygenists. In Crania Aegyptiaca; or, Observations on Egyptian Ethnography (1844), Morton argued that each race's cranial capacity and general conformation at least dated back to ancient Egypt. According to Morton, the average "Negro" had crania sized at seventy-three cubic inches and the "Negroid Form" sized at seventy-nine cubic inches, making them much smaller than the "pelagic" group (ancient whites), who had a cranial capacity of eighty-eight cubic inches.[81] Not only were there significant embodied racial differences, but these distinctions also existed at the beginning of recorded history. Writing to Morton in 1842, George Gliddon, Morton's skull collector in Egypt, explained, "You would produce monumental examples to prove, that the Egyptians were not N—rs . . . but that they were not only pure blooded themselves."[82] Using this brand of evidence, Morton argued that ancient Egyptians clearly depicted each race on their monuments. He thus concluded, "The physical or organic characters which distinguished the several races of men, are as old as the oldest records of our species."[83]

Where Morton arranged his works Crania Americana; or, a Comparative View of the Skulls of Various Aboriginal Nations (1839) and Crania Aegyptiaca; or, Observations on Egyptian Ethnography (1844) around limited and specific scientific questions about racial features, the works coauthored by Josiah Nott, a Mobile physician who was briefly an anatomy professor at the

University of Louisiana and later the Medical College of Alabama (which he helped found), and George R. Gliddon, an English archaeologist and U.S. diplomat who also collected skulls for Morton, represented an attempt at syntheses. In *Types of Mankind* (1854) and *Indigenous Races of the Earth* (1857), Nott and Gliddon sought to bring together a wide array of arguments in favor of polygenesis, including differential anatomy, cranial capacity, archaeology, geographical position of each race (this section was written by Harvard naturalist Louis Agassiz), and history. Joseph Leidy, the professor of anatomy at MDUP in the 1850s, even wrote a brief essay for *Indigenous Races of the Earth* arguing that species differentiation should be defined by inherited anatomical traits rather than the fertility of mixed-race people. In short, Gliddon and Nott intended to create overarching reference texts and syntheses for racial scientists that would provide new directions for future researchers. They even based these compendiums on their late friend Morton's notes that he compiled to write his own synthesis before dying in 1851.[84]

Perhaps polygenists' most incisive critic was self-liberated abolitionist Frederick Douglass. Rather than make his own racial science–based counterarguments like Bachman or Prichard, in a commencement address at the Western Reserve College, Douglass countered polygenists through pointing out the illogic already built into their claims. Douglass noted that in Crania Americana; *or, a Comparative View of the Skulls of Various Aboriginal Nations*, Morton's "contempt for negroes, is ever conspicuous," which led Morton to be blind to the contradictions in his own argument about the race of Egyptians. Critical to Morton's argument is the notion that the ancient Egyptians, a supposed point of origin for European civilization, were totally distinct from Black Africans. Quoting Morton's own morphological descriptions of ancient Egyptians, Douglass explained, "'*Complexion brown. The nose is straight, excepting the end, where it is rounded and wide; the lips are rather thick, and the hair black and curly.*' This description would certainly seem to make it safe to suppose the presence of '*even* some negro blood.' A man, in our day, with brown complexion, 'nose rounded and wide, lips thick, hair black and curly,' would, I think, have no difficulty in getting himself recognized as a negro!!"[85]

Rather than counter Morton on his own grounds and validate his methods, Douglass emphasized the inherent contradictions within polygenesis. Despite critiquing northern polygenists like Morton and Louis Agassiz, the abolitionist associated polygenesis almost exclusively with the politics of southern slavery. Thus, due to his immediate aims of abolishing slavery, Douglass mostly ignored polygenesis's ability to bolster northern white supremacy. This decision was both politically expedient given his white northern audience and probably necessary, but it also kept scrutiny over racial thinking aimed at southern slaveholders and not American scientists and doctors more generally.[86]

The writings of polygenist medical professors were influential in medical schools and among the public. In *Types of Mankind*, Nott and Gliddon caused significant controversy in the United States, unlike previous public reactions to ethnological works. Public interest was heightened to the point that in Philadelphia at least one song was written in defense of the work. The lyrics play on the biblical story of David and Goliath, framing polygenesis as a Goliath with the outraged local ministers appearing as David, slinging mud instead of rocks and failing to defeat this scientific giant.[87] Despite evidence like this song, historians sometimes frame racial science and polygenesis as a primarily southern phenomena with authors stoking the fires of proslavery thought. However, for many, like the writer of this melody, polygenesis asked key questions about the origins of humanity and the role of religion in science.[88] Likewise, in the spring of 1854, northern newspapers echoed the general sentiments of the unknown Philadelphia bard (even if they were not always so partisan). Some reviewers argued that the religious narrative of humanity's origins could no longer be trusted, and that perhaps there was not a unified human species.[89]

The national appeal of *Types of Mankind* appeared most clearly in the diverse geographic background of the first edition's subscribers.[90] Forty-eight percent of the more than 900 total subscribers resided in nonslaveholding states or countries, and Philadelphia and Pennsylvania had more subscribers than any other city or state. The geographical distribution of subscribers, combined with reviews in northern newspapers, highlights a need to reevaluate the cultural legitimacy of *Types of Mankind* and the reach of polygenesis as a scientific theory.[91] Historian Terence Keel has argued that to understand the influence of polygenists requires understanding how religion, politics, and science were in conversation in the antebellum era. For Keel, the contention that polygenists were merely fire-eaters in figurative lab coats misrepresents the extent of their influence. Many antebellum scientists did not regard science and politics as inherently in conflict, and Keel explains that polygenists employed science to make racial features "into quantifiable 'objects' of scientific inquiry."[92] Antislavery polygenists like the reviewer of *Types of Mankind* in the Boston abolitionist newspaper the *Liberator* and proslavery monogenists like Bachman underscore a need to understand this debate as not entirely beholden to proslavery politics. It also existed within the world of midcentury science and medicine.[93]

By the end of the antebellum era, polygenists had become the dominant intellectual force in U.S. racial science, thereby influencing how medical professors taught race. This is not to say that most medical professors in the 1850s were polygenists, although it was certainly possible. Rather, polygenists' dominance can be understood through physicians' general adoption of their depiction of race as defined through indefinite and inherited anatomical differences. While the debate over multiple versus singular origins of humanity remained hotly contested at the end of the antebellum era, few white physicians would have argued that Black and white people had a shared anatomy or intellectual capacity. Likewise, with John Bachman, the most prominent American monogenist, ardently supporting slavery, it would be hard to say that a belief in shared origins necessitated opposing slavery in the United States. When it came to defining Black people as inherently different during this period, racial scientists and physicians were actually remarkably consistent and unified.

TEACHING THE DEBATE: POLYGENESIS DURING THE EXPANSION OF U.S. MEDICAL SCHOOLS

In the introduction to the "Report on the Diseases and Physical Peculiarities of the Negro Race" (1851), Samuel Cartwright, a white physician–racial scientist and the chairman of the Medical Association of Louisiana's standing Committee on the Diseases of the Negro, made a significant misstatement. His core complaint that racial difference had not led to "much scientific investigation" and had remained "almost entirely unnoticed" by the field of medical education was false and highly misleading.[94] By the time of the publication of the report, Cartwright had established himself as a prominent physician in both New Orleans and the United States, and he had garnered a wide readership. However, he thought southern doctors could best teach southern students about regional ailments, racial medicine, and southern environments. Cartwright explained, "A radical reformation is greatly needed in our system of education, medical and political, which is so defective as to lead to the fatal error that there are no physical or organic characters in the Ethiopian organization different from that of the European."[95]

Cartwright was likely propagandizing for regional schools, because this idea of race-neutral medical education was a fantasy. In a review of the "Report" in the *Charleston Medical Journal & Review*, the author argued that Cartwright had completely misrepresented northern medical schools' pedagogical approach to race, introducing a political division where none existed. The reviewer explained that he had attended medical school in the North, and he declared, "We never once heard a Professor term the negro a 'lamp-blacked white man;' we never heard a syllable uttered that could be contorted into an attack on the institution of slavery. . . . But we can bear witness, at the same time that we found our professor quite as well acquainted with the anatomy of the negro, as well as with the science of comparative anatomy in general."[96] Despite sectionalist claims by those such as Cartwright, racial science had become an accepted part of U.S. medical education by the 1850s in both the North and the South.

In this era of expansion, many racial scientists also held professorships in medical schools. Physicians who had publicly written pieces on the subject of race taught at schools across the United States, including Hampden-Sydney College, Harvard University, Jefferson Medical College, MCSC, MDUP, Medical College of Alabama, the Medical College of Ohio, the Medical Department of Transylvania University, the Medical Department of the University of Louisville, New York University, the Pennsylvania Medical College, the University of Louisiana, and UVA. For example, going back to 1830, in the introduction to his physiology syllabus at MCSC, Samuel Henry Dickson ranked the races from highest to lowest: "1st, The White; 2d, The Olive, or Tawney; 3d, The Red; and 4th, The Black." Professors held significant positions of influence over their students and brought their expertise on race into the classroom.[97] Certainly, these educators' views were far from identical. UVA professor James Lawrence Cabell advocated for monogenesis, Joseph Leidy (MDUP) and Dickson pushed polygenesis, and Harvard's Oliver Wendell Holmes Sr. appeared to teach the debate between the two theories. By the 1850s, though, physicians clearly saw race as an expected subject of discussion in medical education. Whether in the North or the South, medical students received new insights into seeing and treating African descendants' bodies, and they reproduced these ideas in their practice. Compared to the beginning of the century, a much higher number of physicians had been formally educated in medical theories of race by this time, just as polygenists' influence grew.[98]

As with monogenesis, students wrote about polygenesis throughout the antebellum era, but they did so more often in the 1840s and 1850s. As early as 1829, MDUP student Singleton Jones Cooke of Virginia wrote about the head and the impact of its shape on the "various species of the human race."[99] While Cooke analyzed the physiology and anatomy of the head in general in his thesis, he also described African descendants' heads as closely related to "the monkey tribe," and he stated that African descendants had "always remained in a state of barbarism."[100] In 1837, MCSC student Dyer Ball wrote one of the first medical theses devoted exclusively to the defense of polygenesis. He made clear where he stood in the first sentence, explaining, "Mankind have been divided into five Species." Like other defenders of polygenesis, Ball conceded that the Bible and the existence of mixed-race people still provided significant questions for polygenists. However, these matters did not supersede the embodied anatomical distinctions that made racial difference a matter of observation. In composing their theses, students rarely intended to create new knowledge. Instead, they hoped to show their overall knowledge of a specific medical issue and the ideas of key authorities, making theses inherently derivative.[101] Works like Ball's were important not due to their novelty, but because they displayed how students digested what they learned in lectures and supplemental readings.[102]

In 1855, two southern students at MDUP wrote their theses on polygenesis, and both cited Leidy, stating that anatomical differences necessitated classifying African descendants as a different species.[103] Arguing from the interrelated perspectives of anatomy and environment, Tully S. Gibson of Vicksburg, Mississippi, explained, "A black skin seems best suited for a hot climate; and for this reason we suppose that a special creation of black races took place in Africa."[104] Gibson presented a two-pronged thesis. First, African descendants' skin and the longevity of their anatomical differences made them a distinct species. Here, Gibson relied on the supposed observational evidence that he learned in medical school. However, his second argument, that African descendants were specifically fit for labor in plantation climates, represented the product of both an informal sociopolitical education garnered in the plantation districts of Mississippi, where he grew up, and familiarity with works by those like Harvard scientist Louis Agassiz that argued for the climatological specificity of each race.[105] In his thesis, Gibson framed racial difference not only as scientifically and medically valid but also as central to the health of laborers in the South.

In his 1855 thesis on polygenesis, MDUP student from Alabama John Ramsay McDow cited all of the typical figures in racial science, such as Morton, Agassiz, and Prichard.[106] In their theses, McDow and Gibson demonstrated both the derivative nature of medical student writing and the organic interplay between politics and medicine. Their ideas derived from both science and larger political questions but were then filtered through the knowledge and medical worldview that they acquired at the University of Pennsylvania.

The similarity between McDow's and Gibson's theses points to a shared experience of how students digested ideas presented by racial scientists and professors. The imitative style of their works displays how race itself was taught in medical schools—not as a separate subject from politics. Instead, professors employed medical theory to speak about critical issues in U.S. society. These students wrote about race during the culmination of two major trends in antebellum science: the growing acceptance of polygenesis (before its precipitous decline in the wake of the rise of Darwinian evolution) and the mass expansion of medical education.[107] Students such as McDow and Gibson represented a profession in U.S. society that was growing at a rapid pace. As communication technology improved and education standards became more rigorous, students and professors engaged in a shared medical conversation about race. Debaters rarely came to a consensus, and physicians saw themselves as engaging in an accepted set of questions with a diversity of possible conclusions. These exchanges existed in a professional culture that assumed the significance of race to medical practice. During this period, doctors also increasingly located the defining features of race inside the body as anatomical markers in opposition to earlier skin-deep models. Furthermore, these students spoke to the growing presence of essentialist racial determinism in U.S. politics. As the antebellum period came to a close, medical degree candidates no longer sought a cure for race. Instead, they tried to find the social and physical environments best suited to match the unique insides of Black people's bodies.

In the wake of John Brown's raid on Harpers Ferry in 1859, southern medical students in the North famously departed from their Yankee schools. As the story goes, hundreds of pupils left northern colleges and universities and headed straight for New Orleans, Charleston, and Richmond to complete their education.[108] Despite this tantalizing narrative meant to illustrate how deep sectionalism had fractured U.S. society, these students were more the exception than the rule. More notable than the pupils who left were those who stayed, unconvinced that their loyalty to the South required a southern education.[109] Despite the growing cries of fire-eating physicians like Samuel Cartwright claiming that northern schools preached abolition, many people knew better. In 1861, MDUP still had hundreds of students, including ones submitting their theses from Alabama, Mississippi, and Florida.[110] Such southerners had cultivated a white medical identity during their education that transcended regional boundaries. These institutions and ideas dated back to the eighteenth century, and they allowed southern medical students to remain in Philadelphia for their education after South Carolina had seceded.

While theories of race, blackness, and health were formed as early as the medieval period, during the eighteenth century, physicians began establishing the institutions that would make medical racial pedagogy more homogenous. Specifically, through founding medical schools and journals and studying race, late eighteenth-century professors nurtured the roots of a white medical identity with claims to a special expertise about blackness that would persist well beyond their life spans.[111]

By the end of the antebellum era, physicians defined racialized bodies much more by the permanence or at least longevity of racial traits than they had when Benjamin Rush wrote. Moreover, late antebellum monogenists like Prichard, Bachman, and Cabell conceded one of the central points asserted by polygenists, that Black people's bodies were anatomically different from whites'. On this issue, the difference between the two sides was largely of degree, not kind. These concessions by monogenists displayed the growing influence of polygenesis over racial science discourse. Polygenists like Nott, Morton, and Caldwell were important not just because they had obtained prestigious positions in the 1850s scientific and medical communities, but also because they had shifted this larger racial discourse. By the end of the antebellum era, monogenist views of Black people's bodies more closely approximated those purported by polygenists than they did the ideas of early monogenists like Rush.

These shifts took place in the ever-growing institution of the U.S. medical school. Just as racial science increased in importance during the antebellum era, medical schools grew both in the sheer volume of doctors they produced and their influence over the profession at large. As polygenesis grew in popularity, professors taught that race was permanent (or at least indefinite) and embodied. Professors such as Leidy, Dickson, Caldwell, and Nott, along with monogenists like Cabell and John Augustine Smith, taught that members of each race had markers inside their bodies that were only observable to the trained eye of the physician. This belief was taken to such a point that a person could be Black without having obviously black skin. Finally, the structures emerging in the antebellum era influenced a generation of physicians who firmly believed that race represented an important factor in medical diagnostics and therapeutics. Many of these students would go on to practice in a geographically and racially diverse set of communities, carrying highly developed notions of race and health with them that would not be extinguished.

2

THE

CLINICAL-RACIAL

GAZE

In Paris, I am at home.
—*Josiah Nott to Joseph Leidy, April 12, 1859*

During the antebellum era, in addition to obtaining a degree at a reputable U.S. medical school, many elite physicians traveled to Paris for further medical study, forging and building on transatlantic professional networks. For example, as a student in Paris in 1835, racial scientist and future medical professor Josiah Nott built a professional network that remained strong throughout his career. During his studies, Nott met local notables and countless other foreign medical students who had flocked to Paris for training and prestige. In fact, when he returned to Europe in 1859 to stock the new library and anatomical museum for the medical school that he was establishing in Mobile, Nott required no letters of introduction to Parisian physicians. However, he could not say the same about his professional network in London.[1]

By the time Nott traveled to Paris in 1859, though, he was an established scholar, not the student that had first arrived for further medical study in Paris in the 1830s. During that first trip, Nott sought to further his medical education and gain more practical clinical experience in the city's hospitals. Before going to Paris, he had completed a medical degree at the University of Pennsylvania. Moreover, Nott had been raised by a South Carolina slave owner and judge and educated by religious skeptics at the College of South Carolina. Before arriving in Paris, he had seen his father acquire enough enslaved laborers to work a sizable plantation. Nott was born in 1804, and from 1800 to 1830, his father went from owning seven enslaved people to more than fifty. On his father's plantation and in the growing state capital of Columbia, Nott came of age as a witness to and participant in the local slave system. In the only state with a Black majority, he learned enslavers' methods for evaluating enslaved people's bodies for purchase in the local market. When Josiah Nott arrived in Paris the first time, he was already questioning orthodox religion. He had also obtained a medical degree and gained considerable experience observing people of African descent. In Paris, then, he sought to develop further the clinician's way of analyzing the human body, having already cultivated a fine-tuned racial gaze.[2]

For those like Nott who sought advanced medical education in Paris, the city also had much to offer a student hoping to understand the nature of racial difference. Before the birth of the American School of Ethnology, at the turn of the nineteenth century, the famous Parisian anatomy professor Anthelme Richerand in his *Elements of Physiology* wrote that compared to varieties that were defined merely by superficial changes, the human races comprised a set of "more profound, more essential differences, changes not confined to the surface, but extending to the very structure of the body." MDUP professor Nathaniel Chapman even edited the translation of Richerand's monograph with the express purpose of assigning it in his classes for students like Nott at MDUP. Chapman likely found the endeavor profitable, as the translation went through five printings by 1826. Paris also had been home to perhaps the most influential skull measurer of the turn of the nineteenth century, Georges Cuvier (1769–1832). By the time of his death, Cuvier had amassed perhaps the largest paleontology collection in the world, including numerous human skulls. While he was no polygenist, he did believe whites had the most perfectly symmetrical skulls. In short, for a young, elite, and white American man, Paris was an ideal locale to study diseased human bodies, and those like Cuvier and his successors in French natural history made it a vibrant place to consider race.[3]

Before the U.S. Civil War, clinical and racial methods of analyzing human bodies coalesced in the works of racial scientist physicians like Nott and came to be taught in U.S. medical schools. As this chapter will show, both medical education and theories of blackness were influenced by the growing importance of pathological anatomy in French medical education. Richerand was just one important figure in the trend to center French medical instruction around anatomy and clinical experience. Just as French physicians began dissecting thousands of corpses and aggregating their results to understand the specific seats of diseases, racial scientists dissected bodies and collected thousands of skulls to define difference as mapped onto the skeleton. Through their medical training, American physicians cultivated a "clinical-racial gaze" that allowed them to reimagine African-descended people's bodies' internal structures and biologically bolster white supremacy in U.S. social life.

Specifically, medical educators combined a mastery over the powerful set of optics of the anatomist with the racial gaze that had been evolving in

American slaveholding cultures for centuries. These unified optics constitute what I describe as the "clinical-racial gaze." Upon returning to the United States, physician–racial scientists such as Samuel G. Morton and Josiah Nott joined their clinical experience with their firsthand observations of enslaved people's bodies to create a clinically rooted approach to racial science. Thus, these scientists combined the racial gaze of the slaveholder with the clinical gaze of the anatomist. Using this gaze to claim scientific expertise over the meaning of blackness and race more broadly, the medical profession sought to establish itself as the premier commenters on Black life and death, and therefore deserving of considerable social power.

THE FRENCH CONTEXTS FOR U.S. RACIAL ANATOMY

In the first half of the nineteenth century, opportunities for experience in the clinic and with dissection brought more than a thousand American physicians and students to Paris.[4] Prominent figures James Lawrence Cabell, Charles Caldwell, Samuel Cartwright, William Gibson, Oliver Wendell Holmes, William Horner, Joseph Leidy, Samuel G. Morton, John Collins Warren, and Jeffries Wyman, among many others, all made medical trips to Paris. Some came as students, and some from the older generation came to buy books and specimens for their medical schools. Others, like Nott, eventually came to Paris under both circumstances. The French clinics that drew Americans taught an approach that emphasized practical experience and statistical rigor over theory. From a marketing perspective, the downside of the clinical method was that it cast doubt on the common therapeutics of the antebellum era, such as bloodletting. As a result, Americans left Paris with an extensive knowledge of disease and the internal working of the human body, and a commitment to creating medical statistics. These students and doctors, however, gained few therapeutic improvements to bring back to their patients.[5]

While scholars have explored the construction of racial ideas by Enlightenment-era French naturalists and the influence of nineteenth-century Parisian clinicians on U.S. medicine generally, little attention has been given to how the American School of Ethnology applied the central methods of French clinical medicine to studies of race.[6] Many of the American professors and physicians who taught and wrote about the nature of blackness and race had studied medicine in Paris. This trend illuminates two central facets of antebellum racial anatomy. First, rather than aspiring to be regional leaders in southern medicine, many antebellum physician–racial scientists understood themselves as among a national and transnational elite possessing the best medical credentials in the Atlantic World. Moreover, these physicians saw measuring blackness and race as a route to distinguish themselves in transnational medical circles, making a novel use of elite French methods to study the diverse American population.

Second, rather than being exclusively inspired by the ideologies of slave societies, antebellum physicians constructed their racial medicine through the same transnational, intellectual prisms that called into question the effectiveness of bloodletting and heroic medicine. Piecing together the logic of antebellum racial science requires an understanding of the training that students such as Nott and Morton would have received in the French capital. Moreover, studying the education of those like Nott and Morton illustrates that their theories were hardly an exclusive product of the U.S. slavocracy. Instead, these practitioners formulated and revised their ideas about race through their initial medical education and ongoing evolution as participants in elite transnational medical circles.

To understand the importance of anatomical observation for U.S. racial theory, a focus on the clinics of Paris in the first half of the nineteenth century is essential. During this period, French physicians began to formulate a new approach to the production of medical knowledge. Through training in Paris, elite American practitioners returned to the United States with a distinct understanding of illness and the human body, one that sharply contrasted with the knowledge of the Edinburgh-trained physicians who had dominated late colonial and early national medicine. Parisian clinicians emphasized sensorial observation, and they opposed the systems of medicine that had characterized the Enlightenment. In this paradigm, physicians had to observe how diseases affected certain internal organs and tissues—almost by necessity, dead ones—and abandon speculative theories of disease causation like Benjamin Rush's.[7] Moreover, as the younger generation of French-influenced doctors began to take over teaching positions in antebellum medical schools, students increasingly received a notably French education, one rooted in pathological anatomy, clinical observation, and statistics.

French instructors built the content of their sensory and practical education in the hospital wards of Paris. In 1788, over 20,000 patients resided in the city's almost fifty hospitals. At the end of the eighteenth century and first half of the nineteenth century, physicians used this wealth of bodies to create quantitative renderings of diseases' pathological appearances. French clinicians relied on this access to bodies for dissection and used medical statistics to make the postmortem appearances of a disease its defining features.[8] For example, in the winter of 1801–2, Xavier Bichat, an early advocate of the clinical method, conducted 600 autopsies. Similarly, for his *Studies on*

Pulmonary Phthisis (1810), the French clinician Gaspard Laurent Bayle performed 900 autopsies. Finally, Pierre Louis, who was notably popular among American students and professors including Nott, John Collins Warren, and Oliver Wendell Holmes, used thousands of autopsy records from the Hospital Charité for his works on the pathology of typhoid fever and phthisis.[9]

Through the sheer volume of pathological explorations taking place in Parisian clinics, physicians could synthesize their findings about the natures and seats of various diseases. In Bayle's work on phthisis, he found that the most statistically reliable identifying features of a disease were not the symptoms noted during bedside observation, but organic lesions found on the organs and tissues in postmortem examinations.[10] Using these methods, elite clinicians defined diseases as distinct and locally afflicting specific sites on the body, as opposed to Enlightenment beliefs in the unity of disease. Boston physician and professor of the theory and practice of medicine at the University of Maryland Elisha Bartlett, a chief American proponent of Louis's numerical method, described the unity of disease as "in direct and manifest opposition to all common sense, to all true philosophy, and to all correct observation."[11]

In *An Essay on Clinical Instruction* (1834), Pierre Louis set out the basis of his system of medical training, and what differentiated the clinical lecture from other medical subjects. Of all the French clinicians, American students most readily gravitated toward Louis. They even turned him into the symbol of French medicine in the United States.[12] In this pamphlet Louis explained, "[Clinical medicine] is the period for examination; the point when it is necessary to observe and compare, to oppose facts to theories and general descriptions, to judge of pathology as it exists. It is the most interesting point of medical study, and calls for the employment of the highest faculties of the mind, intelligence and observation, as well as *judgment to generalize the facts observed*."[13] Despite this empirical gloss, Louis actually argued that after gaining clinical experience physicians were able to generalize. Racial scientists found a powerful skill in their ability to leap from supposed observation to generalization. As opposed to Enlightenment-era theorists, empiricists such as Louis aimed to create a synthesis of facts garnered from clinical observation.[14]

While observation at the bedside was a central part of Louis's system of instruction, every form of observation was subordinate to pathological anatomy. In the clinic, external symptoms could be verified through autopsy.[15] As one MCSC student noted in 1839, "The French have arrived at a greater perfection in diagnosis and pathology than any other nation, and it is entirely owing to their having paid greater attention to the post mortem appearances of disease."[16] The critical theorist Michel Foucault explains, "Hence the appearance that pathological anatomy assumed at the outset: that of an objective, real, and at last unquestionable foundation for the description of diseases."[17] Thus, the pathological anatomist had to abandon a focus on symptoms that, according to those like Benjamin Rush, showed the whole body in states of imbalance. Instead, French clinicians understood the body to be diseased in specific internal locations that external symptoms corroborated. A trained clinician could understand the internal damage represented by outward signs on the living patient. These physicians educated their senses to see the body's interior on its surface, constituting what Foucault famously describes as the "clinical gaze."[18] Through this gaze doctors could link afflictions on the body's interior to its outward appearance in clinical observation, a skill that would be notably useful to American racial anatomists.

In Paris, American medical students educated their senses to correlate the outside of bodies to their internal structures—diseased or healthy—through rigorous training in clinical medicine and pathological anatomy. Using the language of the clinic and supposed observation, racial scientists such as Nott imagined a new anatomical map of Black people's bodies.

In the antebellum United States, Louis saw a wide adoption of his numerical method, helping further create a transatlantic medical paradigm. American physicians used statistics to support the efficacy of quinine, examine the mortality rates of common surgeries, and call into question the safety of bloodletting. From French physicians' use of statistics, American racial theorists also learned to study the volume of bodies traveling through and dying in hospitals. In addition to the grisly work of mass autopsy, at the core of Louis's philosophy was a devotion to detailed note-taking. During this period, American printers even marketed numerous forms of record books to physicians, allowing them to emulate Louis's practices. Printed record books helped systematize medical practice and allowed for statistical comparison. When these printed volumes were used to their fullest extent, doctors would record each patient's symptoms, the therapeutics used, and the result of the illness. These record books also demanded demographic data including sex, form of employment, and, of course, race.[19] Simultaneously, enslavers began to adopt accounting books and quantitative approaches to managing their plantations.[20]

In short, in medicine and other professions, Americans increasingly adopted a more quantitative technique for data analysis and record keeping. For physicians, Louis's numerical method inspired much of this trend. Both doctors and enslavers systematized their approach to understanding the human body. Along these lines, physician–racial scientists would use quantitative methods for measuring human difference. The simultaneous popularizing of aggregation among southern enslavers and Atlantic medical practitioners revealed how polygenist physicians developed their theories through a constellation of intellectual movements in the United States and abroad.

Louis's and his American followers' methods were not without significant flaws, and they built many of these shortcomings into U.S. racial science. Beyond just prioritizing pathology and statistics over other forms of medical knowledge such as chemistry, physiology, and therapeutics, Louis's statistics were crude at best. Despite his invocation of large numbers of cases, in practice Louis often derived conclusions from a much smaller and more curated sample, skewing his results. Much the same could be said for skull measuring and race. Ironically, Louis and many of his students paid scant attention to other breakthroughs in statistics occurring in Paris during the first half of the nineteenth century. As a result, "the numerical method," explains historian James H. Cassedy, was "a circumscribed approach to medical numbers." While physicians using the numerical method aided in breaking down some of the most problematic aspects of antebellum medicine, like the heavy use of bloodletting and other heroic therapeutics, in general, antebellum physicians applied statistics to medicine through a deeply flawed approach.[21]

In 1836, when Josiah Nott traveled back to the U.S. South, he, like others trained in Paris, carried a set of methods that would prove essential to the construction of anatomical blackness. Educated to privilege analysis of human anatomy, Nott and other racial anatomists began to define each race by supposed differences in the shape of the organs and structure of the skeleton, as well as in skin color. These physicians and scientists were heavily indebted to the two central methods of the French clinic for their evidence of racial difference: postmortem examination and statistics. Practitioners conjured up a map of the distinct anatomy of African descendants' bodies through their access to a large selection of human remains. Thus, racial scientists created a science that welded together the rhetoric and piercing gaze of the French clinician and the racial gaze typical of slaveholders.

AUTHORING THE NEW RACIAL ANATOMY
By the 1850s, the link between anatomy and racial science, both of which relied on anatomical examination, had been well established in the Atlantic World with the help of French-trained Americans such as Josiah Nott and Samuel G. Morton. As an example of how physicians and intellectuals in the first half of the nineteenth century viewed these two subjects as connected, J. G. Heck devoted a third of one volume of his *Iconographic Encyclopædia of*

Science, Literature, and Art to a section entitled "Anthropology and Surgery."
It is worth noting that Spencer F. Baird—an American physician-naturalist
and curator at the newly established Smithsonian Institute—had translated
the encyclopedia into English from the original German in 1851. In "Anthropology and Surgery," Heck covered brain size and the anatomical roots of
skin color.[22] His encyclopedia and its English translation highlight how this
discourse of anatomical difference developed in an Atlantic World with a
variety of intellectual interests and philosophical underpinnings, and how
these theories traversed geographic and linguistic boundaries. Following
the pattern of racial science's evolution dating back to the late eighteenth
century, American physicians shaped their arguments about race around
shifting transnational intellectual currents. Out of this context, U.S. doctors
used poorhouses and plantations to analyze African descendants' bodies,
filtering their observations through the language of French medicine.

Elite southern physicians such as Nott inherited two different methods
for a sensorial understanding of African descendants' bodies: the racial and
clinical gazes. In the anatomical works of the American School of Ethnology, medical professionals combined these two separate forms of mastery
over the human body into one set of optics. In the slave markets, "slave's
bodies were made racially legible," explains historian Walter Johnson. "The
buyers' inspections, the parts they fingered, the details they fetishized, and
the homosocial connections they made with one another gave material substance to antebellum notions of 'blackness' and 'whiteness.'"[23] White American physicians used both the clinical and racial gazes to demarcate the
parameters and meanings of African descendants' bodies, and they gave the
racial gaze new meaning and scientific legitimacy through the introduction
of the methods of pathological anatomy. No longer was delineating race to
be understood just through the experience of slavery. Instead, physicians
such as Nott turned the study of race into a science of the body, one capable
of the same empirical confidence as the diagnosis of disease.

Both Josiah Nott and Samuel G. Morton had experience with this racial
gaze before they compiled their texts on racial anatomy. By 1850, Nott
personally owned sixteen slaves, and he socialized with elite slaveholder-
politicians including Senators John C. Calhoun, James Henry Hammond,
and Pierce Butler.[24] As a resident of the Deep South and a slaveholder, Nott
had considerable experience in the methods of evaluating enslaved bodies
in the market. Through "gazing, touching, stripping, and analyzing aloud,"
Walter Johnson continues, "the buyers read slaves' bodies as if they were
coded versions of their own imagined needs—age was longevity, dark skin
immunity, a stout trunk stamina, firm muscles production, long fingers rapid

motion."[25] Buyers also analyzed enslaved people's backs for whipping scars to create a history of their behavior.[26] The sensorial experience of the slave market in many ways resembled the invasive probing that defined the new clinical medicine, as well as the numerous autopsies and dissections where medical students crowded around one opened body and examined its internal structure. Moreover, slave buyers at times acknowledged the expertise of physicians in evaluating enslaved bodies, inviting them into the slave pens.[27] As a result, while the racial gaze certainly transcended the borders of the South and other slave societies, it also had an added dimension for those who grew up amid slavery and had closely examined the bodies of enslaved people.

Unlike Nott, who was a native southerner, Samuel G. Morton was a Pennsylvania Quaker who claimed to oppose slavery.[28] In the mid-1830s, however, Morton traveled to Barbados and other islands in the Caribbean just after emancipation had occurred in the British West Indies. In his journal, he provided descriptions of recently emancipated people of African descent, and he evidenced a highly developed racial gaze. He even presaged physician, racial scientist, and provocateur Samuel Cartwright's prescription of the whip to cure his invented slave diseases in the 1850s. Morton explained that the formerly enslaved people "who [were] indolent by nature, require[d] the lash to stimulate their languid limbs to exertion." And with a telling correction, he wrote, "[The] slaves blacks of this island have in my eyes a very repulsive appearance. They have the genuine African face, [were] witless and stupid in their manner. . . . The women, in particular, [were] thin and squalid." This loathing represented more than a racist flourish. Charles Caldwell and James Cowles Prichard had debated whether Black and white people's supposed mutual sexual repulsion or lack thereof made them distinct species. Thus, sexual aversion held weight in defining racial difference.[29] While Morton did not see this as necessarily justifying slavery—quite the opposite—he did believe that emancipation should have been more gradual. He explained, "Notwithstanding the restraint and coercion of the new laws, it is much feared that this fine island will be infested with needy vagabonds."[30]

While Morton claimed to oppose slavery, he certainly did not favor equality. His experience in the West Indies led him to believe that free people of African descent would most likely always require control by white society. Morton and Nott correlated their observation of living people of African descent to their problematic statistical studies of human skulls and anecdotal evidence of differential internal anatomies constructed during dissection. Moreover, Morton's elite white status allowed him easy passage through Caribbean society while traveling the routes of empire to better understand blackness.

Through relatively quick international transportation and correspondence, descriptions of slavery, health, and the bodies of African descendants circulated across the borders of nineteenth-century empires with relative ease. During this period and earlier, anecdotes about race and slavery like Morton's circulated around the Atlantic World. In his 1823 *Lectures on Comparative Anatomy*, Edinburgh's famed surgeon Sir Everard Home gave an account of an inspection of an African-descended woman's body in Dominica by a Dr. Clark. From sexual repulsion to hypermasculine Black women, Clark included many details that would become commonplace in later racial science texts. Providing alleged proof that some ethnic groups had larger clitorises, Home recounted that the woman—presumably forced to strip—"was of the Mandingo nation, twenty-four years of age; her breasts were very flat, she had a rough voice, and masculine countenance. The clitoris was two inches long, and in thickness resembled the common sized thumb." Home, who was "favoured" with this story that initially took place in 1774, highlighted the similarity in approach of the enslaver and physician. As a part of their trade, doctors and enslavers could force African-descended men and women to strip, and they could closely analyze their bodies, taking in every detail to narrate the supposed biological potential of African descendants.[31]

Home and Clark's description of this woman's nude body evidences the degree to which nineteenth-century medicine was shaped by comparatively rapid communication, racism, and toxic masculinity. Clark's delineation underscores three key features of medicine in the ages of slavery and empire. First, Clark, the white male physician, held extreme power over the body of this and other enslaved women in Dominica. Beyond simply forcing her to strip for science, Clark made the woman manipulate herself in ways that were invasive. He either made the woman stimulate her clitoris or did it himself, because he explained that her clitoris at some point "became half erected." While Clark and Home showed no interest in this woman's thoughts and feelings, she likely felt ashamed or abused by the personal acts that Clark made her perform publicly. Second, Clark's descriptions of this woman reveal how physicians and racial scientists often described Black women's bodies as masculine. He made this woman strip and sexually stimulate herself, and then he sent accounts of this interaction to friends and colleagues. In doing so, Clark illustrated his belief in Black women's hypersexuality and immodesty.[32]

Third, these dehumanizing examinations were not just discrete local events. By discussing Clark's assessment in his lectures before the Royal College of Surgeons, Home brought the intimate details of this woman's body before the most prominent professional group in Britain. When the lectures were published, they reached an even larger audience and survived indefinitely. Improved communication technology, the power of white physicians over enslaved women's bodies, and the gendering of racial difference ensured that the invasion of this woman's privacy was not merely the fodder of a local physician's curiosity. Instead, it became part of a transnational medical discourse, reaching the most elite members of the medical profession long after the original event. Clark and Home undeniably brought medical attention and legitimacy to a form of analysis that would not have been foreign to a slave market.[33]

While Samuel G. Morton also used the transnational communication networks of empire and commerce, he focused his racial gaze through Louis's numerical approach, describing his collection of more than a thousand human skulls. Morton relied heavily on George Gliddon for skulls from northern and, to a lesser extent, southern Africa. During the period when Morton assembled his collection, Gliddon served as vice-consul for the United States in Egypt, further illustrating the ties between U.S. foreign entanglements and scientific knowledge production. As vice-consul, Gliddon collected more than a hundred skulls for Morton, at one point having ninety-three examples "grinning horribly their ghastly smiles" in his home, which terrified Gliddon's Egyptian servant.[34]

By the middle of the nineteenth century, European empires intervened in the affairs of African states with growing regularity. For example, while under the leadership of Muhammad Ali, Egypt grew increasingly independent from the Ottoman Empire, but it also came under greater influence from Britain and France. At one point, the Egyptian ruler even hired Gliddon "to obtain information, purchase machinery, &c., in reference to the promotion of the cotton-culture in Egypt." This period marked the early efforts to create the Suez Canal, even though it would not be completed until 1869. More specifically, European empires viewed Egypt and the canal as potential means to increase their influence over Asia. With all of this, it was little surprise that Egypt represented an important collection center for Morton.[35]

Moreover, it was during this period when Morton began corresponding with Gliddon. While living in Egypt, Gliddon obtained skulls for Morton from India and the Red Sea. He usually just received crania as Morton's agent, but on occasion Gliddon also robbed tombs for Morton himself.[36] In addition to Gliddon, James Cowles Prichard, Daniel Drake, and John Collins Warren shipped stolen skulls to Morton. Warren, though, would not trade his "two flat headed Indians," explaining, "They are so different, so peculiar and so useful, that I cannot part with them." These skulls remained at Harvard.[37]

Unwilling to obtain skulls himself, Morton was a sort of armchair medical imperialist using already-existing international networks of naturalists

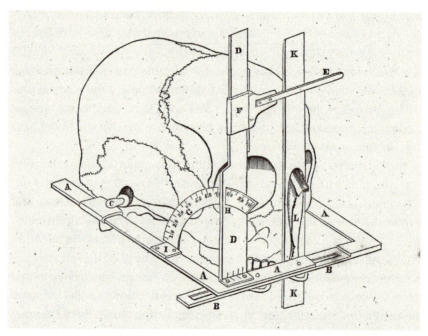

Figure 2.1. An illustration of Samuel Morton's facial goniometer, which was meant to measure a subject's facial angle. Samuel George Morton, Crania Americana; *or, a Comparative View of the Skulls of Various Aboriginal Nations of North and South America* (Philadelphia: J. Dobson, 1839), 252. Photo courtesy of the Huntington Library.

to fill his cabinet of crania. Therefore, his collection would not have been possible without the growing empires that allowed American and European physicians to move across oceans and continents.[38] Morton relied on communication and exchange networks produced by technologies such as the steamship that allowed people to better traverse the globe in the mid-nineteenth century. Through his collectors, Morton created an evidence base that spanned the world, allowing his clinical-racial gaze to compare peoples from every inhabited continent. Skull collections like his thus required the establishment of efficient trade networks. Through curating these representative racial skulls, Morton also used his authority to generalize, shaping at least two other institutions' representations of racial difference. Specifically, he sold sets of casts of idealized racial skulls to Harvard's medical school and the College of South Carolina.[39]

In addition to developing his ever-growing skull collection, Morton used specialized instruments to measure the anatomical dimensions of skulls. He mapped the dimensions of the face, using a facial goniometer (fig. 2.1), which

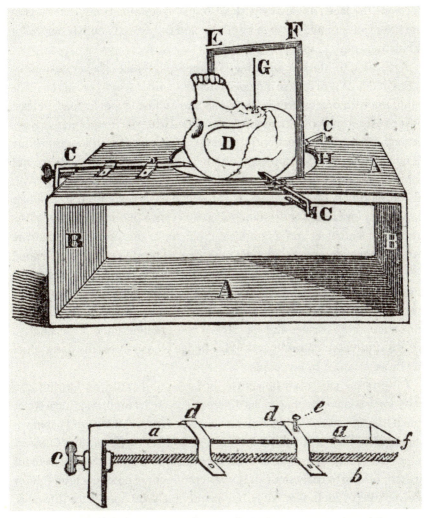

Figure 2.2. An illustration of Samuel Morton's device to measure cranial capacity, also known as a craniometer. Samuel George Morton, Crania Americana; *or, a Comparative View of the Skulls of Various Aboriginal Nations of North and South America* (Philadelphia: J. Dobson, 1839), 254. Photo courtesy of the Huntington Library.

allowed "the facial angle of any skull" to be "ascertained with exactness in the brief space of two or three minutes," and he created another device for tabulating cranial capacity (fig. 2.2).[40]

According to Morton, in order to compare the races, "a very extended series of crania is of course indispensable."[41] In other words, racial scientists could not turn one or even a few skulls into an ideal type. Instead, at least dozens of examples of each group were needed to create representative types through statistical aggregation. By prizing cranial capacity as the cornerstone of racial difference, Morton even situated race as internal to the body, not capable of simply being defined by external phrenological reading. With the development of these methods, the casual observer or even slaveholder could not completely understand racial difference. Rather, only specialists trained in statistical and anatomical medicine could properly demarcate each human race across space and time. Racial knowledge had transcended the experiential basis of the plantation or the slave pen. Like understanding disease, delineating racial boundaries required a technical knowledge not available to the average slave owner or slave trader.[42] Through the introduction of statistics and specialized instrumentation, Morton situated race as a professionalized type of knowledge whose truest meaning could not be ascertained by laypeople.

Despite the supposed objectivity of tables and statistics, Morton also used illustrations depicting racial difference through curating for ideal types, much like the casts of skulls he sold. To some extent, Morton did acknowledge the fallibility of artistic renderings. For Crania Americana; or, a Comparative View of the Skulls of Various Aboriginal Nations (1839), Morton sent his artist to Boston to draw some of Harvard professor of anatomy John Collins Warren's Peruvian Indian skulls, but he ultimately did not use the drawings. He found them too inaccurate. The use of imagery underscored the limits of the numerical method, as a single or small number of images were able to be used as evidence of racial difference. This methodological failing was akin to Pierre Louis's tendency toward generalization and small sample sizes.[43]

While medical textbooks used Morton's data, medical students cited Morton in their theses. Influenced by Crania Aegyptiaca; or, Observations on Egyptian Ethnography, Alabamian and MDUP student J. Ramsay McDow asserted that the entirety of Africa "may be called the land of Negrodom with the reservation of Egypt, the birthplace of arts and civilization." McDow then explained, "Dr. Morton, by measurement of many crania, has shown that the cranium of the Negro contains nine cubic inches less than the white man." On top of his influence over fellow naturalists, Morton and his skull collection oriented much of medical students' transnational approach to race and the anatomy of the skull.[44]

Another example of this distance between lay and technical constructions of race resided in the use of the microscope for hair analysis. While Black people's and white people's hair had long been considered aesthetically different, physicians and scientists used microscopes to prove their allegedly essential divergence. In his 1861 textbook *An Elementary Treatise on Human Anatomy* (he had bound his own copy in human skin), Joseph Leidy explained, "The fine silken hair of the head of the white race is cylindrical . . . , and the head of the negro, is more or less flattened cylindrical." Harvard's Warren Anatomical Museum also had numerous hair samples, highlighting hair's status as a legitimate anatomical object worthy of medical analysis. Moreover, hairs, like skulls, were scientific commodities that traveled widely.[45]

The Philadelphia lawyer and naturalist Peter Arrell Browne took hair analysis to its logical conclusion, conducting a study that mirrored Morton's work on skulls. In the 1840s, Browne collected hundreds of hairs from different races to come to the determination that Black people had wool instead of hair. While African descendants' hair had long been visually compared to wool, Browne contended that these similarities were quite literal. He asserted that Black people possessed hair that was anatomically the same as sheep's wool. He also obtained the hair of notable politicians and scientists, including most of the presidents and even Nott and Morton.[46] Browne concluded, "[Since] the white man has hair upon his head, and the negro has wool, we have no hesitancy in pronouncing that they *belong to two distinct species*."[47] Browne combined both statistical methods and the budding interest in microscopy to prove racial difference. He also showed how the study of racial difference had gone beyond just skull size into other parts of the body. Specialized instrumentation, combined with the importance of statistical methodology, placed racial analysis squarely in the hands of specialists during the antebellum period.

Like Morton, Browne used the routes of empire to obtain his collection. In fact, Nott and Morton helped Browne complete his assemblage. For example, in 1851, Morton sent Browne the hair of an indigenous Brazilian person. In volume 3 of his collection of hair, Browne stored specimens from Greek people, New Zealand natives, and American Indians. In volume 4, he had the hair of Chinese people, indigenous Amazonians (sent by famed naturalist Henry Schoolcraft), Hawaiian hair, and the hair of a "compound hybrid . . . 1/4 Creek, 1/4 African, 1/2 white." Browne then devoted volume 6 to Black and mixed-race people. Volume 9 had animal hair including that of primates, also putting animal bodies in this global trade in anatomical goods. Like the far more common skull series, Browne's collection was built through medical and scientific traders.[48]

In *Types of Mankind*, Josiah Nott also incorporated a novel statistical technique for measuring racial anatomy that required tapping into transimperial networks of knowledge. He explained that while Morton's skull collection was unparalleled, it was also still too small for its results to be absolute truth. Nott did not see this deficiency as immediately curable, but he had a short-term solution—using statistical data on hat sizes to help provide auxiliary evidence to support Morton's claims. Thus Nott turned to hat manufacturers in Newark, New Jersey, and Mobile, Alabama, for information on white cranial size and the hat sizes of Black British West Indian soldiers. He contended that these statistics corroborated Morton's general conclusions that white people had larger cranial capacities than African descendants.[49]

The rise of statistics and an increasingly interconnected medical elite also made studies like Nott's possible. For example, on February 13, 1853, Josiah Nott wrote Jeffries Wyman requesting data on head circumferences from Boston-area hatmakers. Nott even went further in describing his skepticism of Morton's data, saying, "The anatomical collections of races are so small as yet, that all measurements of crania, including those of Morton are very unsatisfactory." The solution was more data collection. In the short term, this need for more information meant hat manufacturing, but in the long run, Nott saw a necessity for even larger collections of human remains. Nott's study of hat sizes and the surrounding correspondence revealed his own reflections on some of the limitations of antebellum statistical studies of human crania, even as he recommitted to the numerical method and its emphasis on large data sets. By utilizing hat store records, Nott underscored another new trend that would become common in the world of statistics: using data for purposes vastly different from their original intent.[50]

Through clinical education, physicians redefined the human body, both in terms of its biomedical functions and the inherited differences of each race. Influenced by Parisian medicine's emphasis on observation, racial scientists measured thousands of skulls, analyzed the internal and external conformation of the body, and laid claim to a distinct black anatomy. While racial scientists employed the language of French medicine, their observations were based on anecdotal and statistical evidence equally often. In the case of measuring skulls, racial scientists shared many of the same methods (and the flaws that came with them) as French clinicians.

Alongside building medical schools and popularizing polygenesis in the United States, leading physicians during this period combined the racial optics of the slaveholder with the statistical and anatomical methods of the clinician. Compounding the generic racism already rife in the United States, physicians created the clinical-racial gaze through the growing influence of French empirical medicine and analysis of human bodies—alive and deceased. As elite U.S. physicians traveled to Paris for training, they learned the numerical method with its emphasis on dissection and statistics. Upon returning to the United States, physicians such as Samuel Morton, Josiah Nott, and Jeffries Wyman applied the numerical method to race, measuring the human body and creating statistical tables that they believed supported the notion that racial difference was biologically ordained. White American physicians used their simultaneous access to enslaved bodies and cutting-edge medical theory to assert a unique expertise for defining and enshrining racial difference.

Not only reserved for elite racial scientists, though, the clinical-racial gaze would emerge as a central tool for medical students to study race. It combined the experiential approach of the enslaver and the clinician, constituting a novel scientific method for classifying race. Professors rooted students' anatomical training in studying the human body through the dissection of cadavers and handling of museum objects. This practical experience combined with course content represented the core features of antebellum anatomical education. Constructing this new approach to the body was just as essential to creating medical schools' racial curricula as the institutions themselves. The clinical-racial gaze was the optics students learned from their professors to describe difference, and it would shape the way prospective doctors practiced medicine after they completed their education. This was the foundation for creating a medical profession with claims to expertise over Black people's and other non-white people's bodies.

PART 2

ANATOMY AND THE EXPERIENCE OF MEDICAL EDUCATION

3 TRAINING ON BLACK PEOPLE'S BODIES

The medical student is thought to spend much of his time in the vicinity of grave-yards; and to have acquired in the dissecting room that relish for mangling the dead, which is inconsistent with the exercises of due benevolence towards the living. His pursuits are associated in the minds of many, only with skull-bones, morbid human preparations, and other equally revolting objects: and they instinctively shrink from intimate contact with an individual, whose social sympathies are supposed to have become perfectly callous, or he could not take an interest in such disgusting enquiries.
—Henry Edwin Morrill, "An Essay on the Formation of Medical Character," M.D. thesis, University of Pennsylvania, 1840

A muscular subject without much fat answers sufficiently well for this dissection; the male black, is therefore, most frequently resorted to in our school.
—William Edmonds Horner, professor of anatomy at the University of Pennsylvania, 1846

Near the beginning of his education at the Medical Department of Transylvania University, Abraham Addams stole a corpse. As he recounted in his 1828 thesis, he and a friend were visiting the house of a local preacher when "a black child, that was not expected to live many hours, was brought by its parents, to be baptized." Addams described the youth as "extremely emaciated, its countenance haggard, its breathing frequent, and anxious, interrupted by a short distressing cough, its pulse small and quick."[1] Articulating little empathy, Addams displayed the extent of his clinical detachment by describing the child as "it" even before the child had died. Throughout the account, Addams neither listed the sex of the youth, nor discussed any attempt to alleviate his or her suffering. Even while alive, for Addams, the child had become an object to dissect, not a patient.

Just a day or two later, "the child died," and Addams and a fellow student put their plan into action. The two "clandestinely, obtained it for dissection." This was no autopsy. Addams and his classmate merely wished to acquaint themselves with the internal structures of the human body. Once again objectifying the child, Addams asserted, "Having other objects in view, the disease of which it had died was forgotten, and the cause of its death overlooked." Only by accident did Addams make any pathological conclusions. When he removed the lungs, "a large abscess, filled with matter, bursted and its contents ran out," thus giving the pupils insight into the youth's fatal illness.[2] Addams's matter-of-fact description of the events shows his own clinical detachment. Indeed, it is a testament to how accepted, even encouraged, a part of medical education body snatching had become that Addams was so comfortable including such a story in his thesis. Though students such as Henry Edwin Morrill argued that medical students were not simply detached grave robbers, Addams certainly fit the stereotype.[3]

Through anatomical education, prospective doctors learned to treat the human body as an object available for experimentation in the name of science. In the case of Black people's bodies, however, students became further detached due to their sense of racial superiority. Historians of dissection have shown that throughout the Atlantic World, physicians preyed on the bodies of the poor most regularly. Anatomists generally focused on the bodies of African descendants and impoverished people because they wished to avoid the social and legal repercussions of dissecting the elite.[4] Moreover, by working on cadavers, students cultivated moral and emotional distance between themselves and their subjects. An able medic needed to be able to work on a corpse without being sickened, frightened, or saddened. Physicians also required this dispassion to perform gruesome surgeries on the living.[5] While dissection cultivated general clinical detachment, the clinical-racial gaze nurtured in medical schools added another dimension to how students treated Black people's bodies. Doctors and students used Black people's bodies due to their inferior social position, and these bodies' disproportionate use as dissection material simultaneously reinforced this subordinated status.

Following the larger theoretical influences of polygenesis on medical education, pupils treated Black people's bodies on the same level as they ranked them taxonomically, between white humanity and the lower animals. As well as comparing white people's and Black people's bodies, medical professionals considered the treatment of African descendants in relation to animal bodies in a manner analogous to their supposed taxonomical position.

Historians such as Stephen Kenny, Todd Savitt, and Daina Ramey Berry have revealed how African descendants' bodies were obtained for dissection. Likewise, southern students and physicians regularly used enslaved people's bodies for dangerous experimental procedures aimed at curing patients.[6]

However, the previously unknown student experiments related in this chapter reveal medical faculty's acceptance of extreme medical abuse against the enslaved. One South Carolina scholar deliberately infected an enslaved man with measles. Another student in Virginia induced nicotine toxicity in a mother and suckling infant to the point where he feared killing the enslaved baby.

Extreme medical racism gestated in antebellum medical schools. This chapter relates how it evolved, showing that students learned medicine on Black people's bodies in light of their animalization by polygenists. Due to availability and lack of legal accountability, medical faculty and students abused Black people with greater ease than they did other socially weak groups like poor whites. In the social structure of obtaining and using bodies in medical education, Black people came to mirror their positioning in racial science as an intermediary link between white humans and the lower animals. Analysis of northern medical schools' early use of Black cadavers underscores how, in many ways, this model for the appropriation of African-descended cadavers for dissection was created in Philadelphia and New York City. Likewise, these schools and their associated hospitals were key sites for the exploitation of African descendants' bodies, like southern hospitals were for the enslaved. Occasionally, students and physicians also used living enslaved people for life-threatening nontherapeutic physiological experiments. By using live bodies, doctors set out a class of tests that they believed were more ethically suitable for African descendants and animals, further highlighting Black people's dual status in the medical system as both animal and human. Through experimentation and dissection, physicians practiced the racial ideology that their professors taught them, making a lived experience of the racist medical mastery taught in schools' curricula.

DISSECTION AND THE EMERGENCE OF A
RACIALIZED CLINICAL DETACHMENT

> *For my part, I very much doubt the medical students having visited . . . [public*
> *cemeteries], for dead bodies; I rather believe, that the only subjects procured for*
> *dissection, are productions of Africa, or their descendants, and those too, who*
> *have no friends, and have been transmitted to gaols [jails], and elsewhere, for*

having been guilty of burglary and other capital crimes; and if those characters
are the only subjects of dissection, surely no person can object.
—Daily Advertiser *(New York, N.Y.), April 23, 1788*

I have enclosed a number of observations on the anatomy of negroes, shewing
how far they differ from whites, this I expect will help you in your justification of
negro slavery which I hope to receive by return of post.
—Newport (R.I.) Mercury, *March 24, 1788*

On August 8, 1861, William Lloyd Garrison's abolitionist newspaper criticized southern medical schools for stealing and dissecting deceased Black people's bodies. The *Liberator* asserted ironically, "What a convenience to possess for scientific purposes a class of population sufficiently human to be dissected, but not human enough to be supposed to take offence to it!"[7] The newspaper highlighted how medical schools' exploitation of Black people represented a significant issue in U.S. racial politics. However, the article also draws attention to how often northern institutions' exploitation of Black people's bodies went unnoticed by contemporary commenters. For example, the article's author needed to look no further than Harvard's medical school to see Black corpses being stolen for dissection.[8] Indeed, during the late colonial and early national era, northern colleges and universities established many of the norms and justifications underpinning medical educators' exploitation of African descendants' bodies, as displayed during the 1788 anatomy riots in New York.

That spring, all along the Atlantic Seaboard, working-class whites were outraged over body snatching from public cemeteries by local medical students and physicians. Citizens rioted over allegations of corpse theft in both Baltimore and New York.[9] For several years before these riots, free Black people in New York had been petitioning the government to legalize the use of criminals for dissection and to punish those who stole bodies. However, legislators only acted when whites rioted upon the discovery of the theft of a missing white woman's body.[10]

When discussing the history of stealing Black people's corpses and U.S. medical education, scholars of slavery and medicine often overlook the New York College of Physicians, Columbia University's medical school, and MDUP, even though both Pennsylvania and New York permitted slavery well into the nineteenth century.[11] Throughout their history, northern schools resorted to stealing white bodies more often than their southern counterparts did. However, since the founding of the first U.S. medical schools in the eighteenth-century North, students and professors had found Black people's bodies to be the easiest to obtain. In the 1810s and 1820s, when southern doctors began founding medical schools in the antebellum South, they already had a model for the exploitation of Black people's bodies. Fittingly, these southern professors were often alumni of northern schools.

In the eighteenth-century North, medical schools set the precedent for the heavy reliance on Black cadavers for anatomy instruction. From the beginning of U.S. medical schools, physicians understood the bodies of African descendants to have a dual purpose. On the one hand, they could be exploited with relatively little popular backlash, and on the other hand, medics' readings of them could be used to justify or oppose slavery. In this sense, physicians understood African descendants' forms as a central battleground over the meaning of social relations in the United States. As can be seen in this section's epigraph from New York's *Daily Advertiser*, in the public, commenters worked to justify body snatching and dissection through claims that only Black people's and criminals' bodies were dissected. This worked to assuage the rioting working-class whites in 1788 by making it appear that their gravesites would be respected, even though their bodies were also routinely robbed.

Through the systematic exploitation of African descendants' bodies for dissection beginning in the eighteenth century, students treated Black people's bodies as inferior to whites' yet highly useful. As the number of venues for medical education expanded in the antebellum era and the popularity of French clinical medicine grew, schools required even more dissection material. The increasing prominence of anatomical instruction roughly coincided with the rise of polygenesis, and medical students learned to use African descendants as they were framed taxonomically by polygenists—as both animal and human. Their bodies could be dissected for understanding a general human anatomy. But due to African descendants' inferior social status, their corpses also could be stolen, maimed, and discarded in far greater volume and with little resistance from the white population. Through postmortem examinations, students encountered Black people's bodies regularly, and these practices empowered future physicians' sense of medical and social superiority toward African descendants. As autopsy increased medics' certainty in diagnosing disease, pupils gained confidence in their ability to explain essential racial differences through dissecting Black people's bodies.

The connection between dissection and the animalization of African descendants was quite literal, as was apparent in the popular press's descriptions of orangutan dissections in 1825, 1826, and 1835. These articles shared a common trait: comparing orangutans to African descendants.[12] Describing the dissection of an orangutan in 1835 at Peale's museum in Baltimore, Charleston's *Southern Patriot* noted, "Almost every person who saw this animal was struck with its astonishing similitude to the negro—its face that of an old man in its eyebrows and mouth—its body and limbs that of a child especially the naked hands and feet, and its use of these members in eating, drinking, &c. and in embracing its keeper around the neck like an infant, moaning and sobbing, expressive of its affection and tender feelings."[13]

These connections between the bodies of African descendants and apes were both structural and superficial for observers. In the catalog for the Boston Society for Medical Improvement's anatomical museum, the curator compared the stolen, desiccated penises of African descendants to the organs of a "chimpanzee (Simia Boglodytest)." Many white physicians and Americans saw African descendants as more animalistic in their nature and in the literal conformation of their bodies, taxonomically confining them to a liminal space between animal and man.[14]

Medical professors routinely depicted African descendants as both animal and human. As Jeffries Wyman, by this time the professor of comparative anatomy at Harvard, explained, "It cannot be denied, however wide the separation, that the Negro and Orang do afford the points where man and the brute, when the totality of their organization is considered, most nearly approach each other."[15] In these respects, the enslaved were dehumanized through the process by which the medical profession appropriated their bodies, compared them to apes, and allowed medical students to hack them apart. Through comparisons to animals, physicians framed African descendants as the closest species to white humans that could be ethically treated more like animals. Practitioners cultivated a detachment to African descendants' bodies through noting their similarity to animal forms, and they acted out this animalization by using the bodies in medical training.

Animal comparisons also explained the seeming paradox between racial scientists' depiction of African descendants as anatomically distinct, and anatomists' use of Black cadavers for dissection to teach universal human anatomy. For MDUP professor Joseph Leidy and other anatomists, the anatomical differences between the races were small but nonetheless significant. For those like Leidy, such disparities were notable enough to require a separate taxonomical position, but not so different as to demand distinct surgical techniques. When dissecting African descendants' bodies, Leidy believed, anatomists could learn about both general human anatomy and the specific anatomy of Black people. He asserted, "One species of felis, ursus, or equus will give the exact anatomy of all the other species in each genus, just as you may study the anatomy of the white man upon the black man."[16]

Leidy showed how Black people's bodies could be imagined as different enough anatomically to make them a distinct species, but also could be used as an object for teaching human anatomy generally. One of the country's leading anatomists at the time, he laid to rest the seeming conflict between using Black people's bodies to understand general human anatomy and depicting them as anatomically distinct. He explained that the types of distinctions that he thought separated Black and white people—and other species—were important to establishing racial difference. However, Leidy also affirmed that Black people's and white people's bodies were similar enough to make their surgical and pathological anatomy largely interchangeable. Thus, animal comparison helped justify using African descendants' bodies in the anatomical theater, even as it further morally distanced white students from their anatomical subject.

When students first entered an antebellum dissecting room, they were confronted with several new experiences that would both challenge their morality and fundamentally change their perspective on the human body. As a student, Joseph Leidy, like many others, found the dissecting room revolting. He explained, "You may think it strange, but I was so disgusted with the dissecting room that after spending the first half day there I went away and could not be induced to return for six weeks and I did not get entirely over the melancholy produced for a year; then the desire to acquire information gradually overcame my repugnance."[17]

Before students even began to dissect, they experienced apprehension, dreading that they might become sick, but they also worried that they might find perverse joy in the study of dead bodies. For example, in 1860, Titus Munson Coan, a student at the New York College of Physicians and Surgeons, confided to his parents that he feared dissection might irreparably change him. Upon entering the dissecting room, he was apprehensive that the body might be robbed of its mystery or that he might embarrass himself before his classmates. Instead, Coan admitted to his parents an even worse result. He found that he enjoyed the potentially immoral act of dissection.[18]

For students such as Coan and the young Leidy, the corpse represented a potential Pandora's box, tantalizing for the enlightenment it could provide and the intimacy with the human body that they might garner. At the same time, aspiring doctors were terrified of how dissection might affect their morals. Critics and even some anatomists believed that through dissecting, students could become attracted to dangerous ideas or fetishes including materialism, misanthropy, and even necrophilia. Most students overcame their dread, as respect and fear turned into gallows humor.[19]

Transcending disdain for the corpse required turning it into an object through the cultivation of a detached clinical gaze. While visiting an anatomical theater just outside Amsterdam in the town of Haarlem, a young

William Horner reacted with disgust at the way the local anatomists callously arranged bodies in the classroom. Horner noted in his diary, "The skeleton of one man in particular dressed up, mounted on a mule with the horn which sounded before him as he went to the execution. This barbarous taste gave a degree of gloominess to the business which I scarcely ever felt on visiting a collection before."[20] Horner's account displays how pervasive gallows humor was among anatomists in the Atlantic World. It also captures how physicians struggled with their morality, attempting to maintain their humanity in the face of the gore that they encountered in their line of work. Nowhere was this detachment between body and physician deeper than in the clinical-racial gaze that medics cultivated toward Black patients, who already existed in a subordinated social position.

Written during his tenure in the mid-1840s as the professor of anatomy at Hampden-Sydney College, Jeffries Wyman's correspondence captures the gallows humor surrounding the use of Black cadavers. As a Boston native in slave country, Wyman was fascinated and repulsed both by African descendants and their enslavement. In an 1845 letter, friend and future Harvard philosophy professor Francis Bowen grimly joked to Wyman, "You speak of tobacco crops and the price of n—rs. Of course, you mean the price of *dead n—rs*, they being the only commodity that you trade in. Do tell me, *what is* the cost of a fine, stiff n—r—one that you will *cut up fat* and that doesn't smell strong enough to be nosed a mile off? Do you have a *price current* for such merchandise?"[21] The racism toward African descendants inherent in the use of the word "n—r" was paradoxically accompanied by the two Bostonians' uneasiness with the slave system.[22] Morbid humor and racist language permitted Wyman to distance himself from both from the slave country and from the African descendants' bodies that he exploited as a professor.

Along similar lines, dissection photographs from the early twentieth century provide some insight into how pupils might have incorporated race into their morbid pranks. In 1902, medical students from the College of Physicians and Surgeons of Baltimore staged a photo in which they gathered around a presumably Black cadaver. The cadaver lay on a dissecting table, and the students held bone saws and scalpels. They had written in large print on the table, "All Coons Smell Alike to Us."[23] Likewise, in 1924, Wake Forest University medical students captioned their dissection photo with "sliced n—r."[24] These photos provide rare insights into dissection-room high jinks, and how they were at times quite racialized. While these images postdate the period of this study by more than forty years, antebellum students undoubtedly subjected African descendants' bodies to similar final indignities.

While the story of the appropriation of enslaved bodies by southern medical schools is widely known, historians have paid far less attention to the consumption of African descendants' bodies in northern schools.[25] In northern cities such as Philadelphia and New York, where the populations of free Black people were quite large, white physicians particularly preyed on the Black population.[26] Moreover, in places that were often sites of body snatching, such as Philadelphia's almshouses, Black people were overrepresented compared to their proportion of the city's population.[27] Like slave hospitals in the Deep South, northern almshouses shared the bodies of the dead with local medical schools.

In his 1828 thesis, "An Inaugural Essay on Ulceration of the Intestines," MDUP student George S. Bettner narrated how students at the Philadelphia Almshouse conducted autopsies on the bodies of the Black and immigrant poor. The almshouse's wards were segregated both by race and gender, solidifying these hierarchies into the very structures of the institution. In this respect, northern institutions reflected the segregated establishments of the South.[28] In Bettner's essay, he recounted the autopsies of five patients suffering from inflammation of their gastrointestinal systems, two of whom were free Black people.[29] William Gwathmey, another MDUP student working in the almshouse, conducted autopsies on two Black infants who died from cholera infantum. In addition to dissecting their gastrointestinal systems, Gwathmey opened the cranium of one of the infants, which would seem unnecessary in the autopsy of a cholera victim, a fact that Gwathmey tacitly acknowledged by not performing the procedure in both cases.[30] These northern students systematically exploited African descendants' bodies during their medical education, as did their southern counterparts. Like plantation physicians, northern poorhouse physicians exercised heightened levels of control over the most socially and economically dislocated patients, who were the easiest prey for the anatomist's knife.

Just as in the South, African descendants in the North had every reason to dread that medical professionals would take advantage of the bodies of their deceased loved ones.[31] While the Black population was smaller in Boston than in New York or Philadelphia, Black patients in the almshouse had to fear physicians, too. During his tenure as the professor of chemistry and materia medica at Harvard in the 1810s and 1820s, John Gorham also served as a surgeon at a Boston poorhouse. In his communications on "Morbid Anatomy" in the *New England Journal of Medicine and Surgery*, Gorham related conducting the autopsy of a syphilitic "negro of an athletic form" and of "Richard Johnson, a negro" who suffered from *phthisis pulmonalis* (tuberculosis).[32] On a similar note, in May 1860, Harvard professors paid a local funeral home to exhume the body of a Native American from Mount Hope Cemetery in Boston for use in their dissecting room.[33]

While differences certainly existed between the quantities of Black and other racially subordinated people's bodies available in the North and the South, physicians in both regions shared a plan for the appropriation of dissection materials. They illegally took white bodies when non-white ones were unavailable. This need for white bodies, in addition to non-white ones, was common in northeastern urban centers due to the high demand of competing medical schools and private anatomy classes. Likewise, students' accounts of racially targeted body snatching reflected MDUP anatomy professor William Horner's bald assertion in his textbook that at MDUP "the male black, [was] therefore, most frequently resorted to" for dissection.[34]

In northern medical schools and their partnered hospitals, aspiring physicians not only garnered mastery over corpses, but also obtained increased expertise on African descendants' bodies. The case of the famous scientist Louis Agassiz captured this systemic relationship between racial science, dissection, and northern medical schools. According to Boston physician Augustus Addison Gould, upon Agassiz's arrival from Europe to the United States, he became "much interested in the dissection of a negro (he had never seen one till he arrived in Halifax)." Gould continued, "He [Agassiz] says the [negro] brain is a genuine *human* brain, & no mistake, but it is not a *Caucasian* brain."[35] Physicians and scientists such as Agassiz envied Americans' access to African descendants' bodies, which allowed them to understand African descendants' supposedly distinct biology better.

The stark reality of the medical profession's open use of Black cadavers must have come into full frame for free Black people when, in February 1836 in New York City, P. T. Barnum arranged for the public dissection of the "161 year old" enslaved woman Joice Heth. Heth's dissection underscores a theme that will unfold in greater depth later: the close connections between popular and professional anatomy. Just before Heth had died, Barnum had taken her on a tour through the Northeast. To witness the final exploitation of her body, over a thousand New Yorkers purchased tickets at fifty cents each.[36] New York College of Physicians and Surgeons professor of surgery David L. Rogers performed the dissection to discern whether Barnum's claims about Heth's age were true—which, of course, they were not. As one newspaper noted in the wake of the dissection, "It turns out, as far as can be judged from physical appearances, that Joice Heth's wonderful old age was only a wonderful humbug."[37] The presence of Rogers, a local anatomy professor, also seemed to publicly reinforce the notion that medical schools exploited the bodies of

Black people for the white population, even if the truth was that poor whites' bodies were also targeted by grave robbers.[38]

Perhaps no other event better encapsulated the unequal treatment of white people's and Black people's bodies after death. In 1788 and regularly thereafter, white people rioted when a white body was found stolen and dissected, but they paid to see this deceased enslaved woman as spectacle. Heth's story highlights the growing presence of dissection in American popular culture during this period. While anatomy riots were common after revelations of stolen white bodies, Rogers sliced open Joice Heth's body before thousands at the City Saloon.[39] Heth's story underlines how the white American public's adversarial relationship with anatomists largely counted for white bodies only.

This blatant exploitation did not mean that African descendants did not resist medical students and professors' greed for their community members' bodies. Archaeological reports of New York City's eighteenth-century African Burial Ground indicate that the city's African and African-descended population actively resisted physicians' and medical students' assaults on their loved ones' bodies. As mentioned earlier, in the decade leading up to the 1788 anatomy riot, free Africans and their descendants had actively petitioned the local government to legalize the dissection of criminals to prevent corpse theft. Local Black leaders even threatened a violent response if the prospective doctors continued to raid the graveyard.[40]

While they did not riot like whites, members of New York's Black community did not passively allow physicians to raid their sacred spaces. In two cases, archaeologists of the African Burial Ground found human remains that had experienced postmortem violence characteristic of autopsy and dissection, but the bodies were interred after the fact. As it is unlikely that the doctors would have returned these bodies themselves, it seems plausible that Black New Yorkers confronted the dissectors, retrieved the corpses, and returned them to their proper resting place. As Warren R. Perry, Jean Howson, and Barbara A. Bianco, the authors of this portion of the archaeological report, explain, "Because we know that African New Yorkers assumed active vigilance over their dead . . . , it is not unreasonable to hypothesize they made efforts to retrieve bodies, which then would have been afforded proper burial." While confronting elite white physicians supplied many potential dangers, African and African-descended New Yorkers met the theft of their community members' and family members' remains with resistance, not passivity.[41]

That Black New Yorkers found body snatching an important issue to coalesce around also reveals the degree to which burial grounds were a vital space for community and identity formation in the local African diasporic population. Despite the diversity of ethnic backgrounds among New York's African-descended population, the burial ground revealed a remarkably unified culture in terms of interment. African-descended communities formed shared cultures despite comprising people from diverse ethnic backgrounds. The vast majority of Black New Yorkers buried in the eighteenth century had coffins and shrouds, and they were placed supine and with their heads facing west. Until the city's common council outlawed the practice in 1722, burials probably took place at night, a custom that was routine among many West African societies. This law also reveals that whites feared the cultural formation taking place around the burial ground. The history of the African Burial Ground thus exposes the fact that eighteenth-century Black New Yorkers understood a proper burial as an essential rite. They viewed the burial ground as a sacred center for their community. Understanding the meaning of burial for African descendants in early America draws attention to the magnitude of the crimes being undertaken by medical students. Body snatching was not just a material theft. It also represented a cultural attack on Black communities in the United States and the Atlantic World.[42]

Crimes such as these were not just confined to urban centers and southern plantation districts. Cases of stealing Black cadavers also occurred in rural districts in the North. In a chapter entitled "The Pioneer Doctor in Northwestern Pennsylvania—Brookville's Pioneer Resurrection; or 'Who Skinned the N—r?'—the True Story of the Origin of the State Anatomical Law," physician W. J. McKnight recounted in his history of northwest Pennsylvania how he and several local physicians had stolen a Black cadaver when he was just an apprentice. Along with his cohort, McKnight thought dissection was necessary for surgical experience. Thus, on Halloween night in 1857, the group exhumed the body of Henry Southerland, a recently deceased Black man and the descendant of a self-liberated, formerly enslaved man. Like the students at Transylvania University, one of McKnight's friends believed Southerland's death "was a good chance for a subject."[43]

However, rumors of the grave robbing spread throughout the town almost immediately, and the townspeople believed the doctors were behind the theft. Ironically, given medical professors' growing claims that Black people could be identified through their anatomy, the physicians decided to first skin the corpse so that it could not be identified as Southerland. They then planned to dump him into a local creek. To maintain their own reputations, and seemingly with little remorse, the doctors disfigured the corpse. The second half of the medics' plan failed, as someone discovered Southerland's skinned body. McKnight eventually plead guilty for the crime and was fined twenty-five dollars.

While McKnight ostensibly faced some repercussions for stealing Southerland's corpse, his punishment was light compared with the riots that took place in the wake of stolen white bodies.[44] McKnight told this story publicly as it related to his role in the fight to legalize dissection in Pennsylvania in 1883. Narrating these events as evidence of the terrible lengths that physicians were forced to go to while learning their trade, he shed light on another aspect of medical history—the ubiquity of postmortem racism. Anecdotes such as his reveal how grave robbers targeted Black people across the nation, even in rural western Pennsylvania, where the Black population was quite small. McKnight's story portrayed the medical profession's exploitation of Black cadavers as a national issue defined by the supposed exigencies of medical training that built on the horrors of the slave system.

In the process of obtaining their medical education, students learned to think of the human body as an object. In both the North and the South, aspiring doctors stole the corpses of Black and white people, subjecting the dead to their unskilled hands while hacking them apart in the name of clinical training. While northern students appropriated white bodies in greater numbers than free Black ones, they stole the bodies of Black people with greater impunity. By targeting African descendants' corpses first, northern medical professionals reinforced the United States' racial hierarchy. This reinforcement was likely more incidental rather than intentional. Black people's bodies were stolen with greater frequency because they had less social power across the United States. In the South, enslaved Black people's position was especially weak, as they lacked legal rights or significant social power outside of dangerous collective action like revolt. Even though most northern Black people were legally free, they were still the least powerful group in society and thus the most vulnerable to the medical schools that consumed corpses at an alarming rate. The disproportionate theft of Black corpses reinforced the social structure, but the goal was to obtain dissection materials with minimal resistance or potential social backlash. In a racially and economically stratified society where they possessed little economic or social power, Black people were the easiest targets for grave robbers.

In Philadelphia, with the secret consent of the mayor, the local medical schools stole and divided between themselves nearly all of the bodies buried in the potter's field each year, about 450 corpses.[45] In fact, in 1832, James Webster, a private anatomy instructor in Philadelphia, wrote a pamphlet complaining that William Horner and MDUP used their power and prestige to take more than their share of the city's dead.[46] The superintendent of Philadelphia's public graveyards only hired security to protect against unofficial body snatchers who would not pay the city for the corpses. New York City had a different arrangement, where grave diggers placed the bodies safe for theft in field number two.[47] Through stealing and purchasing the corpses of their inferiors, medical professionals perceived themselves as having proprietary rights to the bodies of the socially disenfranchised. This systematic exploitation of the bodies of Black and poor white people created a medical profession that understood itself as socially superior to the lower classes of the population.

While northern schools in cities with large populations of impoverished whites and African descendants stocked their dissecting rooms locally, other schools had to look beyond their poor and disenfranchised neighbors for corpses. When the Black Liberian American Samuel F. McGill journeyed to New England from Baltimore in 1837 to begin his medical studies, he brought two Black cadavers. In undertaking McGill as a private student, University of Vermont medical professor Edward E. Phelps required him to bring his own subjects for the dissecting room. Even though McGill became the first Black graduate from a U.S. medical school, he could not escape the white supremacist norms of the nation's system of medical education.[48]

McGill's story illustrates the reliance of northern medical educators on Black people's bodies, and it even reveals a traffic in Black people's flesh going from the South to the North in the antebellum era. After working with Phelps for a year, McGill went on to study at Dartmouth College's medical school, where he eventually received his degree in 1839. In the spring of 1838, McGill hired a Black resurrectionist in Baltimore to steal two more bodies from the local cemetery. After being shipped to Boston, the corpses of two young Black women went on to be dissecting material at Dartmouth. By obtaining the cadavers, McGill was admitted to Dartmouth's dissecting room and employed by the school's anatomist. Based on statements from Phelps and Dartmouth professor Rueben Mussey, local anatomists had been importing Black people's bodies for some time. While ostensibly unique as the first Black graduate of a U.S. medical school, McGill had an education that sometimes resembled the white student experience. Through selling bodies to the North, southern and northern medical schools were connected in both ideas and a trade in Black people's bodies. Perhaps nothing better illustrated the degree to which American physicians were united in their willingness to take advantage of the country's racially stratified economic and social system. Even if some doctors disagreed over the future of the slave system, they all engaged in the exploitation and degradation of African descendants.[49]

While African descendants' bodies were disproportionately used by northern and southern medical schools throughout the antebellum period, southern programs publicly announced their appropriation of Black corpses. As the 1840–41 circular for MCSC advertised, "Subjects for dissection are obtained in ample number, chiefly from the black population, and at far less expense, it is believed, than in any other Institution in the country."[50]

Southern schools also played a significant role in the disciplinary regime of the slave society by dissecting the bodies of executed enslaved criminals. Newspapers around the country regularly recounted the execution of the enslaved and often noted that the "body was given to surgeons for dissection."[51] Upon receipt of the corpse of an enslaved person executed for murder in 1847, Jeffries Wyman's students at Hampden-Sydney expressed a "great desire" to have the body galvanized (electrocuted). Wyman refused the request, having conducted the experiment previously and finding it "too barbarous."[52] Despite his refusal, this anecdote uncovers American medical students' casual mistreatment of enslaved bodies. Dissecting enslaved criminals occupied only a part of southern anatomists' active role in maintaining slaveholder power.

The most glaring example of the medical profession aiding and abetting the disciplinary regimes of slavery comes in the case of slave revolts. According to the *Liberator*, among other sources, in 1831 a local Virginia medical school dissected the rebel Nat Turner's corpse.[53] Free Black people opposed dissection partly because they understood it to reinforce their connection to slavery and inferior status.[54] For enslaved people in the antebellum South, however, this relationship was quite literal. Through dissection of enslaved rebels, medical schools engaged in the process of restoring white rule that occurred during the aftermath of slave revolts. Any enslaved people considering rebellion likely knew that their bodies would be dissected or otherwise desecrated.[55]

Through reporting on these stories, medical schools played an active role in the narrative of the restoration of white rule. John Brown's raid provided another instance of using dissection as a response to an uprising. In this case, rather than just one would-be rebel, a school took almost the entire cohort of rebels. The *New York Tribune* explained, "The colonel in charge at Harper's Ferry tells me that the bodies were all hurriedly and loose'y thrown into the ground, but were exhumed the same night, and carried away for dissection at a medical college in a town not far distant—Winchester, I believe. I understood from his manner of speaking that this disposition of the bodies was not objected to by the authorities but was readily favored by them."[56]

Through these practices, medical professionals directly contributed to the maintenance of the slavocracy. Schools benefited by having legal channels to obtain corpses for dissection—although they nonetheless regularly resorted to extralegal methods. Similarly, the political authorities profited from having an added punishment on top of execution. Dissection caused the dismantling of the bodies of offenders against the slave system, symbolically and literally destroying the would-be insurgent. The enslaved also knew to fear the medical school generally, because their bodies could end up there after death.[57] Through dissection, medical professionals gained intimate knowledge of Black people's bodies and further legitimated their authority in the South. While slavery did not define the practice of the U.S. medical profession's appropriation of Black corpses for dissection, cases of slave revolt certainly imparted added meaning to dissection. In the most notorious rebellions of the antebellum period, dissection represented the final step in the restoration of white rule, with the literal destruction of the offenders' bodies.

Slavery shaped much of the racialization of African descendants' bodies in the seventeenth and eighteenth centuries, and the growing debate over the abolition of slavery certainly fertilized the ground for the flourishing of racial medicine in the nineteenth century. Once these ideas became codified in science, however, they took on a life of their own, where many of the theoretical underpinnings had as much to do with medical practice as with overarching political debates.[58] Furthermore, slave-state physicians were not solely responsible for the emergence of a racialized clinical detachment. Instead, physicians across the country cultivated a callous approach toward Black people's bodies in how they appropriated them for dissection. As essentialist racism gained legitimacy in medical circles throughout the Atlantic World, racial science also defined how white medical professionals used African descendants' persons. Through the act of dissection, physicians furthered the objectification of Black people's bodies, which was in many ways the theoretical project of racial science.

Through the disproportionate use of African descendants' bodies for dissection, physicians enacted the clinical-racial gaze that they cultivated in racial theory. Through body snatching, the medical profession reproduced Black people's social inferiority in the North and South in terms of bodily autonomy. While historians have shown that schools used social class as another essential factor to determine whom to dissect, doctors generally saw African descendants' bodies as more easily accessible than whites'. In northern cities, white working-class people had greater social power through crowd action, and thus stealing bodies of the white poor was a risky if unavoidable part of northern medical education.[59] Through the schools' use of African descendants' bodies, students learned to treat African descendants in a manner analogous to how they were framed in racial theory—as an intermediary link between white humanity and other mammals. Dissection only represented the beginning of this story. As experimental methods became more prominent, physicians began to conduct experiments on animals at a furious pace, along with occasional dangerous experiments on the enslaved.

EXPERIMENTING ON AFRICAN DESCENDANTS

In his 1855 memoir, John Brown, a self-liberated man then living in London, gave a rare insight into the extremes of how the medical profession experimentally used and abused living Black people's bodies. Without Brown's memoir, his story would likely have gone unknown to historians, and he revealed how enslaved people's lack of bodily autonomy abetted southern experimentalists. Specifically, in Jones County, Georgia, Brown's owner, Stevens, lent Brown to Dr. Thomas Hamilton, who had recently cured Stevens of a life-threatening illness. Hamilton, an MDUP graduate, asked to borrow Brown for a series of experiments on sunstroke and more. The physician asked for Brown because he was "a strong and likely subject to be experimented upon." Stevens never asked Hamilton what he intended to do to Brown, and Brown only learned in the moment.[60]

In Hamilton's first experiment on Brown, he hoped to find a cure for sunstroke. Hamilton had said nothing of his intentions, and Brown watched in horror as the doctor had "a hole to be dug in the ground" and "into this pit a quantity of dried red oak bark was cast, and fire set to it. It was allowed to burn until the pit became heated like an oven, when the embers were taken out. A plank was then put across the bottom of the pit, and on that a stool." After making Brown swallow an unknown medicine, Hamilton then ordered him to sit naked in this makeshift oven. Brown had to stay in the hole until he fainted, at which point he was removed and revived. Hamilton repeated the experiment on Brown "five or six times"—with days of rest between each trial—until he found his cure, a "cayenne Pepper tea."[61] Yet the physician had more experiments in mind for Brown.

After giving him a few weeks to recover, Dr. Hamilton then commenced with bleeding Brown regularly until his health again began to fail. Having learned what he wanted from the experiment, Hamilton allotted Brown more time to recover, not wanting to kill an enslaved laborer whom he did not own and still hoping to conduct yet another round of tests.[62] The last experiment that Brown detailed—the others he "refused to dwell upon" in his memoir—involved a series of invasive and painful tests to ascertain the depth of his black skin. Hamilton blistered Brown's "hands, legs, and feet."[63] The experiments lasted for a total of nine months. Hamilton only stopped once

Brown's owner, Stevens, intervened, having realized the damage that Hamilton had done to his enslaved property. Moreover, and not coincidentally, Brown attempted to escape slavery soon after he was returned to Stevens.[64]

Access to enslaved patients—who had virtually no legal rights—for experimentation represented a significant difference between northern and southern physicians. Precisely, it allowed southern practitioners to conduct unethical nontherapeutic tests like those done on Brown. Despite southern physicians' access to enslaved people's bodies, stories such as Brown's remain rare in the historical record. All such cases of testing on enslaved people that have been discovered occurred at schools in the South. During the antebellum period, the voices of enslaved people were scant in accounts of therapeutic experimentation. In comparison, though, stories such as Brown's remain difficult to find, even from the perspective of physicians.

Thus, most previous histories of experimentation on the enslaved have largely focused on cases of therapeutic surgical trials, such as J. Marion Sims's use of enslaved women to practice and perfect a surgical cure for vesicovaginal fistulas.[65] In these accounts of testing on enslaved people, physicians filtered the entire experience through their perspective, with patients mostly appearing as passive objects.[66] While Sims aimed to cure his patients, he did not believe Black people required anesthesia, as he claimed that they were largely insensible to pain.[67] Medical professionals found experimental surgeries to be a more acceptable form of medical testing than Dr. Hamilton's endeavors. Just as with dissection, Black people experienced more than their share of these risky surgical procedures as compared with whites. Through life-threatening physiological experiments, however, physicians literally enacted polygenesis through tests that were too dangerous for whites. Medics further displayed this dynamic in how they experimented on animals as compared with humans.

While in rare cases physicians conducted life-threatening nontherapeutic experiments on enslaved patients, more commonly doctors used animals in tests where subjects had little hope for survival. In their use of animal bodies to understand human life, physicians depicted the difference between animal and man as occupying a spectrum rather than being categorical opposites, much like they were framed by taxonomists. Where Black people's corpses were made to stand in for white corpses for anatomical instruction, animals were commonly used for physiological experimentation.

During this period, French physicians regularly used animals to understand the moving anatomy of humans, in keeping with the contemporary obsession with pathological science. Simultaneously, American students became fascinated with animal experiments by those such as French physiologists François Magendie and Claude Bernard and Philadelphia physician Silas Weir Mitchell. Just as Parisian physicians emphasized dissection and clinical medicine in the first half of the nineteenth century, a budding interest in experimental physiology had also developed, largely on the back of animal and occasional human experiments. In the first half of the nineteenth century, French physiologists such as Magendie and Bernard attempted to map the inner workings of the live body. Where anatomists were interested in the location of organs and diseases' effects on them, physiologists analyzed how organs and tissues worked in concert, and thus these physicians required live subjects for their experiments.[68] Influenced by comparative anatomy and the opposition to systems popular among early nineteenth-century physicians, Magendie and other experimental physiologists saw animal bodies as analogous to human bodies.[69] As a result, they could infer information about the actions of the human heart from exposing a dog's heart, just as MDUP student Charles Schaffer did in 1858.[70] As another inherent part of this worldview, Magendie saw types of animal life as existing on a spectrum, where meaningful connections existed between the physiology of dogs, for example, and humans.[71]

By the end of the antebellum era, American medical students regularly cited Magendie due to his eminence in the field and the knowledge he produced. However, students also were drawn to the transgressive nature of the French physiologist's experiments, finding them both tantalizing and horrifying, much like dissection. Multiple pupils quoted one of Magendie's more disturbing experiments, which proved the stomach's active role in vomiting.[72] In his thesis, MDUP student John W. Caruthers described Magendie's removal of "the stomach from a dog, [after which] he attached to the esophagus a pig bladder filled with liquid, and then injected the veins with tartar emetic, and found that vomiting occurred, just as though the stomach remained uninjured."[73]

In some cases, American medical students conducted their own vivisections, but during the antebellum period, the works of French physiologists would have been more influential than the rare case of a student who had conducted a vivisection himself.[74] Through reading works by experimentalists such as Magendie, prospective doctors were introduced into a new way of seeing animals and their relation to humans. The divisions between different types of life were of degree, not kind. Moreover, through these works, American medical students became acquainted with the benefits and methods of live experimentation.

Physicians used enslaved bodies with little power to protest since most white patients would not consent to life-threatening nontherapeutic experiments. In its 1847 code of ethics, the American Medical Association provided no guidelines for human experimentation, just as it did not discuss animal experiments. The code contains seven "duties of physicians to their patients," and none of them address experimental therapies, much less nontherapeutic experimentation. However, in his tests on John Brown, Dr. Hamilton certainly did not fulfill the duty that "every case committed to the charge of a physician should be treated with attention, steadiness, and humanity."[75] In fact, the American Medical Association did not amend its code of ethics to include rules regarding human experimentation until after World War II, in spite of decades of public outrage over human and animal experiments dating back to the 1870s.[76] During the antebellum period, physicians rarely undertook human physiological experiments, but students who conducted dangerous nontherapeutic tests on human subjects did so on enslaved people's bodies.

This was largely due to the potential outrage experimenting on whites would have garnered, not to mention the fact that whites had legal standing to defend themselves from physicians' dangerous experiments.[77] For example, when Boston dentist William T. G. Morton attempted to test ether on dockworkers in exchange for payment, they refused to submit to the doctor's request.[78] Analysis of physiological tests on whites reveals a stark contrast in the types of experiments that physicians could conduct on white versus Black people and the repercussions a physician could face for casually endangering the life of a white patient.

In the late 1820s and 1830s, the U.S. Army surgeon William Beaumont did engage in many physiological experiments on the white French Canadian Alexis St. Martin. St. Martin had a permanent fistula in his stomach—the result of a gunshot wound treated by Beaumont—that gave the surgeon unusual access to observe and experiment on St. Martin's digestive system. From 1824 through the early 1830s, Beaumont conducted hundreds of tests on St. Martin. For example, he extracted gastric juice from the fistula, and he dipped foods into it to observe the role of the juices in digestion.[79] Unlike physiological experiments on enslaved people, however, Beaumont's tests included pay for St. Martin. Likewise, St. Martin had the ability to abscond, which he did in 1825. He only returned when Beaumont's agents found him, but unlike Black subjects vulnerable to slave catchers, St. Martin could choose not to come back. Beaumont explained his actions in 1829 upon hearing that St. Martin was in Canada: "I made arrangements with the agents of the American Fur Company, who annually visit Canada for the purpose of procuring voyageurs, to find and engage him for my service, if practicable. After considerable difficulty, and at great expense to me, they succeeded in engaging him, and transported him from Lower Canada, with his wife and two children, to me."[80]

While invasive and most likely painful, Beaumont's tests differed from physiological experiments conducted on the enslaved in two important respects. First, the surgeon did not intend to risk his subject's life. Second, while St. Martin's relationship with Beaumont appeared to be contentious at times, Beaumont relied on some manner of St. Martin's consent to conduct his experiments. While economic incentives and class differences likely exercised subtle coercion on St. Martin, he did have the ability to say no, unlike John Brown. As a result, Beaumont could publish his observations to great professional acclaim. In contrast, Dr. Hamilton experimented on John Brown without his consent and most likely knowing that he was endangering Brown's long-term health.

One of the most significant moments of public outcry over human experimentation during this period occurred in Paris, and thus provides the best example of the type of scandal that life-threatening experiments on unconsenting whites could garner. In 1859, two Parisian doctors intentionally infected four of their patients at the Hôpital St. Louis with syphilis to determine whether the disease was contagious in its secondary stage.[81] The French government had given hospital physicians far greater power than their American counterparts to treat patients as experimental objects, but directly infecting patients with harmful diseases went well beyond normal medical ethics. Public protest over the experiments caused the French government to reform nonhospital physicians' access to patients, and both doctors faced criminal investigations.[82] The French public found these experiments so shocking because the physicians directly intended to harm the subjects for purely scientific knowledge.[83] In contrast to these French patients and self-liberated people like John Brown, the enslaved still in bondage could be easily silenced by physicians, minimizing the chances for a scandal to occur.

Having access to enslaved people for these types of experiments represents one of the few instances of marked difference between students' experiences in the North and the South. Physiological tests on enslaved people were both similar to and distinct from therapeutic and surgical tests on the enslaved. In both types of experiments, physicians asserted that Black people and other socially inferior groups such as Irish immigrants were safer testing grounds than native white patients. Moreover, therapeutic and nontherapeutic experiments on Black people's bodies medically enshrined the inferior social position of Black people. However, physicians undertaking nontherapeutic physiological trials distinguished themselves in one significant respect: they directly intended to harm, not heal, the patient. In conducting experimental trephinations on Black patients at Transylvania University, Benjamin Dudley intended to alleviate their epilepsy.[84] Likewise, J. Marion Sims aimed to cure his enslaved and Irish patients when he engaged in experimental gynecological surgeries. Sims chose his patients because, if the tests failed, he would face few if any repercussions. Far from being clandestine, like Beaumont, Sims published his experiments and became famous as a result.[85]

Unlike therapeutic surgical experiments, students' and physicians' dangerous physiological trials on enslaved people were rarely brought before the public. In their unpublished theses, however, a few students narrated how they used living Black people's bodies to understand the transmission of disease and the effects of certain drugs. Pupils' physiological experiments corresponded to the nascent influence of physiologists such as Magendie and Bernard. By deliberately conducting potentially fatal experiments, these aspiring doctors treated the enslaved more like animal test subjects than humans. Without legal standing in courts, enslaved people were far more vulnerable to dangerous medical tests than even poor whites or free Black people in the North. Enslaved people's legal status coincided with the growing perception among many medical professionals that their bodies were inferior to whites'. In this respect, Black people were seen as objects of learning for human physiology in general, but experiments and dissection also shed light on their differential racial status. Through physiological experimentation, physicians, like enslavers, treated enslaved people as chattel, not only through the commodification of their bodies as experimental objects, but also in performing tests that would be ethically acceptable only on Black people, convicts, and animals.

While physicians had been performing nonlethal experiments on Black people's skin for centuries, the student experiments of the 1840s and 1850s had a different and more dangerous character.[86] In his 1858 thesis, MCSC student Peter Horn reported a trial similar to those performed in Paris a year later. During Horn's first year of medical school, measles had broken out among his father's enslaved laborers, and the young student/scientist saw an opportunity to see whether this illness was contagious. He also hoped to discern whether the seat of measles and scarlatina was in the blood, like smallpox and in contrast to yellow fever, which was the subject of his thesis. Regarding the method for testing the contagiousness and seat of the illness, Horn noted, "In these diseases, as well as in small pox, transmission can be likewise artificially produced, as the following authentic statements will indicate."[87]

The fact that medical practitioners could intentionally infect patients with smallpox, a practice known as variolation, dated back to at least the seventeenth century. Enslaved Africans brought this technique with them to the Americas, a medical practice that white physicians had appropriated. Variolation acted as a rudimentary form of vaccination before Edward Jenner began vaccinating people with the far less dangerous cowpox in 1796.[88] As a result, when Horn conducted his tests, he had significant precedents. As with the French syphilis experiments, Horn hoped to discern how the disease was transmitted. While his test predated the Paris trials, his choice of an enslaved subject ensured that the story of his experiment remained between him and his professors. Moreover, Horn's experiment underscored that this student saw the body of the enslaved man who was his subject as expendable in the name of knowledge production.

To conduct his test, Horn first isolated one healthy enslaved man from those already taken ill. Horn explained that the man "had not been at all exposed" to measles. He "was afterwards carefully protected from contraction from any other source"—besides Horn's syringe, of course. Horn planned to make a blood transfusion, injecting measles-infected blood into the healthy enslaved man. Relating the experiment to his professors, he explained, "Having drawn a drachem or two of blood from the arm of a negro labouring under the disease, I injected it by means of a small syringe into the circulation of" the isolated man. Horn believed that his experiment proved contagion true, as the man was almost immediately suffering from measles. The effect of the disease on the enslaved patient was devastating. He suffered one of the worst cases of measles on Horn's plantation during the epidemic. As Horn related, "In a few days, the ordinary symptoms of measles manifested themselves which were soon fully developed, and the case subsequently became one of the most obstinate with we had to contend though it terminated successfully."[89] The enslaved man was lucky to be alive in the wake of this student's test, and Horn had an exceptional piece of scientific data to relay to his professors. Moreover, Horn graduated from MCSC, highlighting that his professors did not disapprove of his experiment, or at least not enough to fail him.

While Horn's experiment was not typical, it also was not completely unique to South Carolina medicine. Horn came from the Colleton District, just south of Charleston on the state's Atlantic coast. He explained that he had repeated the test of an acquaintance who "employed a like experiment in a case of scarlatina, under similar circumstances and with corresponding results." Horn gleaned from the result of both trials that the seat of the disease was in the blood and contagious, unlike yellow fever, whose seat was in the liver. Horn explained why he believed it important to prove measles contagious and yellow fever not: "Contagious diseases are not limited by latitudinal demarcations . . . and attack all complexions and races." As a result, when he found that yellow fever was not contagious, he upheld the notion of innate Black resistance and white vulnerability to the ailment.[90] In his findings, Horn highlighted the dual purpose of experiments on Black people's bodies. Their persons provided medical data on the nature of humanity in general, while also supplying knowledge of the alleged essential differences between white and Black people.

In 1846, C. Caldwell Higgins, an MCSC student from Virginia, also conducted a series of physiological experiments on local enslaved people. His first set of experiments was most likely physically harmless although potentially frightening for the infants involved. Higgins wrote his thesis about the skin's ability to absorb outside materials, and both of his tests were related to this question. In the first trial, he hoped to see whether the skin's ability to absorb water diminished with age. He submerged four infants, ranging from two weeks to one year old, in bags of water up to the neck for durations of fifteen to thirty minutes. With these tests, Higgins proved his thesis correct, as the two-week-old took on the most water during this period.[91] While this first series of experiments was innocuous enough, by choosing to use the enslaved exclusively as his subjects, he further positioned them as specifically fit for experimentation. Like Abraham Addams describing the child cadaver, Higgins decided not to mention the children's sex, instead referring to each one as "it."

Higgins's next experiment caused far more damage to his subjects and thus prevented the student from conducting multiple trials. This test required an enslaved mother and a suckling child. Higgins first intended to see whether tobacco could be absorbed through the skin. He isolated the woman's head by putting it through a "broken pane of glass." Higgins then sealed the area between the glass and her neck with pillows "so that she could not inhale the particles of tobacco fumes." Once the woman was ready, Higgins spread moist tobacco all over her limbs and stomach. She remained in this state for nearly a half hour, "when she complained of being quite sick." Higgins then cleaned the woman's body, removing the tobacco.[92] Through her illness, he proved the skin's ability to absorb tobacco.

Having verified his first point, Higgins then set out to see whether the toxin could be transmitted through breast milk. After having been washed, the woman "still complained of being sick but did not vomit. [Higgins] immediately applied the child to her breast." Once again, he guessed correctly. He explained, "In a short time afterwards the child began to vomit. In fact for a while I was afraid it was going into convulsions but luckily for me it did not."[93] In the aftermath of these tests, Higgins displayed the complicated nature of the physician's morality when dealing with the enslaved as experimental objects. On the one hand, Higgins did not repeat the test, "thinking it a sin to cause innocency [*sic*] to suffer."[94] However, he was more than willing to risk the enslaved infant's life once to test his suspicion that the toxins could first be absorbed through the skin, then transmitted through the mother's milk. Moreover, he chose not to continue his tests only after he had obtained proof of his theory. Higgins and Horn displayed a willingness to use Black people's bodies as experimental objects and, when necessary, to significantly endanger the lives of the enslaved in the South.

The regularity of experiments such as those by Higgins, Horn, or Dr. Thomas Hamilton remains difficult to discern. Although they were certainly not typical, both students appear to have passed their exams and graduated from MCSC without raising ethical concerns. During this period, physicians began to set the precedent for medical professionals' use of Black people's bodies to gain experimental knowledge, just as they articulated a vision of race rooted inside the body and biologically determined. Unlike the Tuskegee experiments in the twentieth century or the two French hospital patients that caused controversy, the harrowing experiments conducted on Higgins's and Horn's enslaved workers would have been known to few people. As many physicians increasingly considered Black people essentially different from whites, the medical profession enacted these differences through how they treated their bodies experimentally.

Medical students revealed how they were trained to see African descendants taxonomically through the routine ways that they dissected and experimented on Black people's bodies. Essentialist racial medicine justified the brutal usage of African descendants' bodies. Conversely, medical professionals' power over African descendants gave further credence to racial science. In fact, through their intimacy with Black people, racial scientists justified their theories. Unlike the white people's bodies in Paris, African descendants' bodies—those of the enslaved in particular—were safer targets for both experimentation and dissection without risking the medical profession's reputation. Through their use of Black people's bodies for dissection and testing, white physicians engaged in the objectifying and disciplinary practices inherent to the chattel system. Physicians simultaneously extended the commodification of African descendants into their death and treated them as a literal link between white humanity and the rest of the animal kingdom.

By stealing Black corpses and dissecting them, medical students increasingly treated Black people as a medical underclass. In the dissecting room, pupils garnered a clinical detachment toward patients, and this relationship was only magnified by racial science. Students strategically targeted Black people for corpse theft because they were particularly vulnerable. Through their empowered position in relation to corpses, pupils increased their sense of mastery over African descendants' bodies. The relationship that students developed with African descendants' bodies also shaped Black people's role as experimental objects. By systematically exploiting Black corpses in northern and southern medical schools, students learned to see African descendants as inferior, compounding their legally codified status as enslaved.

More than any other factor, rare instances of dangerous nontherapeutic experiments represented the material culmination of the new pedagogy of racial medicine. African descendants' bodies were anatomically different, but not so much so as to necessitate different surgical treatments. The white medical profession used African descendants' bodies as objects to produce knowledge, just as they situated them rhetorically and socially as inferior. White students used Black bodies in ways that were characteristic of how medical professionals used animals. This choice made Black people's degraded status quite literal and solidified their liminal position between white humanity and the rest of the animal kingdom. Through these experiments, students enacted the racial science that they were taught in lectures, understanding Black people as defined by both human and animal features. Moreover, prospective doctors presaged the now-famous twentieth-century cases of racial science–informed experimentation that occurred in Tuskegee, Alabama, Nazi Germany, and elsewhere. These experiments on the enslaved highlight the continuity between racial science in the nineteenth and twentieth centuries. Medical practitioners viewed racial science as informing both the medical treatment of African descendants and their social position.

4 MASTERING ANATOMY

Anatomy is a liberal pursuit, holding out the highest incentive to exertion and has been injured and rendered odious in the eyes of mankind by the laws confounding it with criminals.
—*William Horner, later the professor of anatomy at MDUP, 1821*

The advocates for the plurality of races, being met with so many objections, good as well as bad, have attempted to enlarge the circle of their arguments, and, ceasing to make the skull their only study, have proceeded to the examination of the entire individual.
—*Joseph Arthur, Comte de Gobineau,* The Moral and Intellectual Diversity of Races, *1856*

On March 29, 1861, recent MDUP graduate Charles M. Ellis wrote to his former anatomy professor Joseph Leidy. Ellis expected to be called as an expert witness in an upcoming civil case in Baltimore County, where he now practiced medicine. Specifically, one apparently white man had called another a "n—r" and was being sued by the aggrieved party for slander. According to Ellis, for the case to be adjudicated quickly and without the aid of a medical expert, the defendant had three simple routes to prove the plaintiff's blackness. Proving one's whiteness was anything but simple. First, if the plaintiff's mother or father was of African descent, so was he. Second, the plaintiff would certainly be ruled Black if he possessed dark skin and "crisp hair." Finally, if the plaintiff had light skin, "crisp hair," and evidence of "negro ancestry far remote," the court would likely rule in the defendant's favor.[1]

The plaintiff must have appeared white, because Ellis did not believe one of these simple tests would solve the case. Instead, he prepared to use his medical training to discern whether the plaintiff had any Black ancestry. Ellis had finished his medical degree that spring, and the lessons that he had learned about anatomical blackness remained fresh in his mind. He asked

Leidy, "Can a man having negro parentage on one side several generations since be distinguished from a white man?"[2]

Ellis's questions revealed both the conceptual promise of medical schools' racial pedagogies and their practical limitations. According to professors such as Leidy, medical and anatomical knowledge were key to defining racial difference. Yet in practice, medical graduates could not really discern whether a living patient—whose outward appearance was supposedly white—was Black. Anatomical investigation was the only remaining route to proving a white-looking person was Black. As Ellis fawned, "[From Leidy's] most satisfactory lectures during the past three years, I am well acquainted with points of distinction between the European and African existing on the skeleton." For obvious reasons, however, Ellis could not directly assess the plaintiff's naked skeleton.[3] Still, he believed that there must be a route to proving whether this man was Black. Ellis thus asked Leidy about distinguishing traits other than hair or skin color: "Is there then any other point that can be relied upon to prove that he is or is not a negro? Would it be conclusive if the facial angle is below 75° and the jaw protrudes?"[4]

In preparing for the witness stand, Ellis revealed a great deal about how medical schools taught racial difference at the end of the antebellum era. While somewhat anomalous in possibly being called into the courtroom, Ellis illustrated the nascent success of medical professionals' campaign to market themselves as scientific masters of racial difference. In the early national period, debates over skin color and environmentally generated changes to the body dominated medical racism. By this period, however, medicine was in its "anatomical era," and contemporary racial medicine mirrored this orientation.[5]

Leidy's reply to Ellis is unavailable, but that does not mean his and other anatomy professors' racial pedagogies remain untraceable. By the beginning of the U.S. Civil War, anatomists had built a system of medical education that deliberately trained physicians to describe Black people as physically, socially, and intellectually inferior. Rather than being a profession that universalized humanity, medicine adopted racial pedagogies that became more essentialist as the country grew more divided by slavery.[6]

At MDUP and other schools, anatomy professors such as Leidy used various pedagogical tools at their disposal to teach anatomical white supremacy, including textbooks, lectures, museum displays, and the students' final test, their senior thesis. Reading textbooks and listening to lectures allowed prospective doctors to contextualize the sensory education that they received through museum objects, dissections, and illustrations. These tools constituted what historian Carin Berkowitz describes as medical educators' "system of display." As Berkowitz explains, schools' "anatomical museums functioned alongside books and bodies to form a set of instructional tools and objects of study. Individual elements of display, such as [anatomical] atlases or dissected bodies, were understood to function together as parts of a system that were created and deployed in a particular setting and for a particular purpose. That purpose and setting were classroom based." Employing this system for white supremacist ends, professors used textbooks and the spoken content of lectures to contextualize the active sensory learning that students gained through studying illustrations of racial difference and handling human remains in lecture halls and museums.[7]

Race only represented a small but systematized part of the pedagogy of anatomical textbooks, lectures, and museums. Rather than diminish its importance, this dynamic revealed how embedded race was in medical training. Racial skulls were only a small fraction of the museum's objects. Anatomical lecturers only devoted one or a few lessons out of dozens to race. Professors taught race alongside surgical techniques, disease etiologies, and materia medica. In short, the subject was treated as a normal aspect of medical education that students learned about alongside many other subjects seen as legitimate medicine. This approach gave race the appearance of being as appropriate to medical practice as physiology because professors believed that it was.

By analyzing medical schools' systems of displaying race, this chapter reveals that, rather than being limited to a random aside here or there by professors, racial science and the politics of slavery were deeply entrenched in anatomy curricula. Throughout their studies, instructors reinforced to students the idea that racial differences were real. Those differences could be mapped onto human bodies, and pupils' education made them racial experts. As the first and most passive line of indoctrination, anatomy textbooks routinely taught embodied racial distinctions, including racial discussions of skulls, hair, reproductive organs, and skin. Lectures, moreover, were visual and tactile demonstrations where professors used objects and images from the school's anatomy museum to illustrate perceived points of racial difference. If textbooks and lectures did not satisfy prospective physicians' curiosity and prejudice, then they could venture to the museum. There, they could study the school's racial skull collection, as well as other preserved body parts marked out as not white. These first three pedagogical tools were the most commonly experienced by students, as they were a standard part of the medical curriculum. The final way that some pupils learned about racial anatomy was through researching and writing their theses. All students had the power of racial anatomy reinforced on multiple levels throughout their education. In their theses, though, they revealed how these ideas became adapted and applied to the most important political question of the period: the abolition of slavery. As a result, this pedagogy had a doubly destructive result, shaping medical and popular beliefs about racial difference.

READING RACE IN ANATOMY TEXTBOOKS

"To students of medicine the following pages are most respectfully dedicated," wrote Samuel G. Morton in his 1849 textbook *An Illustrated System of Human Anatomy, Special, General and Microscopic.* Often remembered by historians for his skull collection and racial science texts, Morton was also a medical educator. In the early 1840s, he served as the anatomy professor at the Pennsylvania Medical College in Philadelphia. As the dedication makes clear, unlike his original research in racial science, Morton's *Illustrated System of Human Anatomy* was intended to be read by medical students, familiarizing them with the most basic anatomical issues.[8]

Morton, like many of his contemporaries, saw medical and racial approaches to anatomy as deeply intertwined. *An Illustrated System of Human Anatomy* reflects this imbrication. Morton devoted eight pages and ten illustrations in his textbook to discussing alleged racial differences in the bones of the skull. He ranked each race in descending order by facial angle: "Caucasian," "Mongolian," "Malay," "American," and "Negro." In his primer, he set out his most basic racial science claims for medical students. White skulls (and thus brain size and intelligence) surpassed the size of African descendants' skulls. Other races' intelligence and cranial capacity rested between these two poles. While brief and derivative of his racial science, Morton's inclusion of craniometry in his text implies that he believed the subject should be a standard part of medical education.[9]

When Morton emphasized racial difference in his book, it was hardly an anomaly. In fact, starting in the 1820s, U.S. anatomists began writing textbooks that used cranial analysis and promoted anatomical white supremacy. By the 1850s, this emphasis was no longer novel, but instead had come to typify anatomy curricula. An analysis of three works by MDUP professors Caspar Wistar (1808–18), William Horner (1820–53), and Joseph Leidy (1853–91) draws attention to how nineteenth-century anatomy instructors directly shaped medical and scientific concepts of race. In his 1811 textbook, Caspar Wistar discussed race sparingly, but by the 1861 publication of Leidy's volume, polygenists' depiction of racial difference had a clear role in MDUP's anatomy curriculum. Each textbook went through multiple editions, and as faculty members of the first and most prominent U.S. medical school, the authors of these texts influenced schools across the country. These faculty helped shape the meaning of race for the nation in their primers, influencing thousands of physicians' and racial scientists' approach to race during the decades preceding the Civil War. MDUP anatomists even trained some of the most prominent polygenists of the era, including Morton and Josiah Nott.[10] Thus, when the United States was beginning to break apart over the question of slavery, anatomists had created a medical education system that trained and socialized students to support essentialist white supremacy.

Compared to the textbooks that would come later, in his two-volume *A System of Human Anatomy for the Use of Students*, Caspar Wistar mostly treated the human body as universal except for skin color. While subsequent authors spent pages summarizing the latest advancements in craniometry, Wistar barely mentioned race in his description of the cranium and the brain. In contrast to Horner's and Leidy's later texts, most of Wistar's discussion of cranial difference is cultural. Notably, Wistar emphasized how some Native American cultures bound parts of their heads to manipulate the shapes of their skulls. Generally, though, his treatment of race reflects the influence of physiologists at MDUP. These authors focused their racial discussion on blackness as a potentially curable condition. They did not see blackness as defined by the sum total of perceived anatomical differences. Following Rush's disease theory, Wistar argued that darker skin color signified ill-health. "The Colour of the healthy skin," explained Wistar, "is invariably white, when all the lamellae exterior to it are removed. This is the case not only with the European, but with the blackest African, and the people of all the intermediate colours."[11]

Yet a few casual comments in Wistar's textbook presage the later obsession with skull size, anatomy, and race. Wistar asserted, "The figure of the cranium is somewhat varied in different races of men." He also endorsed phrenology, which was already being applied to racial groups. These passing references reveal how racial anatomy was still in its infancy in medical schools. During the early national period, students at MDUP learned more about race from faculty like Benjamin Rush and Benjamin Smith Barton than from Wistar, the school's anatomist.[12]

Both professional anatomy and the politics of slavery changed precipitously after the release of Wistar's textbook. Wistar taught anatomy prior to the theoretical ascendancy of pathological anatomy in U.S. medicine, a change that was spurred forward by the growing influence of French clinical medicine in the 1830s and 1840s. While later faculty emphasized pathology, anatomists during the early national period focused more on gross anatomy. Rather than providing a theoretical framework for health in the United States, gross anatomists described the geography of the human body. Benjamin

Rush even described the subject as nothing more than "a mass of dead matter." By the 1820s, however, physicians began to embrace anatomy as a paradigm-shaping field because of its perceived ability to describe blackness's and diseases' fundamental effects on the body.[13]

Slavery also defined much of politics when Horner and Leidy wrote their textbooks. Between 1820 and 1860, conflicts over slavery forced festering racial tensions into the political forefront. Rebellious enslaved people and abolitionists confronted enslavers in events such as Nat Turner's uprising and "Bleeding Kansas." Thus, by the time Leidy published his textbook, not only had anatomy become the dominant method for physicians to understand the human body, but the United States had also been undergoing decades of violent political fracture over slavery.[14]

In the second edition of *A Treatise on Special and General Anatomy* (1830), William Horner made it clear that MDUP's racial anatomical pedagogy was changing dramatically under his direction. While Horner gave passing references in his textbook to racial differences in the foot and scrotum, he most clearly revealed the growing importance of skulls and their measurement for understanding racial difference in the United States. In the section entitled "Of the Face, Together with Some Remarks on the Facial Angle, and on National Peculiarities," Horner launched into five pages of discussion of racial distinctions in the skull. Emphasizing facial angles, he asserted, "In European, or Caucasian heads, this angle is about eighty degrees. In the Negro, or Ethiopian, it is about seventy degrees; and in the Mongolian or copper coloured man, about seventy-five degrees." It is worth recalling that, in reference to his potential involvement in a case of slander, C. M. Ellis asked Leidy whether a facial angle of below seventy-five degrees constituted blackness. A later edition of Horner's *Treatise* likely would have been Ellis's textbook.[15]

Facial angles were useful because physicians could easily measure them, and they were falsely thought to dictate a person's intelligence. Explaining this logic, Horner wrote, "The more acute that the facial angle is, the smaller is the volume of brain, and the larger are the nose and mouth." Thus, he made the stakes of African descendants' supposedly smaller facial angles clear: the anatomy of the face and cranium supposedly correlated to brain size, which white scientists thought ordained intelligence.[16] Ultimately, Horner emphasized that while he thought only one human species existed, the anatomy of skulls separated humanity into hierarchical races. In the little more than a decade separating the publication of Wistar's and Horner's textbooks, MDUP's anatomy faculty had adopted a biologically determinist racial pedagogy. Anatomy supposedly proved indefinite Black inferiority.[17]

Building on the groundwork laid by Horner, Joseph Leidy treated racial anatomy as an accepted part of medical thinking that required little explanation. In fact, predecessors like Horner and Morton had made race a typical aspect of anatomy textbooks by the time Leidy published his primer. The work's discussion of the supposed racial variations in the skull captures this stylistic difference. Leidy scattered short asides about racial differences throughout a long chapter on the skull. For example, he noted, "The spongy substance [of the cranium] . . . is more abundant in the negro than in the white race." Eleven pages later, he asserted, "The margin of the *na'sal notch* in the white race is usually acute, but is rounded off to the anterior surface of the alveolar border in the black race."[18] The longest single passage on racial difference in Leidy's textbook, two pages devoted to facial angles and craniometry, also comes in his discussion of the skull. In many respects, Leidy treated race like any other component of anatomical thinking. Through matter-of-fact language, he reinforced the notion that these distinctions were accepted scientific facts because, by 1861, white doctors thought they were.[19]

Leidy even introduced his entire section on the brain through racial analysis. He asserted,

> The *Brain*, the seat of the intellect, the will, the sensations, and the emotions, is the great nervous mass which, with its enveloping membranes, completely fills the cavity of the cranium.
>
> The size and weight of the brain varies with the race, sex, age, and individual. It is the largest in the white race, and, all other circumstance being equal, such as race, sex, age, size of body, and health, its bulk bears a general relationship with the development of intellect.
>
> Its weight in the adult white male averages near fifty ounces avoirdupois; in the female, forty-five ounces.

This passage is remarkable for several reasons. First, it reinforces to students their embodied intellectual superiority as white males. Leidy then revealed the ways in which gender and race intersected. In his hierarchies of brain weight, a white male was superior to a white woman and a Black man to a Black woman. This passage also captures how Leidy differed stylistically from Horner and Morton. Leidy systematized racial discussion in his textbook, introducing race in short bursts of discussion on specific body parts. The collective effect was to depict racial analysis as a normative but essential lens for anatomical study.[20] In employing detached anatomical language, Leidy normalized these ideas for students, a task that he took even further in his lectures.

Rather than exceptions, these textbooks were emblematic of a national and transatlantic trend. For example, in his 1845 work, the British physician Robert Bentley Todd gave numerous examples of European physicians who had dissected African descendants' brains to understand racial difference.[21] Likewise, in the Scottish anatomist and racial scientist Robert Knox's manual on anatomy for artists, he noted, "Each race has been given its own form of body, colour, shape, dimensions, skeleton, muscles, brain, mind. They differ from each other in all these points."[22] In his 1854 primer, T. G. Richardson, the demonstrator of anatomy at the Medical Department of the University of Louisville, devoted four pages of text and images to the racial anatomy of the human skull, routinely citing Morton. Soon after its publication, the University of Louisiana's medical department adopted Richardson's textbook.[23]

By the 1850s, U.S. anatomists promoted racial anatomy by including the subject in their textbooks, standardizing the role of race in medical curricula. Elementary school primers even began including craniometry, raising the possibility that students were familiar with the subject before beginning medical studies.[24] However, this represented a shift in anatomical instruction. As Wistar's textbook illustrated, earlier anatomists in the United States mostly dealt with race in passing. It was not until the antebellum period that anatomists inscribed biologically determinist racial thinking into their curricula. Through their more argumentative styles, Horner and Morton displayed how teaching racial anatomy required some justification as late as the 1840s. By 1861, however, Leidy was able to treat the subject as a standard aspect of the curriculum. Yet textbooks only represented an entry point into racial anatomy, and most authors focused almost entirely on the head. Even so, professors built on this more basic knowledge in lectures, descending down the body to describe a whole host of racial differences.

DICTATING DIFFERENCE IN THE ANATOMICAL THEATER

> Lect. 18th (3d on Races)
> Some account of the Aztec Children. *Further account of the Caucasian family,* Origins *of mankind. Theories of Prichard, Pickering, Agassiz, Smyth, . . . Authorities. Prichard, Pickering, Agassiz, Smyth, Knox. Figure 1. From Layard & Hawkes and other figures from Prichard shown.*
> —*Professor Oliver Wendell Holmes Sr., Anatomy Lectures Notes for the Harvard Medical School, 1850–1851 Session*

By the 1850–51 session at Harvard, Oliver Wendell Holmes had been the professor of anatomy for three years. This term would prove to be a particularly tumultuous one. In that session, Harvard experimented with racial integration when the faculty admitted the abolitionist and Pittsburgh physician Martin R. Delany and two other Black students from Boston, David Lang Jr. and Isaac H. Snowden. Working with the Massachusetts Colonization Society, Lang and Snowden matriculated on the basis that they would practice in Liberia. Despite Harvard's colonizationist aims, this choice was deeply controversial with white students. Perhaps to assuage them, Holmes even increased the number of lectures on racial science that year from one to three. By the year's end, though, the experiment had failed. A paper rebellion by some white pupils ensured that Black students would not be admitted the next year.[25]

Holmes expected students to learn about race both actively and passively in his lectures. He based his lessons on the work of foreign and domestic racial scientists such as Louis Agassiz, Robert Knox, and the American physician and Harvard alum Charles Pickering. Holmes also employed visual and tactile methods to instruct students. As set dressing to his lecture, he surrounded himself with images from the works of the British physician and monogenist James Cowles Prichard. Around him, he arranged stolen human crania from the Warren Museum to illustrate racial differences. If he owned his craniometer by that point, perhaps he used it in his first lecture on race, when he taught students some "modes of examining crania." Moreover, in providing students with an "account of the Aztec children," Holmes displayed the close relationship between popular and scientific forms of anatomical display. Bartola and Maximo, two siblings from El Salvador dubbed by their captors the "Aztec children," suffered from mental disabilities and were the victims of human trafficking.[26] In his lectures, Holmes, like other anatomists, relied on visuals, demonstrations on museum objects, and oratory to depict distinct races. Understanding the power of Holmes and other anatomy professors, then, requires analysis of all three facets of lectures.

In terms of content, lectures on racial anatomy added greater detail to textbooks, and they laid a foundation for students to make their own racial anatomical measurements. In his anatomy lectures at MDUP, Joseph Leidy taught students about supposed racial differences in the cranium, going into depth on facial angles and cranial size.[27] Compared to his textbook, though, Leidy provided many more examples of supposed anatomical differences, descending down the body. He demarcated numerous characteristics supposedly peculiar to African descendants' bodies, including narrower pelvises, longer limbs in relation to the body, "longer foot[,] shorter toes," shorter neck, smaller and longer heel bone, and no arch in the foot.[28] In his lectures, Leidy captured how polygenists had gone beyond just the cranium as the seat of racial difference. Instead, he depicted African descendants' bodies as diverging from whites' forms in their totality. These small differences were negligible on their own, Leidy contended, but when combined, they defined African descendants as entirely distinct.

Writing his friend and colleague Josiah Nott, Leidy described how these small traits supposedly defined African descendants' distinctiveness. He explained his belief that African descendants' bodies differed in the same regards as distinct species of animals in the same genus. Turning British physician, naturalist, and monogenist Richard Owen's own logic against him, Leidy asserted, "A certain fossil horse-tooth, [that Owen] carefully compared with the corresponding tooth of the recent horse, showed no differences, excepting in being a little more curved, he considers it a distinct species, under the name of equus curvidens," but "with differences of greater value in the jaws of the negro and white man, he considers them the same."[29] Appropriating Owen's logic, Leidy contended that these supposed small variations between human races supported classifying them as separate species. As Leidy saw it, the differences that separated species were mostly of degree, not kind. The small racial distinctions that he conjured up for his students were far from trivial, though. Supposedly, they constituted scientific evidence for white supremacy and the permanent subjugation of people of African descent.

Along with enumerating anatomical differences, lecturers employed a visual style that blended oral content with demonstration. In an 1895 essay remembering his experiences as a student at Harvard in the 1860s, Holmes's eventual successor Thomas Dwight recalled, "One of the features of the Harvard Medical School from my earliest recollections was the elaborateness of the preparations for the anatomical lectures. Not only were hours spent, on the dissection itself, but every refinement of neatness, and even elegance—clean sheets, careful draping, effective arrangements of specimens and pictures—received the most careful attention. This arrangement of the amphitheatre with an eye to artistic effect, was the combined work of the professor and the demonstrator [Dr. David Williams Cheever]." In the catalog for the 1850-51 session, Harvard's faculty also portrayed lectures as more than just oratory. They explained, "The demonstrations are aided by a large cabinet (the Warren Anatomical Museum, which is increasing by regular accessions from a fund appropriated to the purpose, and from individual contributions)."[30]

In the introductory lecture to his first session at Harvard in 1847, Holmes plainly explained that his talks would be highly visual. In fact, his motto was "Illustration." He told his students that anatomy was an inherently optical and tactile discipline, and that, in most respects, students learned more from

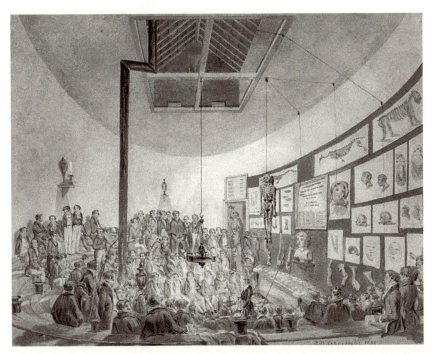

Figure 4.1. A painting of an 1830 anatomy lecture in London. R. B. Schnebbelie, *A Lecture at the Hunterian Anatomy School, Great Windmill Street, London,* watercolor, 1839, Wellcome Collection, Attribution-NonCommercial 4.0 International (CC BY-NC 4.0), https://wellcomecollection.org/works/gb4caj56. Image is also published in Carin Berkowitz, *Charles Bell and the Anatomy of Reform* (Chicago: University of Chicago Press, 2015), 47.

visuals than rhetoric. A professor, "who merely talks about that which he might show to the eye or make palpable to the touch," related Holmes, "fails to give that particular subject the clearness and permanency in the student's mind of which it is susceptible." Holmes's first point on the importance of visuals to anatomical lectures focused on retention. He believed that pupils could understand and retain information about the human body better when it was transmitted through rhetorical, visual, and tactile instruction (see figs. 4.1–4.3).[31]

Holmes argued that the second power of a visually oriented anatomical lecture resided in observation's ability to render anatomical knowledge objectively real. According to Holmes, compared to discussion alone, visuals and models made human anatomy material for students. As he explained, "I have attempted, therefore, to render visible everything which the eye could take cognizance of, and so turn abstractions and catalogues of names into substantial and objective realities." Holmes used images, models, and

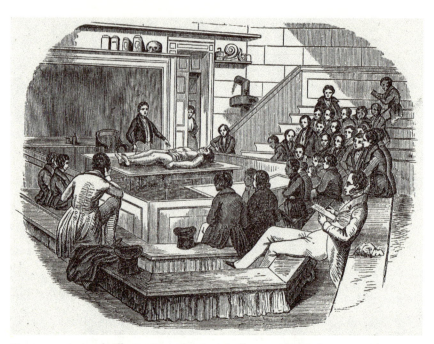

Figure 4.2. A simple illustration of an antebellum anatomy demonstration at the University of Pennsylvania. Henry H. Smith, *Anatomical Atlas, Illustrative of the Structure of the Human Body, under the Supervision of William E. Horner* (Philadelphia: Blanchard & Lea, 1854), title page. Photo courtesy of the Huntington Library. Image is also published in Michael Sappol, *A Traffic of Dead Bodies: Anatomy and Embodied Social Identity in Nineteenth-Century America* (Princeton, N.J.: Princeton University Press, 2002), 75.

anatomical specimens as a part of a larger pedagogical approach to anatomy. He even contacted Louis Agassiz for works from his private collection. Holmes believed that effective anatomical instruction required students not only to memorize written or recited information about the human body, but also to learn human anatomy through sensory experience. The visuals that students eyed and the objects they handled gave antebellum beliefs about anatomy and race the impression of being "objective realities," as described by Holmes.[32]

Essential to Holmes's lessons about racial difference were the images that surrounded him as he explained whites' supposed anatomical superiority. Most simply, when Holmes gave his lectures, he encircled himself with visual representations of racial difference that supported white anatomical supremacy. He used enlarged artistic reproductions of figures from prominent racial science texts like Charles Pickering's *The Races of Man*. Most

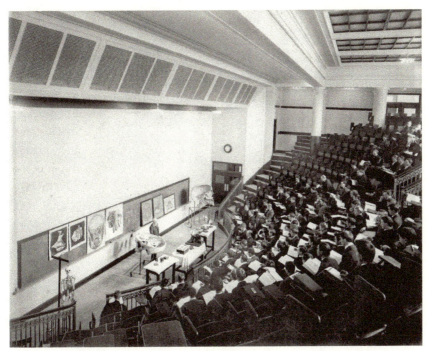

Figure 4.3. A 1906 image of Thomas Dwight, Holmes's successor as the Parkman Professor of Anatomy, as he lectured on the anatomy of the head. "Thomas Dwight lecturing to students in anatomy," Harvard Medical Library Collection, Center for the History of Medicine, Francis A. Countway Library of Medicine, Harvard Medical School, Boston. Photo courtesy of Harvard's Center for the History of Medicine.

visuals in Pickering's monograph are sketches of people that he encountered during the U.S. Exploring Expedition's circumnavigation of the globe. Pickering also created a racial map of the world shaded with different colors so that readers could locate the geographic homes of different racial groups. Maybe Holmes used Pickering's map, or perhaps he displayed an image of "Iolo-Ki, a native of Western Africa who was brought from Mina to Rio De Janeiro" (fig. 4.4).[33]

While Holmes lectured on medical white supremacy, he also demonstrated it. This approach was not unique to the lecture on race; rather, it typified Holmes's pedagogical approach to teaching anatomy more generally. Holmes's lectures on race appeared to be similar before and after the Civil War, making it possible to guardedly use postbellum sources to consider his pedagogy in the 1850s. Notes from the 1873–74 session at Harvard Medical School provide insights into the aesthetic choices underlying

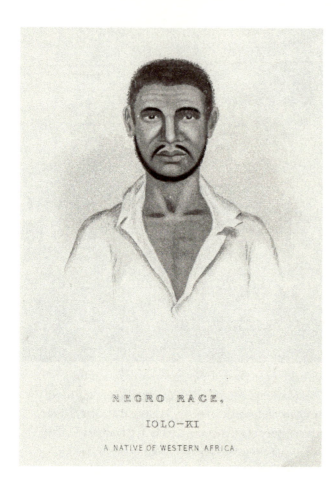

NEGRO RACE,

IOLO—KI

A NATIVE OF WESTERN AFRICA.

Figure 4.4. An example of the illustrations from Charles Pickering's *The Races of Man,* some of which were featured in Oliver Wendell Holmes Sr.'s anatomy lectures. This is an illustration of a man of African descent named Iolo-Ki. Charles Pickering, *The Races of Man: And Their Geographical Distribution*, new ed. (London: H. G. Bohn, 1854), 187. Photo courtesy of the Huntington Library.

Holmes's pedagogy. That year, he explicitly noted using "skulls & casts from the Museum skulls." However, almost every year's notes indicate that he delivered lectures on craniometry. He was likely surrounded by images of white supremacy while handling genuine and reproduced human remains stolen from the around the globe. In possessing Black people's preserved remains, Holmes demonstrated a type of power over African descendants and other non-white people's bodies that was germane to both anatomy's promise of mastery over dead bodies and enslavers' mastery over enslaved people.[34]

Holmes's methods were far from unique, as southern anatomists also analyzed race and used visual and tactile instructional methods. In his lectures at UVA, Professor James Lawrence Cabell delineated three categories of skull shapes in the human species. Though Cabell supported monogenesis, his white supremacist hierarchies of human difference were remarkably similar to those of his polygenist colleagues. In his syllabus, he put Khoisan people ("Bushmen of Southern Africa") on one end of the spectrum of the human species and whites on the other.[35] Likewise, in the 1840–41 *Bulletin* for MCSC, the faculty explained that polygenist Professor J. Edwards Holbrook employed dissection, artifacts from the museum, and reproductions of organs, body parts, and the entire human form in his lectures. Also, James Moultrie, MCSC's physiology professor, explicitly noted that he discussed racial hierarchies, and he, too, used objects from the museum for his class. In the same catalog, the faculty pointed out the museum's comparative anatomy specimens, as well as its "interesting phrenological collections."[36]

Living people of color were even forced into service for lectures, as when Oliver Wendell Holmes discussed the "Aztec Children" with his students. When P. T. Barnum and Columbia professor David L. Rogers publicly dissected Joice Heth for profit and public amusement, they highlighted professional anatomists' contribution to popular abuse of enslaved and colonized peoples' bodies. By invoking the Aztec children Bartola and Maximo, however, Holmes drew attention to the corollary: popular racist exhibits contributed to academic anatomy.[37]

The story of Bartola and Maximo evidences a symbiotic relationship between those like Holmes and Barnum, and it reveals how professors enacted their racial ideas on the bodies of living people. In the early 1850s and into the postbellum period, Bartola and Maximo attracted many gawking customers. Barnum and their manager promoted and displayed them as the last surviving Aztecs discovered in a lost, walled city. Local doctors in Boston and elsewhere, though, knew the tragic past that had brought these children to the United States. In El Salvador, Ramón Selva bought Bartola and Maximo from their mother, and he later sold them to a man named Morris. Morris made himself their manager.[38]

Clearly, Bartola—"from four to six" years old—and Maximo—"from seven to eight years of age"—did not come to the United States of their own volition. This was human trafficking. En route to Boston, Morris even set up a display of Bartola and Maximo in Kingston, Jamaica. On that occasion, they were simply shown as examples of dwarfism.[39] Just as Boston's medical elite taught students racial science, they also exploited networks of human trafficking that turned colonized people into exhibits of the Other.

In an essay about Bartola and Maximo's anatomy, Jonathan Mason Warren replaced the siblings' life story with minute descriptions and measurements of their bodies. As the visiting surgeon at the Massachusetts General Hospital and John Collins Warren's son, Jonathan Mason Warren was an influential member of the medical community. His account likely shaped early medical and racial beliefs about Bartola and Maximo. In his essay, Warren noted that the youths' jaws projected and gave a full paragraph on the children's genitals. Here, he unveiled that he must have closely examined the children naked.[40] Further illustrating his awareness that he was examining individuals with significant disabilities, Warren demeaned the children by comparing them to dogs. In addition, he noted that other people with dwarfism did not have smaller heads like Bartola and Maximo did. These doctors were not ignorant about or innocent of the exploitation that Bartola and Maximo experienced. Physician D. T. Brown expressed to Warren apprehension about the pair's future. He pondered, "When popular curiosity shall have expired, a new question is to arise in regard to them viz.—who is to support them?"[41]

While we know little other than the fact that he discussed Bartola and Maximo in his lectures, Oliver Wendell Holmes most likely was working from a script similar to Warren's. In the anatomy classroom, rather than being understood as victims of popular ethnology's networks of human trafficking, Bartola and Maximo were discussed as examples of indigenous degeneracy, disability, or both. Given medical schools' connections to Barnum exhibits, it was possible, perhaps even likely, that the siblings were exhibited at Harvard during Holmes's lectures.[42]

It is difficult to discern what Bartola and Maximo thought of all their travels. Before arriving in the United States, these two children had been sold by their parents into bondage and shoved onto stages to be looked on as ethnic and medical oddities. Maybe audiences in Boston and Jamaica laughed or jeered at them. Certainly, spectators must have stared. Moreover, what Bartola and Maximo thought of the doctors who analyzed their bodies, fondling, measuring, and describing their most intimate parts, is lost to history. Their story reveals a type of invasive medical analysis that compares to the purchasing, prodding, and poking of the slave market. Bartola and Maximo were bought and sold by popular hucksters, but in the United States, these children were turned into props for medical and racial scientists. Their emotions remain inaccessible, but this whirlwind journey between guardians, stages, ships, and countries must have made for a frightening, insecure, and traumatic childhood. Even as their lives were exceptional, Bartola and Maximo's story underscored how people of color were impressed into medical schools' service. Against their will, they were used to create an anatomistic spectacle meant to prove their own inferiority.

Through spoken content, visuals, and museum objects, anatomy professors created dynamic presentations meant to turn racial differences into corporeal realities. As they lectured on racial difference, instructors like Holmes, Holbrook, and Leidy surrounded themselves with racialized human remains and scientific imagery of white supremacy. Building on their readings, these multisensory talks impressed on students the supposed anatomical reality of racial distinctions, a theory they could pursue further in the museum.

ORDERING RACE IN THE ANATOMY MUSEUM

In the anatomical museum, students and professors engaged in activities that aped many features of enslavers' control over enslaved people's bodies. Likewise, the museum reflected medicine's larger animalization of Black people and physicians' presumptive ownership of their bodies. For example, upon capturing Nat Turner in 1831, white Virginians planned to use his corpse to tell multiple narratives of the restoration of white rule. That year, Turner led more than seventy enslaved people to kill fifty-five whites in a bid for freedom. White Virginians responded with a reign of terror, executing many enslaved people with no connection to the uprising. Turner's punishment, however, did not end with his death. In Virginia, whites used his body as a means to display their power to enslaved people. Taking an approach not unlike a dissection, the authorities skinned and decapitated Turner, mangling his corpse to display their dominion over other would-be rebels. Supposedly, whites even made memorabilia from Turner's skin. The insurgent's body endured yet more postmortem disfigurement. According to local newspapers, medical students dug up Turner's buried corpse, continued with the dissection, and persisted in transforming the remains into souvenirs. How whites treated Turner's body captures this deep relationship between anatomical and white supremacist spectacle. Both relied on the disfigurement of human remains and their display, and both transgressed accepted burial norms in the nineteenth century.[43]

Anatomists and enslavers displayed human remains as signs of mastery. In the wake of a revolt such as the 1811 German Coast rebellion outside New Orleans, whites exhibited enslaved people's heads on pikes. In this case, they depicted the restoration of the social order through the public exhibition of desecrated deceased African descendants' bodies.[44] The clinical-racial gaze further captures the parallel practices of enslavers and anatomists. Like slave markets for enslavers, anatomical theaters and museums represented spaces for the display of human bodies where white men in the medical profession could better understand blackness's supposed embodied meanings.

Just as museums projected on students a broad power over patients and illnesses, racial collections reinforced the anatomical white supremacy outlined in textbooks and lectures. Throughout the antebellum period, southern medical educators routinely harvested anatomical objects from the stolen bodies of enslaved people. Beyond the South, though, museum curators collected the stolen remains of African descendants and other colonized

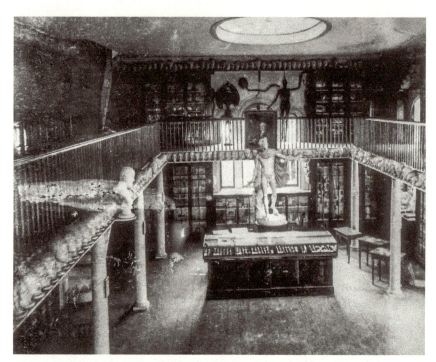

Figure 4.5. An undated photograph of the inside of the Warren Anatomical Museum. This location of the museum was on North Grove Street from 1847 to 1883. Harvard Medical Library Collection, Center for the History of Medicine, Francis A. Countway Library of Medicine, Harvard University Medical School, Boston. Photo courtesy of Harvard's Center for the History of Medicine.

peoples. They used these remains for two purposes: general pathological education and fashioning a white supremacist pedagogy. In addition to large skull collections, museums had preserved feet, reproductive organs, hair, and other body parts—marked out by race. In the museum, students also engaged their senses. They applied the knowledge from lectures and textbooks to seeing and feeling race on human bodies. The pedagogical effects of museums, then, were characterized by what stolen human remains were objectified, how they were curated, and the ways students saw them.[45]

While medical museums grew in importance, size, and scope in the nineteenth century, they already had a long history in transatlantic medical education. Racial collections also had been around for decades prior to the creation of a major anatomical museum in the United States. For example, in the late eighteenth century, the famous British surgeons and brothers John and William Hunter began collecting artifacts from African descendants' bodies. Their museum at the University of Glasgow contained the "mamma of a Negro girl," "the Eye of a Negro split into two halves," an "external Ear of a Negro," numerous pieces of black skin, and the genitals of men and women of African descent. Reflecting the normalization of stealing genitals from Black corpses, in 1799, British physician, polygenist, and former Hunter student Charles White noted, "[Black men's preserved penises have] been shewn in every anatomical school in London.... I have one in mine." Completed posthumously, one portrait even depicts John Hunter sitting in front of an open book featuring a hierarchical skull series and the feet of a hanging articulated skeleton (fig. 4.6). Thus, American curators built on an extant European anatomical tradition of including white supremacist displays in museums.[46]

Following European precedents, U.S. anatomy museums played a crucial role in making race visible on African descendants' bodies. The messiness of dissection made anatomical analysis difficult, even if students obtained symbolic power over bodies through dissecting. Models, large illustrations, and preserved remains provided alternatives to the practice. Both original and reproduced anatomical objects were meant to represent an objective material image of the human body. The faculty crafted a scientific narrative through objects that students could study themselves. In the museum, students held, felt, and manipulated dried bones and desiccated human tissues. They closely eyed preserved organs in jars, and they evaluated the particulars available in models that were not always visible on cadavers. Museum objects allowed students to analyze bodies at a level of detail that was not visible through the gore of dissection.[47]

As sites of curation, faculty at museums such as Harvard's universalized anatomical observations in their displays. These exhibits provided companion curricula to the visual and tactile aspects of lectures. Samuel Morton's model "set of typical skulls" exemplified this approach. In Harvard's crania display, Professor J. B. S. Jackson, curator at the Warren Anatomical Museum (fig. 4.5), placed this set first. Morton curated and cast the typical skulls from his collection at the Academy of Natural Sciences of Philadelphia. The exhibit comprised twelve casts of skulls from around the world, including examples from Peru, Manila, and Germany. Morton created the collection so that students could understand racial difference without dealing with large numbers of skulls. Personally selected and cast, these skulls represented Morton's conclusions about difference and crania. Like the rest of the curriculum, Jackson arranged the museum to depict a curated vision of anatomical difference. As John Collins Warren explained upon donating the molds, "They will, I think, be useful in explaining the peculiarities of form in the different races."[48]

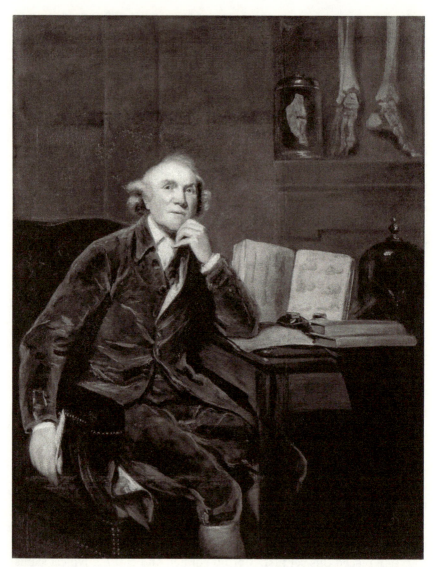

Figure 4.6. A portrait of John Hunter featuring an illustrated series of skulls in the open book and the bottom of a hanging skeleton. Another nineteenth-century painted copy of this portrait is on display at the College of Physicians of Philadelphia. John Jackson, *John Hunter*, 1813, after the 1786 portrait by Sir Joshua Reynolds, National Portrait Gallery, London.

In the next set of shelves, Jackson placed the main set of Eurasian and African skulls, ordered by race. On the top shelf, he positioned whites. Thus, when students studied the collection, they found whites' skulls in a superior position to those of all other races. White skulls were followed by a shelf of Egyptian crania, then by the crania of South Asians or "hindoos." Next were Chinese and other East Asian skulls and casts. Jackson confined African descendants' skulls to the bottom shelf. On the next shelving units, he housed nearly all of the American Indian skulls and a collection of "Bengal Muslim" skulls.[49] The high number of human heads in Harvard's anatomical museum must have projected on students a sense of craniometry's validity and its importance to medical education. Faculty encouraged pupils to handle these remains. Moreover, by placing whites' skulls on the top shelf and Black people's skulls on the bottom, Jackson made a simple visual argument for anatomical white supremacy.

Only objects from non-white bodies were routinely described racially. While northeastern schools invested in racial anatomy displays, most artifacts in their museums were probably from white cadavers. This rhetorically positioned white anatomical objects as normative and requiring no specific racial knowledge, as compared to marking out artifacts from non-whites as racially specific.[50]

In addition to skulls, American curators showed a fascination with Black people's reproductive organs and sexuality. Museum curators made beliefs about Black hypersexuality anatomically ordained. In the collection of preserved male genitalia held at Harvard's Warren Anatomical Museum, the first series of objects had no race denoted in the catalog. However, Jackson made sure to mark the race of Black people's genitals. One entry reads, "[Item] 725. A second specimen: injected by Dr. H. This was also from a negro, and it measures in length, 10 3/4 in. . . . [Donated in] 1847. *Dr. O. W. Holmes.*"[51] Similarly, MDUP had multiple examples of Black people's genitals, including "external genitals of a black hermaphrodite" and the "vulva of a black infant."[52] While other pieces of African descendants' bodies were collected, preserved, and marked out racially, genitalia had an added sexual dimension. White anatomists routinely described Black people as hypersexual and possessing larger genitals.[53] Through preservation practices, Holmes turned the penis of this deceased Black man into a grisly teaching tool capable of telling students about the contours of African descendants' sexuality and its anatomical roots.

Whether through creating reproductions like Morton's casts or preserving original human remains, the museum relied on corpse theft. Curators and collectors rarely seemed to consider the deceased's wishes. For example, in 1822, William Horner exhumed the body of a Cherokee man who had served in the U.S. Army, and he cast the skeleton for MDUP's museum. Like dissectors, museum curators embraced the clinical-racial gaze. White students and professors felt a presumptive right to steal, preserve, display, and racialize people's bodies. While these efforts often targeted African descendants, prospective doctors fetishized the remains of other groups as well.[54]

As well as visually reading the museum, faculty intended for students to produce museum objects of their own. Separate from his textbook describing human anatomy, William Horner also wrote a manual on anatomical methods entitled *The United States Dissector*. Here, he emphasized applied elements of anatomy such as dissecting and preserving cadavers. Horner included instructions and recipes for injecting veins and arteries that would make their appearances stand out in preservations. He also gave recipes for cadaver preservatives, the chemicals needed to make "wet preparations," and the methods for creating the opposite "dried preparations." Thus Horner and other faculty expected medical students to analyze museum exhibits and contribute to them. As Jackson explained in the 1870 catalog of the Warren Museum, while the institution had "a great many deficiencies," he hoped that they could be rectified "by the zeal of the young men who [were] coming forward, and that the profession generally [would] continue to contribute, *as they have heretofore*, until there [was] not common form of injury or disease that [would] not be represented in the collection." Exemplifying this trajectory, many physicians had an articulated human skeleton in their office, as displayed in the portrait of John Hunter. As a matter of fact, an articulated skeleton was the most iconic symbol of the profession during this period (see fig. 4.6).[55]

Thus, professors saw the museum as a space of practice and study, and alumni, students, and professors created its contents collaboratively. Alumni saw donating museum objects as an important rite of passage and a route to becoming peers to their former professors. In letters to Joseph Leidy, MDUP graduates revealed that their relationship to their alma mater's museum was a reality and not just an aspiration. On June 29, 1860, J. H. F. Milton from the class of 1860 sent Leidy a unique kidney that he had found, removed, and preserved from the corpse of a four-year-old boy. Likewise, in 1863, Thomas J. Eastman, an MDUP alumnus from Wisconsin who had graduated in 1854, wrote to Leidy to discuss his dissection of a rooster that had died during castration. Despite his anatomical training, Eastman needed help discerning testicles from kidneys.[56]

By the 1850s, medical professors had developed a clear approach to teaching about African descendants' anatomies. They brought together

three different pedagogical techniques: outside reading, lectures, and tactile engagement with anatomical objects. Educators used objects in museums as adjuncts to the theoretical ideas presented in lectures. By cultivating
this prior knowledge in textbooks and lectures, when students first entered
the museum, they had sensory expectations. There, they used anatomical
objects to connect this knowledge base to tangible artifacts of blackness.[57]
Ideas and material life met in the medical school's semiprivate anatomical
museums and theaters. In museums, pupils and professors projected on
African descendants' bodies an anatomical image of race. All of this worked
to frame race as something discrete, knowable, and controllable through a
system that educated physicians to see race in ways inaccessible to the lay
public. With their new tools for understanding race in hand, some students
went on to narrate Black people's bodies as divergent in their theses.

HOW MEDICAL STUDENTS WROTE ABOUT RACIAL ANATOMY
In his 1855 thesis "An Essay on the Negro and the White Man," MDUP student
J. Ramsay McDow illustrated the profound impact racial anatomy had on an
individual student's worldview. Hailing from Alabama, McDow arrived at
MDUP well versed in the white racist thought pervading slave societies. His
thesis, however, displayed the anatomization of this racial worldview and the
specific influence of his professor Joseph Leidy. For example, McDow para-
phrased Leidy telling the class that Black and white people were anatomically
more different than lions and tigers.[58]

In his thesis, McDow not only parroted Leidy's more provocative lines, but
he also reproduced his professor's theoretical framework. McDow argued
that it was not one dramatic anatomical difference that supposedly made
Black and white people different species. He explained, "The differences
enumerated are small, but they are permanent; and it is also true that many
species in nature, totally distinct and never confounded are not characterized by so great differences as those mentioned." McDow explained that
Black people's classification as a different species from whites was justified by multiple small and enduring anatomical distinctions that could be
mapped throughout human bodies.[59]

Theses like McDow's illustrated the power of incorporating racial thinking
into medical education. For evidence, McDow relied heavily on the word of
his professors and famous racial scientists. He also evidenced how anatomical thinking framed Black people as permanently or at least indefinitely
distinct. Mirroring the style of Joseph Leidy, McDow took it for granted that
race was real and embodied, and he delineated what he saw as simple facts.
When describing his own arguments, he characterized them as "drawn from

well-established observations, from analogies and anatomical peculiarities." Such "well-established observations" included Louis Agassiz's contention that whites had larger brains than people of African descent and Morton's "measurement of many crania" that were meant to prove that "the cranium of the negro" held "nine cubic inches less than the white man's." McDow's lack of originality proved the influence of popular ethnology and medical schools' curricula. He depended on lectures and racial science texts, and he closed his thesis with a disturbing white supremacist prediction that devalued Black life. He asserted, "When the historian shall have chronicled his [the negro's] deeds, he can only say, that he was born; he was wretched; he died."[60]

Theses like McDow's capture a growing anatomical consensus on racial difference emerging at the end of the antebellum era. Just as often as students like McDow weighed polygenesis versus monogenesis, they also delineated what they saw as the contemporary reality of anatomical racial difference. While antebellum pupils clashed over the origins question, they often agreed that anatomical distinctions separated human races. Moreover, they believed that these variations would persist indefinitely. It is no coincidence that the vast majority of pre–Civil War theses focused on racial anatomy were written in the 1850s. In addition to the nation being on the precipice of civil war, professors like Horner and Morton had by this point standardized an approach to race in anatomy curricula. Even though earlier students had written about race and slavery, in the 1850s they routinely put racial questions in terms of anatomy. For drawing medicine and racism closer, this was the perfect storm.

This anatomization of racial difference reflects and builds on what historian Rana A. Hogarth describes as the "medicalization of blackness" taking place in slave societies in the late eighteenth and early nineteenth centuries. Hogarth explains that in "medicalizing blackness," physicians turned race into a pathology that had to be managed. In contrast to practice-based approaches to blackness centered on disease, labor, and the environment, anatomized blackness almost exclusively had social rather than medical cures. Anatomy, as students like McDow saw it, largely could not be changed. Anatomists were much more interested in understanding the geography and inner workings of the body rather than discovering new medical therapies. Thus, anatomization represented a portion of medicalizing blackness that "emerged to advance the standing of medical polities in the Atlantic World and expand white prerogatives," even as it had little therapeutic impact.[61]

Writing their theses at the University of Nashville in the 1850s, Theophilus Westmoreland and Newton C. Miller exemplified the emergence of a national consensus on racial anatomy among medical students. Following the era's racial scientists, Westmoreland and Miller discussed anatomy across the body. They also copied racial scientists' worst methods, relying heavily on anecdotal evidence. Miller noted that Black people had narrower pelvises, bowlegs, flatfeet, and, of course, black skin.[62] In his 1855 thesis entitled "An Inaugural Dissertation on the Anatomical and Physiological Differences in the Ethiopian and White Man," Westmoreland gave a more detailed delineation of African descendants' supposed anatomical peculiarities. He listed additional traits including an anterior center of gravity, larger chest, smaller lumbar, protruding stomach and rear, "kidney footed" appearance, larger genitals in both sexes, longer foreskin of the penis, larger mammae in females, darker eyes, and "ivory looking teeth."[63] It is worth noting that Westmoreland and Miller cited many of the same supposed peculiarities as MDUP student J. Ramsay McDow.[64] Writing their theses in the 1850s, McDow, Miller, and Westmoreland depicted African descendants' bodies as entirely distinct and rooted in their supposed internal anatomical features. Moreover, their focus on skeletal structure allowed for the potential to read these supposedly internal differences through surface examination alone. As C. M. Ellis revealed, though, physicians' abilities to read racial difference on the exterior of living bodies were more aspirational than genuine.

Additionally, Westmoreland revealed how dissections were important sites for racial discussion and the construction of anatomical "evidence" for white supremacy. He wrote, "The brain of the negro is not near so well developed as it is in the white man. It is estimated to weigh from two to three ounces less and to measure less big one sixth. This state will need no confirmation by future physiologists for it is a fact that has been fully demonstrated by actual dissection by anatomists for [the] past century."[65] Westmoreland depicted African descendants' heads as distinct, defined by both their skeletal conformation and their internal contents. His phrasing even implies that students at the University of Nashville weighed the brains of African descendants as a part of their training.

In the 1850s, students' theses made it clear that anatomical racial pedagogy was rigorous, standardized, and deeply influential. In his 1855 thesis, like McDow, Tully S. Gibson of Vicksburg, Mississippi, rested his argument that Black people were a distinct species on "the numerous anatomical differences between the white and Black races, as indicated by . . . Dr. Leidy." Whether in Nashville or Philadelphia, students based their claims about race and anatomy on analysis of the whole body, not just the skull.[66]

In his 1857 thesis, MDUP student Arthur B. Myers argued for both monogenesis and separate anatomical races. Asking and answering his own questions, Myers offered, "Do they [Black and white people] differ intellectually? Certainly, they do!" He went on, "Do the white + the Negro differ physically?

I must admit, that they do." Myers then listed multiple differences that would have been included in Leidy's lectures. In addition to noting the typical variations in skulls that anatomists enumerated, Myers asserted, "The pelvis is more perpendicular in the female negro than in the white, *all* tending to show the degeneration of the negro." He also contended that people of African descent had "long heels," as well as other phenotypical features that typically characterized racial stereotyping, like "thick lips" and "flat noses." In short, Myers felt uncomfortable with the theological issues inherent to polygenesis, but he shared his contemporaries' belief in embodied anatomical racial differences. This belief mirrored the larger centrality of anatomy to U.S. medicine and medical education during this period.[67]

The tension between supporting both monogenesis and anatomical difference defined Myers's conclusions. He clung to the Bible while essentially conceding all the anatomical claims of polygenists. Ultimately, he asserted that simply too little was known for certain about either human origins or biology to abandon a biblical understanding of creation. Myers explained, "In order that ethnologists may establish their grounds, the sacred truths of the Bible must be rejected, and when the day comes for such a rejection, may my time on earth be lived out." He was attempting to restore a confidence in biblical history that he had lost to some extent. Just two pages earlier, though, Myers conceded that he was "to a certain extent undecided" about the origins of the human race. He even complained, "If the advocates of the unity expect to sustain themselves in their opinion of the subject without acknowledging that some points are still dark & obscure, they are greatly mistaken." And he noted, "To say, that the dark coloured African was once a white man is saying very much." In retreating to the Bible, Myers appeared to be attempting to assuage his conscience. In his thesis, he divulged that the core scientific problem for believing in a unified human species was anatomical beliefs (and racism). Of the students who wrote their theses on racial anatomy in the 1850s, Myers was the only monogenist, but that hardly influenced his descriptions of anatomical blackness.[68]

In his 1837 thesis "The Origin of the Different Human Species," MCSC student Dyer Ball revealed how medical students' ideas were shaped by a national cohort of professors. In discussing the supposed brutish qualities of Black people's brains, Ball referenced two influential medical instructors and proponents of racial anatomy: William Horner and Charles Caldwell. In the case of Horner, Ball cited passages from his textbook about the supposed distinctiveness of African descendants' crania. Just as telling, though, is Ball's reference to Caldwell. By the time Ball wrote his thesis, Caldwell had published the first major monograph by an American in favor of polygenesis, and he had also become a prominent proponent of phrenology. Ball's sources illustrate how medical professors influenced their own students and other ones through publishing. Some, like Caldwell and Horner, even shaped these discourses nationwide. Ball's thesis draws attention to how antebellum medical professors were creating a national consensus around race and anatomy.[69]

While theses focused on racial anatomy were not common at any university, they do provide key insights into how a slow-developing interest in racial anatomy morphed into a broad consensus by the 1850s. Much like the popular pro-monogenesis writers of the period, even monogenist students believed that racial anatomical differences existed.[70] Likewise, while none of the theses written on racial anatomy from Horner's period survive, MDUP's assessment records provide one insight into how professors received these types of essays. In 1838, Francis B. Carter of Alabama wrote a thesis entitled "Some of the Physical Peculiarities and Diseases of Southern Negroes." While Carter's work has not been discovered, MDUP professors' assessment of it has survived. Horner appraised Carter as "very highly prepared [for oral exams]," adding, "A good essay on Peculiarities of Southern Negro. Passed [and paid MDUP] $40." While this type of assessment of oral examinations was common in some years, it was not in 1838. Records for that year reveal that Horner rarely complimented theses and enumerated their topics. Given his textbook, Horner's evaluation of Carter is hardly surprising, but it provides greater evidence that racial theory represented an entrenched and important part of antebellum medical education. Likewise, Horner's compliment makes it apparent that theses on race were not viewed as efforts to avoid writing about a legitimate medical topic. Rather, racial science theses could receive some of the highest accolades that faculty gave.[71]

In short, by the end of the antebellum era, anatomical approaches to race had become a standard part of the medical curriculum. The rising sectional tensions and the standardization of racial anatomy curricula in the 1850s even created a spike in the number of students writing about racial anatomy. This moment, however, was built on decades' worth of faculty incorporating race and craniometry into their lectures, nationally influential textbooks, and anatomy museums.

As the case of C. M. Ellis illustrates, the effects of this pedagogy were felt deeply inside and outside medical schools. On the national, local, and individual scales, racial anatomy had a profound impact on how and whether people could access freedom. For example, in a widely reported case in Columbia, South Carolina, in 1854, the fate of an enslaved woman named

Lucy was intimately tied to the testimony of Dr. Robert W. Gibbes, a famous naturalist, MCSC graduate, and former faculty member at the South Carolina College. Lucy had been considered a serial runaway by the time her freedom suit was considered in November 1854. For decades, she acted tenaciously and consistently to escape captivity. Inaluskie, described by Charleston's *Southern Patriot* as an "old Cherokee chief," told locals that in the late 1830s a Lut-se had been kidnapped en route to Arkansas. This event occurred during the Cherokees' genocidal forced relocation known as the Trail of Tears. Upon being kidnapped into slavery as a child, Lucy had routinely told playmates on the plantation that she was an Indian. According to the proslavery newspaper's account, Mr. Darby, Lucy's enslaver, had even pressured her to lie and claim Black parentage. Despite that, locals in the area knew of Lucy as "Darby's Indian." From the beginning of her bondage in the late 1830s, Lucy had ran away regularly, making her captivity untenable. Her struggle for freedom led her to jail in Columbia in 1851. Her trial and ultimate freedom had to wait three more years.[72]

In his testimony, Gibbes gave the jury a lesson in the faulty science of craniometry, and his testimony held considerable weight. Ironically, though he was a proslavery racial scientist, he used his assertions to advocate for Lucy's freedom. As a local commenter put it, "[Gibbes] understands the anatomy of our races as well as I know my multiplication tables." In his testimony, Gibbes directly compared Lucy's head to casts of heads of Native Americans and people of African descent. Further proving how racial science was constructed locally and nationally, these molds were likely identical to the set sent to Harvard that John Collins Warren purchased. The South Carolina College had commissioned Samuel Morton to make its casts in 1849. Based on her hair and skull, Gibbes deemed Lucy a Native American, and she obtained her freedom after years of struggle. Legal testimony about race by physicians like Gibbes made the public's growing confidence in medical professionals' expertise about racial difference abundantly clear. Moreover, Gibbes's testimony reflected the leading medical knowledge of the period and medical schools' typical anatomy curricula.[73]

Cases like Lucy's and the slander trial that possibly brought C. M. Ellis to the witness stand display the broad influence of racial anatomy in the antebellum United States. Racial science shaped medical curricula, national politics, and the freedom of people like Lucy. Racial anatomists, however, rarely used their expertise to free those like Lucy. Instead, anatomists regularly made tacit and direct defenses of slavery and white supremacy, depicting African descendants as anatomically subservient.

Like Ellis and Gibbes, medical school graduates carried their racial anatomy education into their careers as physicians. They learned racial science through textbooks, lectures, and museums. Through this multilayered approach to teaching, professors saturated anatomy training with racial ideas. Like other aspects of medical curricula, this multipronged method gave the theoretical and ultimately false depictions of racial difference a veneer of being based in material reality. These young white students from all over the country read about racial difference. They heard educators describe the supposed anatomical realities of these distinctions. On top of that, they could hold the skulls of Black soldiers, enslaved workers, and mothers whose heads were stolen from around the world. Ultimately, in the anatomy theater, students enacted racial science for themselves. As they held the remains of Black humanity in their hands, they repeated theories that called these people's lives into question. By the time they graduated, these pupils were a part of a community of doctors that claimed to be experts on race. Peering beyond the nation's borders, though, racial anatomists crafted their ideas for a transnational intellectual community. U.S. doctors learned about race and anatomy from European imperial doctors serving in Africa, Asia, and Latin America. U.S. physicians and medical graduates themselves went on to serve in imperial expeditions, and they used racial science to justify local and global systems of violence and exploitation. They collected skulls tied to imperial violence from around the globe. In short, racial theorists not only shaped how anatomy was understood inside the medical school, but also, through creating this cosmopolitan class of racial experts, intimately tied together racial and medical sciences worldwide.

PART 3

EXPANSION AND

RACIAL MEDICINE

5

SKULL COLLECTING, MEDICAL MUSEUMS, AND THE INTERNATIONAL DIMENSIONS OF RACIAL SCIENCE

746. Chinese skull; some of the flesh remains, dried on, also the hair which is long + plaited according to the fashion of that people.
—*"Descriptive Catalogue of the Anatomical Cabinet of the Boston Society for Medical Improvement, ca. 1837–1847"*

In 1843, the Boston Society for Medical Improvement acquired a new specimen to add to its already extensive collection of human crania. The skull had belonged to a Chinese opium smuggler who was decapitated by the Qing dynasty during the first Opium War (1839–42), and it had been put on display alongside the heads of two other smugglers in a cage near the mouth of the Pearl River. The heads were exhibited for at least a year, most likely meant to warn others of the consequences of smuggling opium and breaking the Qing's blockade of Canton.[1] The racial skull collections in antebellum medical schools and societies were the products of a U.S. medical culture increasingly connected to distant parts of the world by capitalism and imperialism.

By the late 1830s, the geographic scope of European imperialism was wide, even if the United States remained in its imperial infancy. The British East India Company dated back to the turn of the seventeenth century, and European maritime trade with China had begun even earlier. Mid-nineteenth-century imperialists and their scientific and medical allies therefore continued the centuries-long process of drawing the world together through violent trade and conquest. This smuggler's head and his postmortem journey to Boston in 1843 only further proved this relationship. The story of this head's collection represents just one short anecdote in Western powers' history of intruding on Chinese sovereignty in the long nineteenth century.[2]

The theft took place on the Pearl River, when three ship captains "made a descent upon [the displayed smugglers' heads] in the night, + each of them carried one off." One captain sent the head he had stolen to London, and the ultimate destination of the other smuggler's head was unknown. The third thief, Boston captain George Kilham, shipped the final head to Dr. Paul Simpson Jr., "by whom it was deposited in the" Society for Medical Improvement's anatomical cabinet. In 1870, the society donated its cabinet to the Harvard Medical School, and within two decades, the collection was completely integrated into the Warren Anatomical Museum. During much of the antebellum period, however, medical students in Boston could have accessed both museums. The journey of the unnamed smuggler's disembodied head from disciplinary display along the Pearl River to anatomical display in Boston evidences the degree to which U.S. medical schools were deeply intertwined with the processes of empire and capitalism in the nineteenth century.[3]

During the antebellum era, American medical students could examine skull collections to understand racial difference locally and internationally, speaking to white Americans' transnational outlook in the mid-nineteenth century. Furthermore, racial skull collections drew attention to how medical schools routinely exploited the bodies of non-whites, and they also mirrored larger trends in the development of natural history and medical specimen collections. Unlike Samuel G. Morton's collection that was built primarily for analysis by scientists, medical school museums, like medical textbooks and lectures, had an added power through their ever-present student audience.[4]

This chapter and the next two examine how medical schools—students, graduates, and professors—shaped and were shaped by emergent international networks of exchange in bodies and discourses about health, race, and imperialism. These chapters build on the approach of the new historians of capitalism, who depict slavery's expansion in the nineteenth century as formative to an increasingly transnational approach to capitalist economic development. In the process of unpacking slavery's foundational function in U.S. financial, academic, and social institutions, these scholars have recast the history of slavery in the South in national, Atlantic, and global terms.[5]

The story of the construction of medical schools and their collections of human remains confirms the need for this national and transnational framing of the history of slavery. Yet, due to their proprietary origins, antebellum medical schools were never as capital intensive as universities and colleges, much less cotton or sugar manufacturing. Despite the lack of a looming story of high finance, U.S. medical schools nonetheless used the increasingly transnational nature of the country's medical culture and nineteenth-century commerce to cultivate their racial pedagogy. This approach ultimately increased schools' competitive power in a medical marketplace that did not require physicians to obtain a diploma to be considered legitimate. Medical racism was capitalistic, then, in the ways doctors used their supposed racial expertise to support the growth of their profession.[6]

Medical school practices even mirrored those of racial scientists. Both Samuel Morton and Josiah Nott produced much of their science in the United States, but they relied on international networks of scholars to trade research, anecdotal anatomical descriptions of African descendants, and human remains. Similarly, U.S. medical schools constructed their racial pedagogy through global networks of grave robbers, who stole the remains of mostly non-white people and shipped them back to institutions like Harvard. While skull collectors and medical museum curators created a scientific undergirding for slavery and imperialism, they also relied on the violence of empires and slave societies to create the contents of these museum collections: human remains. Medical schools, then, were an active part of a racist feedback loop. They used human remains created through the violence of slavery and empire to construct and inculcate thousands of students in a racial ideology based in white supremacy—a central justification for imperialism and enslavement.

Building on the previous chapter's analysis of the organizational system of the Warren Anatomical Museum, the story of Harvard's racial skulls serves as a reminder that medical schools were hardly separated from the racial violence that their pedagogies justified. In the daily operations of the medical school, professors and students interacted, sometimes violently, with peoples far outside their lecture halls. Thus, as well as studying the international dimensions of Harvard's collection, this chapter offers a brief analysis of two human stories behind the university's skulls. These narratives uncover how the school's specimens actively erased stories of great heroism and tragedy that could have subverted the white supremacist narratives being constructed on the shelves of the Warren Anatomical Museum. In short, rather than just telling the story of racial skull collections as they would have been understood by white antebellum scientists, a more accurate reckoning with antebellum racial medicine and the totality of its violence requires examining the individual lives lost to create racist museum displays.

The history of Harvard's collection captures medical schools' active role in the violence inherent to slavery and imperialism. Until he donated them to Harvard in 1847, the national skulls were a part of Professor John Collins Warren's personal anatomy holdings, although the university's students had access to the skulls through much of his tenure. Warren saw the national skulls as a centerpiece of Harvard's anatomical museum. In the earliest catalog of the museum, handwritten by Warren and presented to Harvard in 1847, the skulls took center stage, being the first objects described therein. Among more pedestrian anatomical objects, Warren gifted a total of fifty-six skulls and casts of human crania, including thirteen "Caucasian" heads, thirteen heads of the "Mongolian or Tartar race," ten "Peruvian" heads, twelve Native American heads, and eight "African" heads. Simultaneously, Warren purchased the collection of the defunct Boston Phrenological Society. By this point, Professor J. B. S. Jackson curated both the newly enshrined Warren Museum and the Boston Society for Medical Improvement's collection. As a result, by 1847 Harvard students had access to more than 150 human heads organized by race and nation, some casts and some originals.[7]

Even though racial skull collecting had Enlightenment origins, these collections grew in importance and scope during the nineteenth century through their connections to commerce and colonialism. Medical schools and individuals like Morton created racial skull collections by stealing and purchasing human remains created by what historian Sven Beckert terms "war capitalism." War capitalists had many tools to create new markets and human remains, including "slavery, the expropriation of indigenous peoples, imperial expansion, armed trade, and the assertion of sovereignty over people and land by entrepreneurs." Notably, each of these methods was a context for the collection of specific skulls at Harvard. Physicians benefited from this rapid increase in the quantity of human remains available, which met their growing interest in measuring the supposed racial differences of the dead.[8]

Locally, anatomy museum curators profited from U.S. expansionism in North America by procuring "trophy heads" from people killed in imperial wars with Native Americans. During the Second Seminole War (1835–42), violent suppliers met the demands of skull-collecting race scientists like Morton, whose research helped justify imperial violence. During the war, Morton received thirteen "Seminole" skulls from Florida. Medical schools also contributed to this theft of Seminole remains. In 1841, Dr. Joseph Walker donated the "head of Powhushajo, a Seminole warrior," to MDUP's anatomical museum. Even within North America, medical schools both benefited from and intellectually justified imperial violence.[9]

The theft of human heads during the Second Seminole War existed within a larger culture of taking trophy heads during imperial wars. Apart from expansion based in Manifest Destiny in North America, the Liberia colony, failed attempts to create Caribbean and Central American colonies, and international commercial integration, the antebellum United States aspired to, rather than succeeded in creating, a global imperial footprint. As compared with their European competitors, U.S. medical schools could not rely as heavily on their own government's armies or colonies for specimens. For example, the Department of Anatomy at Oxford University had a substantial collection of human heads collected during British imperial conflicts in southern Africa. As a result, outside of colonial wars in North America and deaths on southern plantations, U.S. medical schools relied on a variety of types of collectors to source their racial skulls, including ex-patriots in foreign countries, sailors, foreign doctors, diplomats, European imperial officials, and other collectors.[10]

American skull collectors operated on many geographic scales, including intranational, hemispheric, transatlantic, and global. Intranationally, by 1847, Harvard owned a cast of the "scull of Pepick, a distinguished Winnebago Chief, who was killed at Chicago, in 1812 . . . by the American troops." Moving out just a bit farther to South America, Dr. H. A. Ward donated to the museum the head of an Incan child stolen from a deserted Incan Temple of the Sun in Peru. Increasing the scale further to the transatlantic for "Object 373a," this skull was that "of a negro, of the race Yolog; dug up in a burial place near the mouth of the Senegal [River]." Finally, during Commodore Matthew Perry's gunboat diplomacy expedition to Japan in 1854, American naval doctor J. H. Otis stole the skull of a person from the island of Okinawa off the coast of Japan. Harvard professors used their extended reach to turn the Warren Museum into a home for human remains picked up from battlefields, stolen from cemeteries, and ripped from sacred sites. Moreover, they relied on the ability of mostly white collectors to obtain specimens from graveyards and battlefields that were controlled by other European imperial powers.[11]

Through creating the collection of racial skulls, Harvard medical professors linked together people whose lives were widely separated by time and space. For example, Jackson displayed the skull of a man from ancient Egypt one shelf away from that of a nineteenth-century Austrian. In arranging skulls by his understanding of race, Jackson made a claim that these specimens— separated by geography and many temporal epochs—were racially the same or almost the same by designating their crania as white.[12]

Not only were the national skulls sourced globally, but the methods used to interpret them were also gestated transnationally. A notable interpretive approach was the numerical method as applied to race by Samuel G. Morton. Dating back to J. B. S. Jackson's 1847 catalog for the Society for Medical Improvement's museum, the Harvard professor regularly noted the internal capacity of the crania. In the 1870 published catalog for the Warren Museum, Jackson went even further. In that volume, he published an entire table of measurements of human skulls. As a result, if students consulted the catalog, they could quickly compare the cranial capacities of the skulls of an Austrian, an Egyptian mummy, an East Indian, a Black African, and an ancient Peruvian, among many others. Due to this organizational and analytical system, professors and students imagined through the racial skulls a new vision of bodily difference and a geography for understanding those variations.[13]

Not just confined to Harvard and MDUP, racial skull collections created through colonial violence were becoming an increasingly normative feature of all antebellum medical schools. Students at departments far removed from the elite institutions of the Northeast could access such collections. For example, when Rubin Mussey, later Samuel F. McGill's professor at Dartmouth, was the professor of surgery at the Medical College of Ohio in Cincinnati, his pupils had access to a groups of national skulls that spoke to an emergent global racial construct. In total, Mussey and the college had seventeen human skulls, including crania from Malaysia, Java, China, Suriname, India, and New Hampshire. Thus, like medical students at Harvard, these students in Cincinnati were learning how to conceptualize race as an international ordering principle. They learned on human remains from diverse locations, specimens whose creation and collection were tied to European empires.[14]

In their theses, students used the clinical-racial gaze and the availability of human remains to compare geographically disparate groups racially. As an example, medical students showed a wide fascination with stereotypes of Khoisan peoples from southern Africa, known colloquially by the racial slur "Hottentot." Throughout much of the antebellum era, medical students had been discussing their perceptions of Khoisan people as a route to creating a global model of racial difference. For example, in 1827, white MCSC student Samuel D. Holt noted, "The Children of Hottentots and Esquimaux are as commonly as stupid, while those of the English and French are as usually as sharp as their parents." On a similar note, in 1836, MCSC student Joseph G. Gaffney asserted, "There is ever a corresponding relation between the organizations of the brains and the faculties of minds, the minds of the Indian and Hottentot is inferior to that of European, which originates from an imperfect development of the brain."[15]

In addition to their fascination with Khoisan people, Holt and Gaffney compared ethnic and national groups from three continents, although their descriptions of these groups reflected stereotypes rather than reality. Holt and Gaffney highlighted how aspiring doctors' racial models encompassed geographies and peoples that they most likely had never personally encountered, evidencing their reliance on racial science and transnational collections of skulls and other body parts being displayed in medical school museums like Harvard's.

Like the racial scientists of the period, medical students measured crania to locate diverse peoples within an international racial hierarchy. In 1829, Virginian and MDUP student Singleton Jones Cooke asserted, "The skull of the Grecian makes nearly a right angle; that of the European of colder climates is something less; the savage and the Hottentot have their gradual approaches to an acute angle, in consequence of the greater or less protrusion of the bones of the face; the ape, the dog and the swine makes a still more acute angle." Cooke depicted Khoisan people as a missing link between whites and other Mammalia such as apes and pigs. Moreover, Cooke's, Holt's, and Gaffney's theses illustrate students' considerable interest in defining race and ethnicity beyond the borders of southern slavery. Collections of human remains encouraged these comparisons. Just as the slave trade made the bodies of many West and Central Africans accessible to racial scientists, the trade in human remains funneled through the nodes of imperialism and commerce connected Khoisan people to American physicians and their clinical-racial gaze.[16]

Few of the stories of those people whose heads were displayed are reclaimable by historians. However, it is safe to assume that the vast majority of those individuals would not have been willing to have their heads on exhibit.[17] White medical faculty, then, forcefully displayed the remains of non-white people to create a narrative of white supremacy. Like corpse theft for dissection, which has received much more attention from medical historians, the display of stolen human remains in anatomy museums also represented a transgression against the commonly held desire for a proper burial among peoples in the Atlantic World.[18]

Despite the Warren Museum's intended effect of erasing the individual narratives of the people whose heads were displayed, the available records of a few more storied skulls allow for at least some subversion of this historical erasure. No matter how physicians tried to reimagine the meaning of these crania racially, the reductive narrative told by racial skull collections did not represent these individuals' exclusive valuation. Understanding the lives and internal self-worth of people whose bodies were displayed in medical museums destabilizes racial scientists' system of measurement.[19]

Telling the stories of the lives, deaths, and postmortem descriptions of two exceptional people's heads has three immediate goals. First, while these skulls were exceptional in the amount of information recorded about them, they serve as a reminder that skull collections represent the sum total of the lives and deaths of hundreds, even thousands, of people. Moreover, through presenting these human remains as objects that signified essentialist racial differences and erased the individual identities of those on display, medical professionals and students created another layer of colonial violence on African descendants. Despite privileging the voices of white men, their racialization of non-white bodies, and their erasure of the voices of people whose bodies became specimens, the archives of the Warren Museum can be used to excavate the histories of some people whose bodies were collected. Second, relating even just a few of these stories within the broader narrative of the medical school makes apparent how these institutions intimately relied on the physical violence of imperialism.

Finally, telling these stories works to undermine the historical erasure of individuals at the core of the racial science project. Their histories can shed light on moments of power, dignity, and tragedy lived by those people whose skulls were stolen. The narratives further draw attention to how the display of human remains represented a distinct type of museum attraction that drew on epistemic and physical violence. Any telling of the history of anatomical museums would simply be incomplete without some attention to the people whose bodies populate these spaces.[20]

The story of a Khoisan man named Sturmann, including his journey to Boston, his teenage suicide far from home, the production of death casts of his head for museums, and the ultimate description of his skeleton for racial scientific ends, epitomizes a case of a person whom white scientists tried to fashion into an image of Black inferiority. Sturmann's life reflects aspects of the famous Sara Baartman's experiences as a living exhibit. Baartman was dubbed by whites the "Hottentot Venus," and she toured through Europe in the early nineteenth century before dying of an unknown illness (probably pneumonia) in Paris in 1815. Throughout much of his life, Sturmann, like Baartman, found himself deeply affected by processes of empire. Where Baartman died of disease and poverty in Paris, Sturmann committed suicide just a year after being put on display in Boston's Aquarial and Zoölogical Gardens in 1860. Sturmann's name, of Dutch origins, also reflects southern Africa's deep history with European imperialists.[21]

In describing his early life to the promoters of his exhibit, Sturmann wove a tale of dislocation, scarcity of food, and fear of whites. Born in the early 1840s, Sturmann and his family lived a relatively nomadic life in Little Namaqualand (near the borders of contemporary South Africa and Namibia) when he was a child. He and his relatives hunted and gathered for sustenance, and they actively avoided contact with whites. White genocidal violence against the Khoisan in this region had been occurring intermittently since the beginning of the eighteenth century.[22]

Attempting to discern more details about Sturmann's identity also reveals the complexity of reading this archive. The term "Khoisan" is a compound word to describe an amalgamated set of identities in southern Africa (which comprised, before colonization, countless independent but connected cultures and languages erased through colonialism and genocide). Khoe groups, usually cattle-herding pastoralists who were more settled, were most often described by whites as "Hottentots." San groups, often nomadic hunters and gatherers, were most often called by whites "Bushmen." Sturmann was called a "Hottentot," but his family hunted, fished, and gathered for sustenance. Both Khoe and San groups lived in Little Namaqualand, and some Khoe groups who lost their cattle and grazing lands during colonial wars certainly adopted hunting and gathering as a way of life. Therefore, it is difficult to conclude with any certainty whether Sturmann was from a Khoe or San group. Either way, before leaving for Boston, Sturmann and his family found that their way of life had undeniably been altered by more than a century of colonial violence in Little Namaqualand.[23]

Sturmann's arrival in Boston was the product of the ever-expanding shipping routes of the nineteenth century and the dislocation of many Khoisan people by centuries of white incursions in southern Africa. At an early age, perhaps five or six, Sturmann and his family migrated from inland to the Atlantic coast in search of food. According to the pamphlet advertising his display at the Boston Aquarial and Zoölogical Gardens, Sturmann explained to his promoters that at this time his family went to the coast "to look for something to eat, and for beads and clothes; for they were often very hungry. They travelled nearly half a moon, when they came to much salt water, and saw ships and white men; and the white men came on shore, with guns, and made them much afraid." To eat during this period, Sturmann and his relatives relied on begging for food from dangerous whites, catching fish, and hunting penguins. Thus, before the age of ten, Sturmann was already living an itinerant life, moving regularly to survive.[24]

After a nomadic and difficult childhood, Sturmann left his family when he was a teenager. He journeyed approximately 1,000 miles to Port Natal on the coast of the Indian Ocean, where he led white hunting expeditions. While Sturmann's account often lacks details like dates, it is possible, perhaps even likely, that it was the genocide of the San, or "Bushmen," in Little Namaqualand in the 1850s that caused him to migrate. In 1863, Louis Anthing, the colonial magistrate of Namaqualand, explained, "During the last ten years a wholesale system of extermination of the Bushman people [the San] had been practiced." While it is unclear whether Sturmann was in fact Khoe or San, his status as a hunter-gatherer could have made him a target in either case.[25]

However, during the approximate beginning of this genocidal period in the history of the Northern Cape, Sturmann moved to Port Natal, with the promise of food and clothing. In an account mediated through the promotional pamphlet, Sturmann explained that as a teenager, he left his family and home country, and he "went to the country of the Boers, near Port Natal, and travelled with the Boers and other white men when they went out hunting elands (a kind of antelope) and springbok and other animals." Thus, before leaving for Boston as an adolescent, Sturmann had relocated from inland to the coast with his family, and he had traveled all the way from the Atlantic coast to the coast of the Indian Ocean on his own. As Sturmann had been born into a seemingly dislocated existence, his decision to travel to Boston, where he would end his own life, becomes less surprising.[26]

In light of his tragic childhood, the promoters who convinced Sturmann to come to Boston appear all the more predatory. By now in his mid- to late teens, Sturmann supposedly agreed to the offer "of a white man Mr. Dillingham." Based on the published account, Dillingham allegedly "asked [Sturmann] if he would like to go over the sea to America, and have plenty of fine clothes and food, and earn plenty of money, to bring back to his own country." In accounts from Boston newspapers, however, the colonial government in South Africa, not Sturmann, appeared as the financial broker of Sturmann's arrangement with the Aquarial and Zoölogical Gardens. The *Congregationalist* reported, "Messrs. Cutting and Butler [of the Aquarial and Zoölogical Gardens] are under bonds to the English Colonial Government in South Africa." Thus, the proprietors' only clear financial obligation was to the colonial government, not Sturmann.[27]

The exhibit itself was curated and promoted by P. T. Barnum decades after he had first made a name for himself touring with Joice Heth in the 1830s. Much as Sturmann's body would be donated to and then dissected at Harvard, Barnum had Heth's corpse publicly dissected by a medical professor. Thus, Sturmann's and Heth's fates reveal the intimate relation between popular display and professional anatomy, and how Sturmann's treatment from display to death was far from unprecedented.[28]

At least some white Bostonians seemed to feel uneasy about how much Sturmann's story resembled that of a man forced into slavery and brought to the center of U.S. abolitionism amid the secession crisis. Sturmann came to Boston as a part of a party of five Black men from southern Africa, each representing a different ethnic group from the region, and all displayed together. The Aquarial and Zoölogical Gardens and the local newspapers rhetorically attempted to differentiate their trade in African people from that of slavers. In an article entitled "Five Native Africans," the *Congregationalist* went to great lengths to show how Sturmann's story was not akin to the slave trade, attempting to assuage Bostonians of any guilt for putting his body on display. On January 25, 1861, the newspaper explained, "Last spring Messr. Cutting and Butler, well known as the proprietors of the Aquarial Garden in Boston, sent an agent to South Africa for the purpose of securing some natives to bring to this country, not after the manner of the slave traders, but with their own consent, and for exhibition as specimens of the wild men of that country." Moreover, the paper related that the men had been visited by numerous local clergy. Enslaved or not by the Aquarial and Zoölogical Gardens, Sturmann and his cohort experienced many indignities while on display.[29]

At the Aquarial and Zoölogical Gardens, Sturmann and these four other men from southern Africa were forced to dance for crowds and fulfill stereotypes of Black indigeneity. In the *Boston Evening Transcript*, an advertisement for the exhibit described the group as *"fresh from savage life."* This notice also gave a sense of what the exhibit looked like in practice and the performative demands put on Sturmann and the four others, named Machiado, Mauolo, Macorino, and Quaggu. The advertisement explained, "They will appear through the day, clad in their native dresses of skins, ornamented with beads, feathers and porcupine quills, and every evening will go through the war, love and festive dance,—(armed with their spears, clubs, shells, and other weapons of war and the chase,) and will also sing the national songs of their several tribes." Depicting the men as one of many animalistic specimens on display, the next paragraph described the aquarium's "educated seals Ned and Fanny." Thus, just months before the outbreak of the Civil War, and even though Bostonians were quick to point out that these men technically had not been bought as slaves (even if they appeared to be rented from an empire), Sturmann, Machiado, Mauolo, Macorino, and Quaggu were being publicly displayed and forced to perform a racist image of African "barbarity" for white amusement and miseducation.[30]

On April 28, 1861, less than a year after he arrived in Boston and while he was still a teenager, Sturmann killed himself. On that day, his four companions from southern Africa were attending church in East Boston. While they were gone, Sturmann ritualistically assembled all of his belongings in a separate room, and in the small tower room where he and the other men had lived in the Aquarial and Zoölogical Gardens, he hanged himself. According to the *Boston Traveler*, Sturmann's "associates displayed the greatest sorrow on learning of the suicide." Another article about Sturmann's death explained that he had been acting odd for days. While meant to racialize the young man as lazy, the description of his demeanor in the original promotional pamphlet for the exhibition made it appear that Sturmann was deeply unhappy. The brochure explained, "[Sturmann] possesses the native indolence of his race, and passes much of his time lying about and sleeping." Thus, rather than a spur-of-the-moment decision, Sturmann's suicide appeared to be long considered, deliberate, and a response to his unfree existence.[31]

Due to the extreme level of colonial disruption of Khoisan cultures, piecing together Sturmann's beliefs about suicide is nearly impossible, but attention to historical context can provide some potential meanings for what he might have thought about his death. First, Sturmann most likely believed in an afterlife.[32] He even might have seen his suicide as an attempt to escape his current condition, rather than just an act of desperation. Also, unlike Christianity, not all African religions saw suicide as immoral. As historian of slavery and suicide Terri Snyder explains, enslaved Africans in eighteenth-century North America "exhibited considerable variance in their views toward suicide. Among early modern Yoruba and Ashanti, for instance, suicide was deemed a praiseworthy and honorable response to peril, disgrace, and a life that had become burdensome. In other nations, the act was condemned." Recently, historians of slavery like Snyder have argued for the need to see enslaved suicide as a potential act of agency that could have positive spiritual meaning. Likewise, it could have been a route to simply escape a life of limited options. Sturmann certainly experienced emotional trauma throughout his life. However, it is worth considering the fact that he might have hanged himself in an effort to control his own life and destiny. His suicide might not have been one final desperate decision. Instead, Sturmann might have seen himself as making a positive change, leaving behind racism and display in Boston for an afterlife of his choosing.[33]

Like Sara Baartman, who was dissected by the famed French naturalist Georges Cuvier and whose remains were displayed in many museums in Paris until being repatriated to South Africa in 2002, Sturmann continued being displayed and exploited following his death. Soon after his suicide, casts of Sturmann's head were made and distributed to numerous local museums. Death casts of his head were exhibited simultaneously in at least two Harvard museums: the Warren Anatomical Museum and what would become the Peabody Museum of Archaeology and Anthropology.[34]

In addition to being a teaching aid in the Warren Museum, Sturmann was further immortalized by Jeffries Wyman's racial typing. The professor and physician described the youth's skeleton for the Boston Society of Natural History in 1862 (the account was later printed in the society's proceedings). In a pamphlet, Wyman erased the complexity of Sturmann's life, reducing his biography to the following: "The subject was nearly adult, and came to his death by suicide." Wyman omitted Sturmann the person, and he instead defined the young Khoisan man through a series of measurements including body height, hip width, foot length, and, of course, cranial capacity. Using the numerical method, Wyman argued that Sturmann was taller than the average Khoisan man. Wyman even gave minute descriptions of many different cranial bones. Perhaps even more dehumanizing, Wyman created a table comparing the measurements of the pelvises of Sturmann, two Europeans, a chimpanzee, and a gorilla. Wyman's pamphlet represented a final attempt by whites to colonize Sturmann.[35]

Sturmann grew up in a social and political space disrupted by European empires. Like many other Khoisan people, the young man found his entire life disrupted by European migrations and territorial wars in the Northern Cape of southern Africa. Then whites took Sturmann to the United States, and they made him display his body as evidence of his supposed inferiority and African oddity. Whether out of desperation or aspiration to begin an afterlife, Sturmann hanged himself. Afterward, whites in Boston continued to use his body to craft a narrative of white supremacy. According to the Warren Museum's records, Sturmann's skeleton was put "under Prof. [Louis] Agassiz's care," and at the medical school, the cast of Sturmann's head became object number 3237. Despite Sturmann's literal objectification in the museum, a reckoning with his life and the circumstances of his death unveils medical schools' symbiotic relationship with colonial violence, and the youth's own repeated attempts to wrest control over his existence, culminating with ending his own life.[36]

Skull collectors and medical schools also benefited from the violence of enslavers, even using the heads of enslaved rebels to teach racial difference. In one specific case, Harvard held the skull of a leader from one of the largest slave revolts in Brazilian history, the Muslim uprising, which took place in Salvador, Bahia, in 1835. The Society for Medical Improvement first received the skull from a Boston lawyer Gideon T. Snow, who had relocated to Salvador and sent the specimen to Boston doctor J. C. Howard. In contrast to descriptions of Sturmann emphasizing his allegedly demure stature and inferiority, the doctors attributed physical strength to the unnamed Muslim revolt leader, as well as noting his cranial capacity. According to J. B. S. Jackson, the man's cranium was "strongly marked" by "the characteristics of brute force." In the initial morphological description of the man's skull, Jackson reduced the insurgent to his supposed racial and ethnic characteristics. Moreover, by associating the man's morphology with ferocity and physical strength, Jackson emphasized the violent aspects of rebellion rather than political agency. Even though this man and other participants in the Muslim uprising had planned a complex political attack on the local enslaver regime, Harvard students and professors read his skull for signs of animality and physical strength.[37]

Despite—or more likely because of—the racial essentializing, Jackson held the man's skull in high regard. The man's participation in a slave revolt seemed to prove his physical prowess and added to the cranium's uniqueness. Like descriptions of Sturmann, Jackson's depiction of the unnamed enslaved rebel's skull clearly fetishized the specimen. In the catalog, Jackson devoted nearly half of the object's unusually long description to an excerpt from Gideon T. Snow's letter that had accompanied the skull. According to Snow, the enslaved leader "was a genuine African, of the Nago [sic] tribe, esteemed above all other blacks for their tall stature, breadth of shoulders, symmetry and strength of limb." Snow continued, "This was the tribe which revolted here last January (1835), and this was one of the chiefs in the affair. He was killed after a most desperate contest, the courage of this tribe being fully equal to their Herculean strength." Snow's letter, along with Jackson's reading of the skull, sought to further fetishize the skull through the physical prowess of its original inhabitant.[38]

A retelling of the Muslim uprising unveils the profoundly important cause for which the unnamed leader gave his life. It also reveals the power of the clinical-racial gaze and its ability to replace an individual's identity, as defined by profound leadership skills and heroism, with a priori assumptions about racial difference. Rather than a case of physical triumph, the Muslim uprising is the story of ethnic and religious solidarity combined with rigorous planning. The Muslim uprising also provides another example of the immense difficulty of arranging and carrying out a revolt in a slave society.

Like Sturmann, the Nagô rebel's skull came to Boston as a product of complex political shifts unfolding around the world. Unlike in the United States and British Empire, in Brazil, the transatlantic slave trade continued unabated well into the nineteenth century. With enslaved mortality rates running high and sugar plantations requiring laborers, Brazilians in Bahia continually imported enslaved West and Central Africans during this period. In fact, despite officially banning the slave trade in 1831, slavers still openly engaged in the trade in Salvador. As further proof of the trade's continual influence during this period, a majority of the enslaved population of Salvador were African born. Many enslaved people like the Nagôs came from Yorubaland and Hausa people from Hausaland (spanning modern-day Nigeria, Togo, and Benin), which had growing Muslim populations. As Islam expanded in this part of West Africa, West African Muslims came into violent conflicts with local political leaders that subscribed to traditional West African religions like Orisha.[39]

As a result of these conflicts, local leaders forced West African Muslims into the slave trade at increasingly high rates. Muslim Nagôs newly arrived to Brazil used their religion to create a sense of solidarity and an identity that they would preserve in the face of enslavement, and they helped shape a broader local African diasporic culture. As further evidence of the centrality of Islam to the uprising, the rebellion took place during Ramadan. The Islamic faith and an emerging, shared West African identity forged in transatlantic and Brazilian slavery represented essential touchstones for the movement. Enslaved Muslim Nagôs also made up the majority of the leadership. The rebels used these cultural ties to bind their movement together. This understanding of the revolt as built through ethnic and religious solidarity defies J. B. S. Jackson's racialized depiction of the rebellion as an extension of the Nagôs' supposedly violent and warlike nature.[40]

In carrying out a large-scale attack on enslaver control, the leaders of the Muslim uprising required secrecy, intelligence, and a well-developed organization. As the uprising's most notable historian, João José Reis, explains, the leaders "put together a shrewdly organized revolutionary structure" without publicizing a date for the revolt far in advance. This strategy allowed the rebels to grow their ranks before committing to a date for the rebellion, which limited possibilities for the details of their plans to be uncovered. Thus, a significant portion of their strategy lay in movement-building, as well as military tactics.[41]

The rebellion took place on January 25, 1835. As was the case with so many other slave uprisings in the Americas, enslavers used police-state tactics to suppress the revolt. The rebel leadership was discovered by police in the early morning of the twenty-fifth in Salvador, just hours before the rebellion's planned commencement. As a result, the revolt began early, with the leadership attacking the police as they tried to enter the rebels' headquarters. The early start upset the leaders' well-laid plans and certainly took away the insurgents' element of surprise. Before being suppressed, approximately 600 enslaved people joined the uprising taking place in the streets of Salvador, facing off against at least 1,500 national guardsmen. It is also reasonable to infer that, had the rebels not been discovered early, even more people would have joined their cause. At the end of the uprising, fifty African rebels and nine of their opponents lay dead. The leader whose skull made it to Harvard died from wounds in a local hospital. Apparently, in a desperate struggle for freedom and his life, he suffered a fatal blow from the butt of a musket. Like most other slave revolts, the Muslim uprising ended in the restoration of enslaver rule, but the rebels' ingenuity, intelligence, and solidarity nonetheless provided an essential counternarrative to the racist depictions of West Africans being propagated by medical professors in the United States.[42]

This story of political agency and the various Black identities created by the African diaspora in Bahia, however, was mostly unknown to the medical students who would handle the Nagô leader's skull. Students would have most likely seen this man's head as just one more African skull on a shelf full of Black people's crania.

By the end of the antebellum era, racial medicine was globalizing at a rapid rate. As was the case with the Chinese smuggler who opened the chapter, Sturmann, and the Nagô rebel, many of the skulls collected in Harvard's and other museums were the products of a world uprooted by enslavement and empire. The methods for understanding race had been developed in the Atlantic World, but the objects that medical students and professors analyzed spanned an even larger geography. In the antebellum era, students at Harvard touched, measured, and manipulated the remains of those killed by American, British, French, Portuguese, and Spanish imperial troops. Pupils could compare the skull sizes of supposed different West African ethnic groups while using the numerical method to link these diverse peoples together into a single racial category. As a result of racial skull collections, even though most medical students went on to be local practitioners in the United States, their training allowed them to think about the world more broadly. Other pupils even obtained influential professional roles, applying further the racial ideologies constructed in and disseminated through sites of racial pedagogy like the racial skulls in the Warren Anatomical Museum.

Moreover, as a routine component of their education, medical students contributed to a transnational history of violence against people of color. Students examined the heads of people from six continents whose remains were stolen from battlefields and graveyards as trophies. They replaced people's life stories with simple and deeply flawed racial categories. When prospective doctors measured and handled these skulls to categorize race, they also erased people's individual and cultural identities, producing another form of colonial violence.

By the 1850s, many medical students had even adopted their professors' transnational framework for understanding race. They used methods created through borderless intellectual movements, violently analyzing living people through travel and locally examining dead people whose remains were being stolen and shipped across the nodes of empires. Beyond just the transnational intellectual community, physicians in the United States built the racial science of the antebellum era through their worldwide access to human remains. Harvard obtained, measured, and displayed the bodies of those like the opium smuggler, Sturmann, and the Nagô leader through the increasing power of European empires in global politics. In a world wed together by new technologies of rapid transportation and communication, Harvard accessed with relative ease the bodies of the recent and long-since dead that were made available through slavery and imperial wars. Therefore, U.S. racial medicine's progressively international gaze emerged from the world created by the violence of imperialism and enslavement.

Ironically, these globe-spanning collections of human remains actually erased the diversity of experiences undergirding them. Erasure compounded the physical violence of imperialism. Rather than emphasize the range of their collections captured under varied and complex circumstances, racial skull collectors and museum curators sought to minimize this diversity, instead lumping skulls into a handful of racial categories. The numerical method applied to these objects furthered this erasure by turning the remains of individuals with complex lives and deaths into aggregated data points.[43]

In addition to stereotyping people internationally, this clinical-racial gaze was applied by physicians and medical students to constructing biased narratives of the health of enslaved and colonized peoples around the world. Using the same racial groups supposedly established in skull collections, doctors began to construct narratives of the health of Black people and their fitness for specific types of labor, diseases, and environments. Thus, as well as the hierarchies being revised and reaffirmed by skull collections, physicians employed racial difference as a means to frame colonized and enslaved peoples as improved and healthy, justifying the global spread of white supremacy.

6

JEFFRIES WYMAN, TRAVEL, AND THE RISE OF A RACIAL ANATOMIST

Both clinical and racial medicine in the antebellum United States demanded experience. Through an emphasis on the clinic and observation, experience and education were almost synonymous. From professor to pupil and whether discussing race or pathology, American medical educators trained their students to trust their senses while studying diseases or anatomical objects. The clinical-racial gaze—formed through the confluence of experiences observing enslavement and disease—represented a way of interpreting experiential knowledge, but it was not a substitute for viewing, handling, or treating the bodies of African descendants. For students not from slaveholding states, chances to study and directly observe supposed racial differences were rarer in everyday life than they were for those from slaveholding societies. From international skull collections to professors sharing their experiences traveling amid slavery and observing the health concerns of the plantation environment, transnational systems of capitalism, imperialism, and slavery made experience transportable.

As they grappled with race and their clinical education, students revealed in their theses not only the centrality of observation for discussing race, but also the limits of their personal experiences as youths. In his 1855 thesis at MDUP, Alabama student J. Ramsay McDow revealed the value of being from a slaveholding district for his understanding of race. He also uncovered students' reliance on their professors' experiences with Black people, even for those from slave societies. Arguing in support of polygenesis, McDow cited his supposed experience and others' observations to discount environmental explanations for racial difference. For example, he wrote, "If the Negro has ever been white, if his hair has ever been straight, is it not strange, very strange that during the long period spoken of [from ancient Egypt to the nineteenth century], and the diversified and favorable influences of converting other white men into negroes, and vice versâ, the metamorphosis has never been observed!" Ignoring that cases of vitiligo like Henry Moss's were widely known and written about by multiple former members of MDUP's faculty, McDow emphasized observation to justify his faulty conclusion. If a student like McDow omitted cases of vitiligo as proving racial environmentalism, then his simple explanation held considerable weight. While mixed-race people were prevalent in southern cities and not uncommon on plantations, cases of vitiligo-induced racial change after birth were rare. Despite the desire of those like Benjamin Rush to build a wider understanding of racial change out of vitiligo, antebellum observers like McDow were skeptical.[1]

Observations about racial differences, however, were portable, and faculty incorporated their personal experiences with health and slavery into medical school curricula. Schools had a pedagogy built around giving students as much firsthand knowledge as was practical, but faculty used personal anecdotes to supplement opportunities for experience. In fact, McDow did not rely only on his experiences. He also cited the anatomical observations of Professor Joseph Leidy to support polygenesis. Furthermore, in his thesis, McDow looked to the lectures of Samuel Jackson, the professor of the Institutes of Medicine. Invoking a case of dirt eating, Jackson did not bring up the account to fetishize the practice among enslaved people. Instead, the "girl" had ingested the "ova of a species of the beetle tribe or family." What emerged were typical larvae. For McDow this proved that a change of environment did not change species. "Here was heat, chemical action, darkness, and every conceivable condition which could alter or modify the physical characters [of the larvae]," he explained, "but no such change was observable." While his evidence was far from being typical for polygenesis, McDow captured the profound influence faculty had on students and the transmissibility of observations and experience. For many aspiring physicians, the anecdotal observations of professors like Jackson were as sacrosanct as firsthand knowledge. When discussing anatomy, in addition to his own Professor Leidy, McDow cited Harvard's Louis Agassiz and deceased European luminaries Georges Cuvier and Petrus Camper. In short, for students, medical faculty were significant authorities, but their influence was often rooted in their ability to cite their personal experience, whether with anatomy or theories of race and the environment.[2]

The case of Hampden-Sydney and later Harvard faculty member Jeffries Wyman represents one route for faculty to gain such experience. As professors had more time to hone their observations as well as travel abroad and network with other elite physicians, their experiences were impressive. Wyman graduated from Harvard in 1837, but he only left medical education for seven years, being appointed the professor of anatomy at Hampden-Sydney College in 1843. He finally returned to Harvard as professor of comparative anatomy in the Lawrence School of Science in 1848. Before traveling as a professor to a slave society, Wyman, like other medical students of the period, learned a great deal of supposed facts about blackness and racial difference more broadly in medical school. He could then transmit these experiences to his pupils at Hampden-Sydney and Harvard. By narrating this trajectory, this chapter shows that, in contrast to neighborhood physicians of the eighteenth century who most often learned and practiced their trade locally, antebellum medical students were enmeshed in a much more interconnected and mobile profession through their professors.

Jeffries Wyman exemplified both the growing transnational medical culture of elite professors in the decades leading up to the Civil War, and the ways that U.S. medical professors created networks and experiences that transcended state and national borders, all of which deepened medical racism. As a medical student at Harvard in the 1830s, Wyman had learned about the supposed health of African-descended people in the tropics. He only continued to build his racial expertise while a medical professor in the 1840s at Hampden-Sydney College in Richmond, Virginia, and during a research trip to Suriname in 1857. Wyman revealed how describing, treating, and subjugating African-descended people were becoming routine duties of antebellum physicians, even of Bostonians like him.

The mobility of scientific travelers like Wyman shaped their perceptions of race and slavery. In traveling to Virginia and Suriname, Wyman obtained direct knowledge of slavery and the people making up the system. He and other antebellum physicians used their expertise and transnational networks as a prism for interpreting the social problems of the antebellum United States and beyond. Trips by those such as Wyman revealed the extent to which the Atlantic World allowed for racial science to mature in the mid-nineteenth century. Like skull collecting, travel to slave societies provided for direct interaction with slavery and African descendants, a circumstance akin to the medical profession's emphasis on clinical experience. Through these trips, physicians fashioned themselves as experts in tropical environments and peoples.

For naturalists and physicians, trips abroad had a two-pronged purpose. The first purpose was the professed scientific goal of the trip, but the travelers also wished to gain greater knowledge about the world and its peoples, coming to an understanding of the diversity of global populations and related political questions. As historian Nancy Stepan has argued, the study of the tropics was rooted in three emerging disciplines in the nineteenth century: natural history, anthropology, and tropical medicine. These fields were deeply intertwined, and scholars focusing on one of them often produced data for the other two. Even though Harvard's Jeffries Wyman ended up in Virginia and Dutch Suriname for various other professional reasons, during these stays, he created racial constructs that carried over into his role as a professor and physician.[3]

Wyman evidenced the increased mobility of elite physicians during this period. In addition to making trips to Europe, many prominent physicians traveled to European colonies. For example, Samuel Cartwright and Samuel Morton traveled to the West Indies. When writing *Races of Man: And Their Geographical Distribution* in 1848, Charles Pickering had circumnavigated the world as a part of the U.S. Exploring Expedition. While these trips were not typical for the average doctor, elite physician-naturalists of the 1850s journeyed to the tropics with increasing regularity. As they were professors and influential writers, their accounts undoubtedly trickled down to and influenced medical students. Thus, in addition to an increasingly international data set on race, physicians and scientists could add their personal observations to this discourse.[4]

While some anatomists such as Hermann Burmeister and Louis Agassiz specifically ventured to the tropics to peer on the racial Other, other naturalists and physicians such as Wyman collected racial data more incidentally. The locale, as much as the discipline, defined what types of observations were made. While deeply invested in studying science and race, Wyman only inadvertently found himself observing slavery. His observations underscore how racial knowledge was a part of the fabric of medicine and science. Physicians routinely collected data on race, even when racial science was not their main discipline. Early in his career as a medical professor in Virginia, Wyman had adopted the role of intermediary in correspondence with northern friends and family, communicating his distorted vision of a slave society. Annually returning to Virginia from his summers in Boston, he found the intimate presence of Black people jarring. Accustomed to the largely white northern city, Wyman never became fully acclimated to the racial intermingling of southern slavery. In a letter to his sister in 1844, he described a sense of disbelief that he had truly gone to the South, which was quickly dispelled by "the voice of a *Virginny N—r.*" Apparently, the presence of Black people, whom he loathed, had a similar effect on his return to Richmond in 1847, for the last session he taught at Hampden-Sydney. Wyman's words serve as a reminder that nominally disliking slavery did not mean welcoming formerly enslaved people to the North. Likewise, as much as Wyman and others claimed scientific detachment, their views of race were filtered through both racist and medical worldviews.[5]

Wyman's tales of southern society evidence a disdain for both enslaved people and many enslavers. While visiting Washington, D.C., with an English friend, the two witnessed a Black man being beaten unmercifully in the street by a cab driver. Garnering Wyman's praise, the English friend intervened. He put an end to "the disgraceful conduct" as some *"gentleman slaveholder"* looked on impotently. Unlike in Suriname, where Wyman would seem to empathize with the enslavers, during his first residence in a slave society, he cultivated disdain for both groups and often depicted the South as socially bankrupt. Ironically, Wyman had developed contempt for the slave society while instructing students whose medical practice would be centered on preserving the health of enslaved laborers and the plantation system.[6]

Despite whatever reservations Wyman might have had about the slave system, he saw his time in Virginia as an opportunity to observe African descendants ethnographically. For this, he relied on planters inviting him to visit their plantations. Invitations such as these evidenced both northern and southern hypocrisy. Despite an intensifying sectional conflict, the enslavers welcomed Wyman. Likewise, Wyman's seeming dislike for the slave system hardly prevented him from exploiting the opportunity to study Black people. When it came to racism, northern and southern whites could often transcend the sectional conflict. In 1847, then, Wyman spent one evening witnessing a neighborhood "corn shucking," or "husking." According to the young physician, the local planters turned this annual task into a sort of party for the enslaved. They plied the enslaved laborers with liquor while they worked. Wyman described how the shucking proceeded: "Two or three of the more musical characters mount the pile & lead the singing while the others join in the chorus." Wyman watched the enslaved work in this vein well into the night. When they finished, he explained, the enslaved ate dinner, which was followed by a dance. Before taking up his role as comparative anatomist in Harvard's Lawrence School of Science (his courses were also offered to medical students), Wyman had garnered extensive experiential knowledge about racial difference in Virginia. As a physician and comparative anatomist, he evidenced how racial science and medicine also cultivated a protoethnographic gaze, and how northern physicians relied on the patronage of the enslaver class when working in a slave society.[7]

When observing African descendants in Dutch Suriname, Wyman used the clinical-racial gaze to analyze the enslaved. His depiction of Black people and their relationship to the tropics supports the notion that the theories underlying polygenesis were shared by many northern physicians, even if they rarely applied racial medicine to their practice. In the spring of 1857, Wyman traveled to Fort Amsterdam in Suriname, along with making trips into the "bush" during an excursion down the Suriname River. While there, he commented regularly about the health of the enslaved and their physical conformation. Many of his observations concern enslaved children. First, he explained that they suffered from diseases related to their poor treatment, such as umbilical hernias and protuberant abdomens, which he believed were caused by a diet too reliant on plantains. Commenting on their clothing, Wyman observed, "Nearly all the [young] children of the slaves go naked." At the age of five, the males received a small piece of cloth attached to a string to cover their genitals, which for some would be a lifelong uniform. In contrast, enslaved women wore skirts, and some wore shirts.[8]

Despite depicting the enslaved workers as hardly clothed and their children as ailing and malnourished, Wyman wrote to his brother that the Dutch were so kind to the enslaved that they did "nearly as they please[d]." Moreover, he explained, the enslaved were a "very happy & jolly set." He also noted that in Suriname, planters could feed and house their enslaved workers for virtually nothing—forty cents a week.[9] Without irony, ten days earlier, Wyman had described the hospital on one plantation as "more of a prison."[10] When Wyman traveled to this slave society, he depicted it in a generally positive light, even if he saw the institution of slavery as philosophically unjust. Likewise, he used the prism of health to evaluate slavery, and he captured the seeming ease with which physicians contradicted themselves when describing the condition of Black patients. In the span of two weeks, he described jail-like hospitals and children's distended bellies but praised the health of the institution of slavery generally.

In addition to observations approximating what would become tropical medicine, Wyman depicted the functionality of slavery in racially essentialist terms, situating Suriname's enslaved population as magnificently suited for the tropical climate. Wyman's understanding of slavery in Suriname was rooted in a belief in each race's inherent relationship to specific climates. Located just a few degrees north of the equator, Suriname was in the heart of the American tropics. The tropics held symbolic value for physicians such as Wyman. During the journey, on March 3, he noted in his diary, "22°. Within the tropics!" In his letters home, he depicted the enslaved as simply thriving in the brutal climate. "With no covering not even a hat," he narrated, "the negro stalks about in the full sun & feels quite as grand & perhaps rather more so than most people who require a larger amount of clothing." Wyman's statement reveals his own adoption of a polygenist understanding of race and climate. In this frame, only people of African descent were capable of going naked in the sun because of their skin's ability to withstand the tropical heat. The enslaved acted as a sharp contrast to Wyman's regular struggle with heat-induced debility. Supposedly biologically ordained to live seminude, African descendants were naturally and sartorially better fit for enslavement. In other words, their anatomy enabled them to dress for the tropics. Black skin and constitution worked together to enable African descendants' healthy residence under the direct sunlight of slave countries.[11]

Wyman's account of Suriname also underscores the male sexual voyeurism inherent to mid-nineteenth-century racial science. In Suriname, Wyman gawked at enslaved women's breasts, and he noted their shapes and sizes as supposed anatomical markers of blackness. Staring at enslaved women while they sunbathed, Wyman made detailed observations of their exposed bodies. He evidenced the tendency of white doctors to see Black women's bodies as what historian Deirdre Cooper Owens calls "medical superbodies." Wyman's unquestioned belief in his right to stare at nude Black women contrasted starkly with how he would have approached a white female patient. Cooper Owens explains, "Medical Men generally did not gaze upon their white female patients once they had disrobed except during emergencies. In contrast, white physicians generally shared the assumption that Black women were immodest about the display of their bodies, and medical doctors examined Black women's breasts, stomach, and genitalia without reserve."

Peering on and analyzing Black women's breasts, Wyman evoked the presumptive male ghoulishness of this science. He invaded the women's privacy, gazing on them during a moment of relaxation. Like the racial scientists Louis Agassiz and Hermann Burmeister, who on separate occasions watched non-white nude Brazilians bathe, Wyman saw in nude enslaved bodies another opportunity to point out his perception of their differences. A trip such as Wyman's evidenced the degree to which scientific travel often went far beyond its stated goals. In Suriname, Wyman brought his clinical-racial gaze, which he had begun cultivating as a student at Harvard. He evaluated the morphology of African-descended people, their fitness for the tropical climate, and the specific diseases that they contracted on South American sugar plantations.

As he did in Virginia, Wyman utilized the skill of the enslaved to collect specimens in Suriname. On two occasions in Suriname, enslaved people brought him specimens that he preserved and carried back to Harvard. In addition, enslaved people likely served as crew members during Wyman's journey up the Suriname River, where he hoped to collect more objects and samples. Like planters, Wyman used the knowledge and expertise of enslaved people yet saw them as inferior, as evidenced by his regular use of "n—r" in both his diary and correspondence.[12]

During Wyman's trip into the interior of Suriname, he evidenced scientists and physicians' reliance on planters. With the U.S. flag flying from their ship, Wyman and his crew stayed at plantation after plantation as they cruised upriver. Enslavers gave the Harvard scientist room and board, and enslaved servants waited on him. Further evidencing Wyman's reliance on slave societies' power brokers, the colonial governor arranged for Wyman's trip into the bush to visit the local maroon community.[13]

When visiting the maroon community deep in Suriname's interior, Wyman analyzed the Saamaka racially, rather than noting the magnitude of their achievement in gaining and maintaining independence. The subject of many books by Richard Price and Sally Price, the Saamaka descended from enslaved people who escaped bondage in the late seventeenth century and protected their autonomy through numerous conflicts with the Dutch government into the nineteenth century. Wyman believed the Saamaka proved the negative effects of Black people's autonomy. He explained to his sister, "It is nearly a hundred years since their ancestors ran away from the colonists, & in the mean time they have reverted to a nearly savage life. . . . They are for the most part athletic, go without clothing, exposed to the full force of the sun on the river as well as on land." Wyman saw the opportunity to visit the Saamaka as a chance to observe Africans in what he perceived as a primitive state. His travels to Suriname reveal how scientific journeys to the tropics often led to new observations about slavery and its alleged benefits, underscoring the deep ties of the academic community to slaveholder and colonial power.[14]

Despite his racism, Wyman's account, previously unknown to scholars, also represents a new source for understanding the Saamaka during a period for which few written records exist. The Saamaka's larger history represents one of the most profound examples of Black agency during the age of slavery. The people's culture has now persisted for over 300 years, even as political autonomy eroded during civil war in the 1990s. Saamaka ancestors escaped bondage from the 1690s through the early decades of the eighteenth century. Despite the brutal tactics of the Dutch, the Saamaka survived or won encounter after encounter with colonial troops. In 1762, they signed a treaty with the Dutch guaranteeing their autonomy. Not only did they win, but they even were able to force the Dutch to pay tribute to them. Even Wyman could not miss this profound evidence of collective Black agency, although it did not sit comfortably adjacent to his other descriptions of the maroons. He explained in that same letter to his sister, "[The Saamaka] number about 8,000, are perfectly independent & in fact exact tribute from the colonial government." Moreover, what Wyman described as a return to barbarism actually represented the Saamaka's success in preserving their culture. Despite intense efforts by Moravian missionaries in the eighteenth century to Christianize the Saamaka, most Saamaka continued with their ancestral religion. They worshiped a snake God and other deities represented through nature.

Throughout Wyman's journey, the Saamaka controlled what he saw of their culture and how deeply he got to venture into their territory. He regularly found locked doors in the villages that he visited and nosed around. For a people who prized their isolation, the Saamaka found it patently absurd that Wyman had traveled thousands of miles from his home merely to collect specimens. And once Wyman got to a certain point, the Saamaka cut off his access to further travel without ever formally refusing him passage. He explained, "The Gaaman pretended to be favorably disposed towards us, told us we might go where we pleased, but afterwards we found so many obstacles thrown in our way that it was clear they were determined we should not go a step farther." In short, despite Wyman's claims about the savageness of the Saamaka, they handled his intrusion expertly, only letting him see what they curated for him. Furthermore, the Saamaka's own history of achieving cultural and political autonomy undermined Wyman's depictions of them as inferior to the white leaders in charge of Suriname.[15]

Through his journal entries and correspondence with family, Wyman also revealed that while his perspective might have evolved somewhat over time, many of his observations of African descendants were rooted in ideologies gestating in antebellum medical schools. His account of slavery aroused the medical concepts central to polygenesis, discussing at length the fitness of African-descended people for tropical climates. Rather than adapting his views to local circumstances or new data, Wyman filtered his observations through many of the same ideologies as medical students like J. Ramsay McDow. He depicted African descendants' bodies as uniquely suited to the tropics. When left to their own devices like the Saamaka, he saw African-descended people as inherently barbarous. Wyman's travels underscore how he understood defining race and social relations as an adjunct duty of the medical profession, mirroring medical schools' curricula that he helped shape. Like Nott and many other antebellum doctors, Wyman supposed that physician-scientists had a central role to play in the political future of Black people and their relation to larger institutions that connected diverse peoples, such as slavery and empire.

From venturing to Europe for training to collecting specimens and studying natural history in the tropics, medical professors traveled extensively.

Through travel, faculty created networks, garnered experience, and produced knowledge. This both enhanced their prestige among their colleagues and created a well of anecdotes for lectures and writing. Like McDow repeating the case of the dirt-eating woman as told by Professor Samuel Jackson, or William Stump Forwood repeating Joseph Leidy's anatomical observations about racial difference, students listened. In their theses, they often reproduced anecdotal evidence from faculty.

Learning through secondhand experience was a critical component for cultivating a clinical-racial gaze, but medical schools also provided students opportunities to gain experience firsthand. As clinical methods continued to grow in importance, they became racialized. Many, if not most, U.S. medical students observed or participated in the dissection of a Black person during their education. Southern students and those who worked in urban poorhouses discussed the relationship between health, race, and climate. As the nineteenth century progressed, like skull collections, anecdotal observations and statistics about race and health from slave societies and colonial spaces circulated widely. These worked to bolster arguments about Black people being uniquely suited to hard labor in hot climates. Anecdotal evidence also supplied experiential knowledge about race, health, and climate to those who had yet to or could not observe non-whites in the tropics directly.

7

RACE, EMPIRE, AND ENVIRONMENTAL MEDICINE

In 1851, MDUP student T. G. Henry asserted, "The coast of Africa, which so fatal to whites, is favourable to blacks." And in 1855, William Henry Daughtry, also studying medicine at MDUP, noted that remittent fever had made "intertropical Africa uninhabitable by whites." Finally, writing on the same subject two years later, another MDUP student, Elliott Smith, inquired, "Why does the negro dwell in comparative safety on the coast of his native land[?]" and answered, "Providence placed him there." In these highly illustrative quotes, medical students invoked the increasingly transnational gaze of racial medicine in the United States. For students such as Henry, Daughtry, and Smith, understanding the diseases of slavery required evidence from tropical nations beyond the South. Much as they used skull collections, through concepts of and data about climate, physicians created comparisons between the United States and the rest of the world. In their writings, they conjured up an image of Africa as inherently unfit for whites and a paradise for Black people. Doctors' conceptualization of Africa evidenced the dawn of a new era for racial medicine in the United States. Peering beyond just internal questions of slavery and its survival, medical students interrogated whether empire was sound health policy for the United States. In this sense, in the middle of the nineteenth century, racial medicine was in the earliest phases of morphing into the international frame that became tropical medicine, complementing some proslavery advocates' expansionist vision for the slavocracy.[1]

In many ways, medical school professors' and students' international racial vision mirrored changes occurring in U.S. culture more broadly. These changes illustrated how the boundaries of U.S. racial thinking had been expanding, tracking alongside the increasing globalization of imperialism and capitalism. As historian Sharla Fett explains about this political frame, "Despite U.S. historians' tendency to tell a domestically focused story of 1850s sectional politics, U.S. newspapers in the period regularly covered all aspects of the clandestine transatlantic [slave] trade." Here, Fett is discussing the growing popularity in the 1850s of what she calls "slave trade ethnography," but the same could be said about medical literature about race. Like Fett's work, recent scholarship by Manisha Sinha, Gerald Horne, and Matthew Karp has emphasized that as much as the sectional crisis over slavery might have caused some political actors to focus on domestic debates, it also led many others to contrive of new imperial schemes to preserve the slavocracy.

Whether discussing the forced exportation of enslaved people to Brazil or reopening the transatlantic slave trade, white antebellum Americans increasingly understood slavery and racism as parts of an international array of economic and political forces. In short, antebellum whites were almost as interested in their position within global racial hierarchies as they were in questions about preserving slavery in the South.[2] In a development rooted in this broader shift, medical students and professors began to depict the relationship between race, health, and the environment on a global scale. They believed that their research could shape the future of slavery, as well as the United States' potential evolution into an imperial power.

During the last decades of the antebellum era, medical professionals crafted new arguments about the health of southern slavery, just as they constructed novel evidence about non-white bodies in the tropics that contributed to a global data set about race, health, and imperialism. American physicians helped develop this new data set even as they relied on it. Inherent to depictions of the South as climatologically sound for African descendants' bodies were theories of race, place, and health that spoke to a world progressively more interconnected through trade and imperialism. In this frame, Africa and the U.S. South were united in their populations, their exploitation by people of European descent, and the tropical aspects of their climates. Both comparing and contrasting the region with tropical zones, white physicians depicted the South as a liminal space for Black people's and white people's bodies due to its mix of the features and diseases of temperate and tropical climates. Where white people's bodies were well suited to temperate ailments, doctors believed that African-descended people were protected from tropical diseases. For example, physicians considered enslaved African descendants as inherently resistant to malaria and yellow fever but highly susceptible to pneumonia. The opposite was supposed to be true of whites, whose constitutions were best suited for temperate ailments and supposedly required acclimation to the southern subtropics.[3]

At the core of these late antebellum therapeutics and pathologies resided racial theory and polygenesis. During the late colonial and early national periods, physicians who supported monogenesis saw race as a minor factor in medical practice. In Benjamin Rush's disease theory of blackness, bodies moving out of balance produced both race and disease, and all bodies were healthiest in a temperate environment existing between the extremes of the tropics and the tundra. However, like with anatomy and the numerical method, many antebellum American physicians embraced the French-touted climatologically specific medicine.[4] As well as treating it as a theory of human origins and the natural social position of each race, physicians used polygenesis to shape concepts of medical environments and therapeutics. Along these lines, doctors fundamentally altered their views of the health of certain body types and their relationship to the environment. The tangled web of medical, environmental, and racial thought emerging in this period meant that polygenesis could not just be seen as politics or natural history influencing medical education. Instead, theories of race were practice centered during the antebellum era.[5]

This chapter traces how medical schools came to teach the relationship between race, health, and the environment, with a specific focus on how racial science shaped and was shaped by ideologies of practice, disease causation, and a transnational medical profession linked together through networks of correspondence and print culture. In the early nineteenth century, professors such as Benjamin Rush taught that the human body had similar reactions to environments mostly devoid of racial difference. Students largely concurred with this worldview, most often attributing higher rates of enslaved people contracting diseases to poor living conditions.

As the antebellum era progressed, however, racial scientists and medical professors began to argue that Black people were built for the southern environment, having natural resistance to tropical diseases that were understood as the South's worst ailments. Due to African descendants' supposed protection from hot temperatures, sunlight, and illnesses such as malaria and yellow fever, physicians saw Black people as least vulnerable to the dangers inherent to laboring on southern plantations. Students also adopted much of polygenists' depiction of the relationship between blackness and climate. They depicted enslaved people's bodies as well suited to the oppressive heat and deadly diseases of the tropics and subtropics. Using data created through global empires and U.S. racial science, antebellum medical professionals believed the Deep South was the healthiest place for enslaved African descendants in the United States, as it closely resembled whites' impressions of West Africa.

As anatomy made distinct Black people's bodies, concepts of health and the environment framed how they should be managed. From specific therapeutics and plantation management to domestic and foreign policy, racialized concepts of health defined how Black and other non-white people should be treated. Racial concepts of health and the environment shaped arguments for and against imperial expansion and whether formerly enslaved people should be admitted into "free states" in the North. In short, proponents of racial medicine hoped to frame Black people's bodies as different through anatomy and to manage the bodily and social health problems that arose from these racial differences. In this way, doctors used race to carve out a position for themselves as an emergent managerial class in the United States, wielding their expertise to control and define Black people's bodies on behalf of the white population.

ENVIRONMENT, RACE, AND HEALTH IN THE ERA OF MONOGENESIS

Monogenists, like their successors, influenced the nature of medical practice, affecting how physicians approached Black patients. At the beginning of the nineteenth century, most white doctors and scientists contended that specific environments created races that were degenerated or elevated from an original type.[6] Influenced by medical thinkers such as Benjamin Rush, physicians largely treated each race the same in terms of therapeutics. They believed that people, devoid of race, reacted to specific environments in ways that were largely universal, even if each individual's body was uniquely shaped by its natural history. As a result, early national physicians saw individual human bodies as being altered by and adapted to external and internal factors ranging from education to diet or even climate. Birth was relevant but not fundamentally deterministic. For Rush and other physicians during the early national period, environments had both climatic and social implications.

Rush's disease theory of blackness mirrored larger questions that he harbored toward the relationship between bodies and environments. As detailed earlier, Rush argued that leprosy caused blackness, and that curing this racial difference was essential to proving that Black people were at their core the same animal as whites. This, he believed, undercut arguments that "qualify them [Black people] for labor in hot and unwholesome environments."[7] However, Rush's model reflected broader medical ideas about the health effects of the environment on the body. According to Rush and his students, heat, diet, and "deficiency of labour" in Africa created much of the culture of Africans, instead of an innate nature dating back to creation as asserted by polygenists. Bodies and environments existed in constant states of flux, resulting in cyclical relationships of mutual influence. Under Rush's formulation, blackness could be contracted in much the same way as any other disease.[8] Rush's theory of blackness mirrored his larger conception of the human body and disease, which was rooted in his early studies under

William Cullen in Edinburgh in the 1760s. Rush believed that actions of the body were "all effects of stimuli acting upon the organs of sense and motion." In this model, Rush depicted the environment as having immediate effects on the body. As examples, he cited the absence of sunlight causing depression, a loud noise "resuscitating a person who was supposed to be dead," and certain scents possessing restorative powers. Thus, the body existed under constant forces of alteration from external influences. Blackness, supposedly like other diseases, was the product of this fluid relationship between body and stimuli that had gone awry.[9]

External forces could be invigorating or harmful, but in Rush's theory, there existed an essential human body being shaped and acted on by a variety of natural and social environmental influences. Disease was the product of the body in disrupted states outside the healthy equilibrium. Thus, most diseases were not unique vectors but instead the result of external stimuli acting on the body's natural state.[10] For example, a young William Horner explained in his notes from Rush's lectures, "[Three] different stages of society or civilization influence the pulse, it is slower in savages than in persons brought up in a civilized society. Savages want [for] the numerous stimuli of thought, conversation, etc. which civilized people enjoy, hence too the pulse is less frequent in countryman than in townspeople." Likewise, emancipation "produced fainting in a negro who was unexpectedly set at liberty." For Rush and his students, the environment represented a wide range of factors that affected the body, both in terms of immediate health and race. Moreover, Rush and his pupils saw environments and bodies as complex and ever changing, locked within constantly evolving relationships.[11]

Rush's approach to medicine and its attendant theory of race posited a vision of slavery and human existence in which Black people were superficially degenerated due to slave labor in unhealthy climates. Rush did not depict Black people as inherently inferior and fit for slavery. While his vision of racial improvement meant curing blackness and thus turning all people white, he also provided a vital antislavery medical therapeutics. Unlike later physicians, Rush did not believe slavery was the cure. Instead, he saw slavery as residing at the root of the illness causing blackness. Despite his antislavery stance, Rush was quite literally a white supremacist, defining white skin as the ideal and arguing that aberrations from it had to be cured.[12]

In contrast with some polygenists who saw slavery as important to the health of the nation, Rush saw slavery and the slave trade as one of the country's gravest ills. His universal vision of embodied health spoke to questions of the soundness of society as a whole, arguing that the free circulation of goods and people in the Atlantic World was central to the wellness of the young and fragile U.S. republic. For Rush, a healthy republic resided in its existence within the flow of goods and people in the Atlantic World if its harmful elements like the slave trade were contained.[13]

Rush presented race as the product of social, cultural, and environmental factors that affected the body's state of balance, and his conceptions of health and race greatly influenced his students. Following Rush's lectures, students attributed Black people's increased likelihood to contract certain ailments such as tetanus, typhoid fever, and other fevers to social and environmental factors, not race. From Rush's era to the late antebellum period, the discourse over race and predisposition represented a significant shift in how physicians conceived of racial difference. Late antebellum physicians expressed a vision of race as biologically determined through their depiction of African descendants' bodies as inherently resistant or susceptible to certain ailments. In contrast, early national physicians believed that built environmental factors caused differential rates of disease contraction.[14]

In theses written during the early national period, medical students frequently rejected contentions from West Indian physicians that African-descended people contracted tetanus more frequently because of their constitutions. Embracing Rush's logic, MDUP students ascribed differential rates of disease contraction on plantations to material conditions rather than inherent predisposition. Moreover, prospective physicians engaged in an Atlantic debate about the meaning of race in medical practice. In 1807, MDUP student Thomas Bryant explained that it was not innate disposition that caused Black people to regularly contract tetanus on plantations. He argued instead, "Its [tetanus's] frequency among them [enslaved people] is owing to their being much more exposed to the causes which produce it; as bad clothing, going barefoot, [and] frequent wounds received in their various occupations."[15]

As late as 1825, MDUP students were disavowing constitutional explanations for Black people's supposedly higher rates of contracting tetanus and, like Bryant, blaming the social and physical environments of enslavement. In 1825, MDUP student Gilbert Heston wrote that high rates of tetanus on plantations did not arise "from any constitutional predisposition, but from [slaves] being more exposed to punctures and wounds in the feet from usually going barefooted." Inherent to pupils' formulation of the relationship between race and tetanus were both a rejection of polygenesis and an accusation that white planters were treating their enslaved human property poorly. These students argued that inattention to clothing—shoes in particular—made tetanus a serious problem on plantations, not the bodies of the enslaved themselves.[16] The rejection of differential disease resistance represented a conception of bodies different from the one common among medical students in the latter half of the antebellum era. These later students attributed higher rates of typhoid fever in enslaved people to constitutional peculiarities.[17]

As the antebellum era progressed, students increasingly saw the health of Black people as a product of their natural organization and relation to distinct environments. Discussion of slaves' clothing and nutrition, however, persisted, even as they became secondary themes in discussions of enslaved people's health. This shift resulted not so much from a lack of interest in the material conditions of the enslaved as from the theoretical divorce of built and natural environments. At the turn of the nineteenth century and into the 1820s, Rush and other physicians grouped as "stimuli" the influence of social and material environments. Such stimuli could be altered. Instead, late antebellum physicians saw the relationship of climate to bodies as inert, inalterable, and causing poor or good health. Dietary or sartorial concerns were largely secondary. In addition to changing medical concepts of the body and disease more broadly, imperialism created an ever-growing body of data on non-white health. By the 1850s, U.S. physicians could compare their accounts of Black people in the South to monographs by European physicians in India, Africa, and Latin America. Considering these intellectual shifts, doctors began to argue that they must treat white and African-descended bodies as distinct organisms.

POLYGENESIS AND THE ENVIRONMENT IN
ANTEBELLUM MEDICAL THOUGHT

In addition to perceiving polygenesis's more overt sociopolitical meanings, antebellum physicians also understood it as a theory of the environment and the health of human bodies. In his 1852 collection *Essays on Life, Sleep, Pain, Etc.*, Samuel Henry Dickson, an MCSC professor who at different times served on the faculty at the New York University Medical School and the Jefferson Medical College, explained, "Providence has allotted to the several varieties of human kind their respective places of abode." Dickson indicated how antebellum racial science had reframed the perceived association between bodies and their connections to specific environments, replacing more fluid notions of degeneration and change with hardened rules about certain races' relationships to climates. The darker races remained healthy nowhere "except under the hot sun of the South," according to Dickson. Nor could the "northern tribes" live in the "Gold Coast." Explaining what happened when these laws were transgressed, he stated, "We encounter a host of difficulties in the deadly pangs of sickness and the tortures of fatal disease." Polygenesis and the relationship between race and environment represented a vital piece of medical theory for Dickson. Understanding these relationships was "the lot of [the medical] profession."[18]

Works such as those by Dickson evidence that during the antebellum era physicians defined racial science and medical practice through a multitude of human types, illnesses, and environments. Doctors approached disease through the triangulation of these factors toward the right treatment for each unique patient. Through their practice, Dickson and other physicians gave underlying support to the polygenetic notion that each body was suited for a specific climate. While subscribing to this concept did not require belief in polygenesis, physicians' belief in unchanging organic relationships between bodies and environments was logically consistent with the notion of distinct human species. Furthermore, by applying polygenesis to medicine, doctors further shaped African descendants' bodies as physically and intellectually fit for the toil of slavery. The hardening of medical theories of race occurred alongside global imperialism and escalating antebellum political tensions between the North and South over the future of slavery. Finally, as polygenesis supplanted monogenesis in scientific thought in the 1840s and 1850s, white medical practitioners gave both tacit and direct consent to polygenesis's ascendance through their understanding of disease in the bodies of their patients, white and Black.

As with anatomy, French empiricism influenced how American physicians approached environmental medicine. The importance of the Paris schools for the purposes of climatically and racially specific medicine resided in its opposition to systems, created by Edinburgh-trained physicians such as Rush, that universalized bodies, diseases, and places. In the wake of Rush's generation's decline in influence, two interrelated therapeutic approaches emerged: medical regionalism and the principle of specificity. Specificity, medical regionalism, and polygenesis acted as mutually bolstering sets of ideas that physicians used to align African-descended people's bodies with hot, potentially malarial climates and requiring specific treatments.

Through the principle of specificity, physicians argued that not all treatment and therapy plans worked equally well for each patient. Instead, doctors had to account for individuals' "Age, Sex, Colour, Climate, and Occupation" when making treatment decisions. In the antebellum period, therapeutic specificity became the reigning approach to medical practice, largely supplanting the therapeutic universalism of Rush and his contemporaries. Physicians came to believe that medical practices useful in one type of person or climate were not always effective in others. Likewise, medical professionals risked their reputations when they did not consider the particularity of patients and places. Following the logic of specificity, Samuel Henry Dickson explained in his 1855 synthetic tome *Elements of Medicine*, "Original predisposition may be—1. Idiosyncratic, or personally constitutional. 2. Parental, or hereditarily constitutional; and 3. Tribal, or derived from the characteristics of race." Specificity and polygenesis captured a shifting perception of the body in antebellum medicine. Physicians' understanding of the human body was that, instead of existing in fluid and evolving relationships to the environment, it had fixed intercourse with its surroundings. Doctors made it their duty to comprehend these supposedly static connections between bodies and places that dated back for millennia.[19]

Specificity also set the theoretical groundwork for medical regionalism, which built on the notion of racial disease resistance and certain climatic intolerances. Better known in southern medicine as "states' rights medicine," medical regionalism's proponents, building out of specificity, argued that medical therapeutics had to be catered to the exact climatic and epidemiological peculiarities of each region. Practitioners in the Old Southwest as well as the South subscribed to medical regionalism.[20] Northern physicians also believed in the theoretical underpinnings of medical regionalism and the principle of specificity. However, since they practiced in temperate climates, they shared a similar set of therapeutics with European doctors, as opposed to their southern counterparts. Thus, northern physicians had little need to create a distinct system of practice.

On the one hand, medical regionalism was a rebellion against the power of the northern profession. By embracing the logic of environmentally specific medicine, on the other hand, southern physicians rooted this rebellion in values shared by medical professionals throughout the United States. Medical regionalism was hardly just politics masked as medicine, but rather a part of the ideological matrix central to the Francophone period in U.S. medicine. French skepticism was rooted in a belief in the power of nature and a reaction to those rationalist physicians like Rush who had argued that doctors could and should control natural bodily processes. Southern physicians had embraced the French skepticism toward therapeutic universalism, arguing that proper medical treatment required specific observation and knowledge of local peoples and climates.[21]

Despite claiming to oppose the universalizing tendencies of early national medicine, specificity and medical regionalism universalized peoples and climates, just along racial lines. For example, regional medicine tended toward treating the South as a medical monolith, but the unifying feature of medical practice in Maryland and Florida was slavery rather than common diseases. In general, this lens was built on a larger political context where many white southerners saw slavery as a unifying principle for their culture. Moreover, during this period, many elite white southerners began to see themselves as intimately connected to various American slave societies. As historian Matthew Karp explains about enslaver foreign policy, "Southern elites showed special concern for their fellow slaveholding societies in the hemisphere, especially Cuba, Brazil, and the independent republic of Texas." In short, the late antebellum period was characterized by an increasing understanding of the slave South as intimately tied to the remaining slaveholding countries in the Americas.[22] Medical regionalism and specificity adopted a similar lens where most slaveholding societies shared similar environmental, medical concerns.

As with polygenesis, medical regionalism and specificity imagined bodies and environments as increasingly locked in webs of entanglements based on individual immutable attributes. MDUP student Joel Lewis explained, "In the slave holding states of our Union, commonly called the 'Southern States[,]' the Practice of Medicine and its kindred branches is widely different from the practice of [it in] the North." Physicians changed their practice on southern whites as well, although less radically. Lewis also advocated for the creation of a systematic treatise on treating Black people in the South. Through medical regionalism and specificity, late antebellum physicians undermined hopes for improving African descendants' bodies and controlling environments. In this frame, medical and social uplift became purportedly implacable in the face of nature due to a polygenetic view of race and place.[23]

Dickson best illustrated this sea change in medical and racial thought. By the 1850s, despite his increasingly unfashionable commitment to humoralism, Dickson supported many of the central concepts of antebellum medicine, including belief in the doctrine of specificity and medical regionalism. Throughout the antebellum era, he continued to cling to many of his humoralist ideas. Still, he viewed the relationship between bodies and their environment in vastly different ways from those like Benjamin Rush.[24] Having graduated from MDUP in 1819—six years after the death of Rush—Dickson represented a transitional figure between those educated in the late eighteenth century and students who graduated in the 1850s. Through teaching and publishing, Dickson helped shape the racial medicine of the 1840s and 1850s, and he illustrated how physicians' ideologies were often complicated and even contradictory during this period. Belief in polygenesis did not always constitute support for southern secession or empirical medicine, and regional identity often clashed with the cosmopolitan self-image of physicians such as Dickson.

Like racial anatomy, theories of race and the environment entered the antebellum medical classroom. In his 1830 physiology course syllabus, Dickson explained, "*Malaria* probably acts upon the skin primarily. Thus we account for the insusceptibility of the Negro race, who differ from the white more in this point than any other."[25] While Dickson later came to see people of African descent as containing a more elaborate set of differences than just the skin, even in 1830, he declared that inherent difference had caused each race to possess unique relationships to diseases and environments.[26] As with malaria, in the case of yellow fever, Dickson again argued that Black Creoles were less liable to contracting it than whites. He declared, "No African is known to have been seized with it [yellow fever]."[27]

For Dickson, Black resistance to yellow fever proved that it was a distinct disease from dengue fever, another virus plaguing Atlantic ports in the nineteenth century. Disagreeing with Dr. David Osgood of Havana, Dickson explained that because native Africans were wholly insusceptible to yellow fever, and since dengue struck every race equally, dengue fever was therefore a distinct disease.[28] Dickson's dispute with Osgood also evidenced the existence of a transnational discourse among physicians in slave societies where Cuba and South Carolina were climatologically and medically linked. Finally, in his 1830 syllabus, in cases of typhus fever on the plantation, Dickson suggested moving the slaves out of their old quarters and into "new huts" for both "remedial and prophylactic" purposes.[29] When writing for students, professors such as Dickson naturalized slavery without overtly discussing mainstream politics, instead prescribing treatments that assumed the alleged inherent health of enslavement on African-descended bodies.

Physicians also used environmental specificity to directly comment on politics, and this went beyond just southerners and proslavery medicine. In a series of letters to retired Harvard anatomy professor John Collins Warren in 1851 that were published in the Whig Party–leaning *National Intelligencer*, Ohio physician Daniel Drake laid out an environment-oriented case for prohibiting free Black people from entering free states. During his life, Drake traveled throughout the South and taught medicine at Transylvania University, the Medical College of Ohio, and the Louisville Medical Institute. While nominally opposing slavery through support of colonization, Drake focused on the supposed utility of environmental racism for northern segregation. He specifically argued that, whether born in the Americas or Africa, Black people "would perish from disease if suddenly carried into latitudes where the white man flourishe[d] best." Citing Dr. J. W. Lugenbeel, Drake explained that this resistance to tropical fevers existed in Africa as well as the Americas.

Lugenbeel was hardly a disinterested commenter. Instead, he was a colonizationist who aggressively pushed free Black people into immigrating to Liberia for the American Colonization Society. Whereas whites were especially vulnerable to disease in Liberia, Drake explained that people of African descent found these diseases to be "generally mild, and when, attended to in time, [were] seldom fatal."

Drake's letters evidence two key features of environmental approaches to race. Like racial anatomy, these physicians looked beyond the South for evidence of racial difference. They understood that creating medically ordained racial difference required observations beyond just southern plantations. Likewise, the implications of racial medicine transcended the immediate questions of the 1850s, such as the abolition of slavery. Racial medical discourses informed the politics of segregation and empire as well as the peculiar institution. Those like Drake used race as a scientific undergirding for state-level exclusionary policies.[30]

Of all the white racial theorists, Josiah Nott most clearly wedded specificity, medical regionalism, and polygenesis together. As a leading physician and racial scientist in Mobile with strong connections to northern medical professors, Nott's influence was wide. While scholars have written about him as a proslavery theorist, they have paid scant attention to how he rooted his ideas in medical theories popular throughout the Atlantic World and in the reputation of his works among medical students. Nott's scholarship was circulated widely, and his extensive connections to prominent professors such as Joseph Leidy, John Collins Warren, and Oliver Wendell Holmes, to name just a few, meant that his ideas undoubtedly influenced medical school curricula nationwide. Nott's 1857 essay "Acclimation; or, The Comparative Influence of Climate, Endemic and Epidemic Diseases, on the Races of Men" encapsulates the collision of medicine and polygenesis. Print works by Nott, Dickson, and Drake provide important sources for understanding how medical schools taught race, because students read these works and used them to frame their approach to practicing medicine on Black people. In his essay, Nott set out to study race and "Medical Climate, [which referred] to climate in its effects on the body, whether in preventing, causing, or curing diseases." His concept of medical climates highlighted the organic relationship between medical and racial theories and how the environment played a key role in both.[31]

While Nott did not completely dismiss the ability of each race to adapt to new climates, he argued that the capacity for adaptation—or acclimation—had racially defined limitations and was therapeutically secondary to ensuring the health of African-descended people. Nott contended that each race was created for a specific medical climate with geographically "pre-scribed salubrious limits." Whites could survive in the tropics and the tundra, but their life span would be significantly limited outside a temperate climate. People of African descent achieved optimum health only in the tropics but could survive in temperate zones. In Nott's model, the South represented a liminal space in terms of medical climate, perfect for neither Black nor white people, but healthy enough for both races' sustained residence. Physicians framed the South as an ideal space for plantation slavery, fit for the occu-pational health of each race's constructed role, the planter and the slave.[32]

According to Nott, Black people's bodies were almost impervious to heat. He described the habits of African descendants in their native coun-try: "[They allegedly go] naked in the scorching rays of the sun, and can lie down and sleep on the ground in a temperature of at least 150° of Fahren-heit, where the white man would die in a few hours." However, the opposite was true of cold weather. As Nott explained, "In America, the Negro steadily deteriorates, and becomes exterminated north of about 40° north latitude. The statistics of New England, New York, and Philadelphia, abundantly prove this." In fact, Nott solicited such information from northern members of the medical fraternity. In 1845, on his older brother's behalf, James E. Nott wrote John Collins Warren. James Nott sent Warren a copy of Josiah Nott's *Two Lectures, on the Natural History of the Caucasian and Negro Races*, and he asked Warren to send him public statistics on the effects of cold climates on mixed-race people. Once again, Josiah Nott evidenced how the medical construction of racial difference represented a project for the national med-ical profession. Through correspondence and print, physicians such as Nott connected their local observations to much larger sets of ideas put toward constructing universal concepts of race and difference. For Nott and other polygenists, not only was southern enslavement healthiest for Black people, removal from (sub)tropical zones could also bring about significant public health risks. Medicine must therefore be tailored to the specific congregation of bodies, diseases, and climate(s) that the local physician encountered.[33]

Nott depicted temperature as only one part of the medical climate, and like each race had its own relationship to hot and cold, white and Black people also had unique connections to the diseases that characterized each climate. When Nott discussed the association between race and disease, the complex entanglements between specificity and polygenesis became most apparent. In "Acclimation," Nott harkened back to his early medical education as a student at MDUP in the late 1820s. He explained that one of his professors, Benjamin Rush's eventual successor Nathanial Chapman, had told the class, "*The negro is much less subject to inflammatory diseases, with high vascular action, than the whites.*" That racialized bodies reacted differently to diseases further proved their innate distinctiveness, Nott argued.[34]

Beyond actual differential labor ability, many physicians argued that Black people were most suited to southern labor regimes because they could survive the inherent climatological dangers. According to Nott and Dickson, African descendants could labor amid malaria in South Carolina's rice swamps with little complaint when whites grew more vulnerable to the ailment. Writing to Nott, Dickson explained "The [white] people living in our low country grow more liable to attack year after year, and generation after generation." While African-descended people were generally seen as physically more fit for labor than whites, physicians often framed darker bodies as better laborers in the southern subtropics due to their protection from the sun and tropical diseases. Dickson also reinforced the notion of whiteness as intimately tied to the temperate climate of Europe. Drawing on the global data set that physicians such as Dickson used as evidence of Black resistance to tropical diseases, Dickson cited imperial records from Algeria, the West Indies, Corsica, Sierra Leone, and India in his letter to Nott. Dickson told Nott that whites were twice as likely to be struck by yellow fever as African descendants in the West Indies and sixteen times more likely to contract the disease as Black people in Sierra Leone, citing various European medical and imperial texts. Observations such as Dickson's and Nott's were only possible due to the increased involvement of physicians in the slave trade and in West African slave ports in the nineteenth century.[35]

While racial medicine might have appeared to be particularly southern or American, Nott's essay points to a global concept of climatic health that transcended the South. In an Atlantic World characterized by empire, migration of peoples, and mobile diseases, Nott used sources that situate the concept of medical climates on a global stage, considering accounts of the health of people of color in the tropical holdings of the French and British Empires.[36] This information constitutes what could be called an emergent global data set of health statistics—created through international imperial expansion—that scholars like Nott were able to consult to create arguments about race and health that transcended national and imperial boundaries. For example, Nott heavily cited French physician Jean Christian Marc Boudin's 1853 statistical study of the colonization of Algeria, *Histoire Statistique de la Colonisation et de la Population En Algerie* (see fig. 7.1). He likewise directly reproduced

"TABLE EXHIBITING THE ANNUAL MORTALITY IN DIFFERENT COUNTRIES IN
EUROPE.

In Sweden	from 1821 to 1825	1 death in	45
Denmark	" 1819	"	45
Germany	" 1825	"	45
Prussia	" 1821 to 1824	"	39
Austrian Empire	" 1825 to 1830	"	43
Holland	" 1824	"	40
Great Britain	" 1800 to 1804	"	47
France	" 1825 to 1827	"	39.5
Canton de Vaud	" 1824	"	47
Lombardy	" 1827 to 1828	"	31
Roman States	" 1820	"	28
Scotland	" 1821	"	50

"The difference of twenty-eight and fifty is considerable; but even the latter rate of mortality is considerably greater than that which the data collected by M. Moreau de Jonnès attribute to Iceland, Norway, and the northern parts of Scotland.

"In approaching the equator, we find the mortality increase, and the average duration of life consequently diminish. The following calculation, obtained by the same writer, sufficiently illustrates this remark:

LATITUDE.	PLACES.	ONE DEATH IN
6° 10′	Batavia	26 inhabitants.
10° 10′	Trinidad	27 "
18° 54′	Sainte Lucie	27 "
14° 44′	Martinique	28 "
15° 59′	Guadaloupe	27 "
18° 36′	Bombay	20 "
22° 33′	Calcutta	20 "
23° 11′	Havana	33 "

"It has been observed that, in some of these instances, the rate of mortality appears greater than that which properly belongs to the climate; as some of the countries mentioned include cities and districts known to be, by local situation, extremely unhealthy.[15] In some, the mortality belongs, in great part, to strangers, principally Europeans, who, coming from a different climate, suffer in great numbers. The separate division from which the collective numbers above given are deduced, will sufficiently indicate these circumstances.

In Batavia, 1805	Europeans died	1 in 11
"	Slaves	1 " 13
"	Chinese	1 " 29
"	Javanese, viz., Natives	1 " 40
Calcutta, 1817 to 1836	Europeans and Eurasians	1 " 28
"	Portuguese and French	1 " 8
1822 to 1836	Western Mahommedans ⎤	
"	Bengal " ⎟	1 " 36
"	Moguls ⎟	
"	Arabs ⎦	

[15] A striking proof of the difference between a malarial and non-malarial climate, in close proximity.—J. C. N.

Figure 7.1. A sample page illustrating the geographical breadth of Josiah Nott's use of imperial data to make his argument about race and health in the global tropics. Josiah Nott and George R. Gliddon, *Indigenous Races of the Earth* (Philadelphia: J. B. Lippincott, 1857), 371. Photo courtesy of the Huntington Library.

pages of comparative national mortality statistics, created by France's chief statistician in the 1830s and 1840s, Alexandre Moreau de Jonnès.[37]

Not just reliant on data from one empire, Nott cited 1840 statistics from a Major Tulloch about health in British "stations" in western Africa, Saint Helena, the Cape of Good Hope, and Mauritius. This data had been published in the influential journal the *Medico-Chirurgical Review*. These examples represent just a small sampling of the sources that Nott accessed to make his comparative analysis about race and health. For cosmopolitan and multilingual scholars like Nott, by the 1850s, the rise of statistics, transatlantic print culture, and imperial expansion made available a previously unprecedented amount of quantitative data on race and health on a global scale. This information—a by-product of imperial and economic expansion—made studies like Nott's possible and functioned as a novel data set for researchers studying race and health in the nineteenth century.[38]

As historian Walter Johnson points out, the 1850s represented a time when southerners were looking to Latin America and the Caribbean for possible routes of expansion. Nott's international gaze corroborated enslavers' interests in Latin America. In this framing, some southern planters hoped to annex Cuba, seeing the island as a route to extend the boundaries of the southern slavocracy. Nott both echoed and opposed this southward gaze of white planters in the Gulf states. While interested in the tropics, Nott believed that further migration of peoples and races could provide significant dangers to the future of the United States' racial public health. He portended racial decline from Atlantic and global migrations when empires did not account for race and environment.[39]

Despite pessimism about imperial expansion, Nott's essay reflects the emergence of this global data set on race, health, and the environment. Physicians like Nott used this data set to contextualize local racial differences within larger trends. As an example, Nott discussed a British colonial force consisting of white and Black West Indian soldiers serving in Gambia. While nearly all the 300 white soldiers died, the Black regiment only lost one soldier. Nott explained, "These black soldiers, too, had been born and brought up in the West Indies; and according to the commonly received theory of acclimation, should not have enjoyed this exemption. No length of residence acclimates the whites in Africa." Rather than reinforcing the impartiality of statistical data, Nott and these colonial statisticians underscored how quantitative and qualitative data were both filtered through the popular racial assumptions typical of much of antebellum white culture. As Nott saw it, acclimation could not overcome the purportedly organic links between racial health and the environment dating back to creation. Ignoring these relationships meant considerable danger to people in an increasingly mobile world.[40]

For his essay, Nott also solicited information from physicians around the Americas, attempting to underscore the fact that issues of race and climate were a hemispheric, if not Atlantic, problem. Highlighting medical professionals' transnational perspective, Nott received a letter from Dr. J. Mendizabel, who wrote, "The coolies are, in this place (Vera Cruz), as well as in the West Indies, exempt from yellow fever."[41] While supposedly South and East Asians thrived amid yellow fever in Central America, whites were not shielded from tropical ailments. Nott then discussed the case of French Algeria to provide further evidence that whites were unhealthy in the global tropics. Whites in Algeria suffered a terrible mortality rate that was only increasing, he contended. These high mortality rates supported his supposition that acclimation was of minor influence on the health of the migration patterns that characterized the Atlantic World.[42]

Nott based his arguments on a truly global data set. In addition to cases from Mexico and various African colonies, Nott listed mortality statistics from India, Martinique, and Batavia (fig. 7.1). In short, Nott did not write only for the South, but he intended to create a global image of the supposed connections between race, climate, and health. While Nott certainly focused on the health of Black and white people in the South for his immediate agenda, his article points to the biological association of certain races and environments as a health concern for an emerging global society being wedded together by imperialism and capitalism. In short, as much as Nott was crafting a local narrative of the health of southern slavery, he understood the enslaver economy as deeply integrated into the emerging global capitalist economy.[43]

Here, Nott fit neatly within larger southern trends. In his popular eponymous magazine, James De Bow argued that southerners should be shipping their goods not just to Europe, but to India and East Asia. Like Nott, De Bow relied heavily on statistical data and pushed for the region to industrialize and become more integrated into the global economy. Unsurprisingly, Nott published regularly in *De Bow's Review*. Thus, Nott and other physicians wrote for a readership that was exposed to an increasingly expansionist and globally interconnected vision for the future of the United States.[44]

Despite his global framing, Nott actually harbored great cynicism for the future of human mobility and European imperial projects connecting lands and peoples that he believed should remain separate. Nott thought the connections created by international commerce and migration defied "the laws of God, both natural and revealed." Civilized man, he asserted, was "the most destructive of all animals," whose greatest accomplishments resided "in blowing out the brains of his fellow-man."[45] Nott believed that Europeans had endangered their lives and that of lesser races by entering *"climates that nature never intended [them] for."* He characterized civilization and mobility as a great tragedy, asking of the American colonial experience, "Who will undertake to estimate the amount of human life sacrificed, since the discovery of Columbus, by attempts to colonize tropical climates?"[46] Nott's conclusions that the American colonial experience represented a transgression against the natural boundaries that segregated the races represents an unlikely critique of empire. This anti-imperial statement also highlights the dichotomy of Nott's racial politics. Nott was highly skeptical of the processes of empire that caused American slavery to emerge, but, as a multicultural democracy was unimaginable to him, he also believed slavery to be the only healthy social and economic structure possible in the multiracial subtropics.[47]

Sharing Nott's view of empire and climate, the Scottish anatomy professor and ethnologist Robert Knox—best known for his involvement in Edinburgh's Burke and Hare murders in 1828—argued that non-whites' last bastion of safety from Anglo-Saxon empires would be Central Africa. While predicting the inevitable extinction of most of the "dark races" around the globe, Knox asserted, "Within the tropic[s], climates come to the rescue of those whom Nature made, and whom the white man strives to destroy." Knox and Nott shared a cynicism that allowed them simultaneously to describe slavery or near extinction as natural, even necessary in many places, while thoroughly criticizing the hypocrisy of the rhetoric of empires as benevolent. Ironically, they also obtained data for their more isolationist racism through the growing web of empire that they criticized.[48]

The mutually constituted theories of polygenesis, specificity, and medical regionalism created a pedagogical approach to practice that was defined by understanding the innate features that characterized bodies, places, and the relationship between the two. In addition to their observations about race and health locally, racial theorists such as Nott shaped their arguments through new data sets created by imperial expansion and distributed through an emerging international medical print culture. Nott's essay reflects the globalization of racial scientists' arguments. Moreover, as with racial anatomical collections, increased data on race, climate, and health did not lead to moral or medical enlightenment. Instead, these new data sets were filtered through the same prejudices as well as scientific ideologies. By internationalizing his racial science, Nott helped ensure its utility beyond slavery. In addition to those such as Nott who benefited directly from new knowledge being produced about race and health in the tropics, the writings of those like Nott, Drake, and Dickson had a profound effect on the ideologies being disseminated in medical schools. During the antebellum period, medical students increasingly saw the health of Black people in terms of the global tropics. Students linked African descendants to hot weather and tropical diseases, and they carved out distinct therapeutics for Black people.

UNHEROIC MEDICINE: STUDENT CONCEPTIONS OF BLACK HEALTH
For antebellum medical students, works like Nott's essay on acclimation built on a decades-old medical discourse on race and disease resistance in Atlantic medicine. In the case of tetanus, medical students had long been grappling with arguments by West Indian physicians that Black people were innately more liable to falling ill. Compared with students in the early national period, antebellum students were more likely to link certain diseases to innate racial differences. In 1821, one MDUP student from New York explained about tetanus, "The nervous system of negroes who are more liable to this disease [tetanus] than whites is also peculiarly excitable." By 1835, these views undoubtedly had become a part of MDUP's curriculum, as Professor George Bacon Wood made a similar claim in his two-volume *A Treatise on the Practice of Medicine*, which went through multiple editions during this period.[49]

While some students in the 1820s and 1830s continued to argue that built environmental and sartorial factors caused increased rates of contracting tetanus, Wood and the aforementioned MDUP student revealed a growing willingness among physicians to see Black people as having a constitutional susceptibility to the disease. In 1860, MCSC student W. J. Bull Jr. argued that the environment had little to do with the increased rates of tetanus among Black people. He contended, "It is pretty well ascertained that negroes are more liable to tetanus than the whites are. Some have ascribed this to the better living and less exposure of the latter, but when negroes and whites have been exposed and treated in the same manner after being wounded, the negro has suffered the most."[50] While the cause of purported differential rates of contracting tetanus remained a subject of debate throughout the antebellum era, in the case of other ailments, physicians came much closer to consensus on the role of race in causing health disparities, further naturalizing the notion of African descendants as essentially distinct.

When discussing a racial practice in their theses, students echoed significant medical texts on race. They looked at the relationship between race, environment, and specificity-based practice through two interrelated approaches: the environmental health of each race and distinct therapeutics. Like Josiah Nott, some students considered the question of race and health through larger questions of migration, or what I call a "racial public health" model, understanding themselves as social as well as medical doctors.[51] In this approach, pupils considered the dangers of migration into unnatural climates, including the potential psychological and embodied damage that was supposed to face Black people's and white people's bodies outside their natural climatic zones. As a subset of their racial worldview, students regularly considered the differential resistance and susceptibility of each race for certain diseases tied to specific climates. Analysis of race and disease underscored the natural fitness of each race for certain climates and occupations. Outside slavery and the tropics (or the southern subtropics), African descendants were in grave danger.

Other students, however, focused less on the larger theories of the social and climatic health of Black people. Instead, they theorized about the role of the physician on the plantation, and the way in which the doctrine of specificity and polygenesis created the need for alternative medical therapeutics for African descendants. Racial theory and practice on Black patients were important topics for medical education across the United States and had a profound effect on plantation therapeutics. Finally, physicians' distinct approaches to Black health aided in the naturalization of Black people as an essentialist underclass in the United States, meant specifically for only select occupations and geographies that could not be subverted.

In the case of diseases such as pneumonia, consumption, yellow fever, and malaria, students linked innate resistance or susceptibility to Black people's relationship to hot and cold climates. In particular, African descendants' supposed inherent resistance to yellow fever and malaria made them ideal for toil on plantations in the U.S. South, among other slave economies. Students argued that African descendants could better withstand or even thrive in what Nott called "*malarial* climates," which included all of Africa and the "low lands" of the South.[52] In the 1856 letter to Nott printed in his essay on acclimation, Samuel Henry Dickson explained that while whites could never acclimate to malaria, African descendants were mostly protected from the disease. Only a change in location could make them slightly susceptible. He elaborated, "If a house negro be sent to a rice-field, he may be attacked."[53]

Dickson and Nott characterized African descendants as exceptionally fit for the toil of slavery in the southern subtropics, and antebellum students almost unanimously agreed with them. MDUP student Elliott Smith of Mississippi inquired in 1857, "If persons can become acclimated, why are many who have been raised in the midst of marshes yearly attacked? And why also can not the white-man become acclimated and dwell in security on the coast of Africa?"[54] Smith intended these questions to be read as rhetorical, and he considered the reasons for health disparities as obviously rooted in racial difference. By invoking white health in Africa, Smith positioned race as essential to the healthy navigation of the international tropics. Of the twenty-eight MCSC and MDUP students who discussed differential resistance to bilious fever or malaria, only four believed that Black and white people were equally susceptible. Likewise, of the seventeen students who discussed yellow fever and racial resistance, sixteen argued that Black people were less susceptible than whites or that when Black people got yellow fever, their symptoms were much milder.[55]

Students believed that African descendants possessed constitutions that protected them from the worst diseases of the plantation South. In 1850, MCSC student J. P. Bonner argued that African descendants' protection from tropical fevers was vital not only to the plantation South but also to the entire Atlantic economy. Bonner explained, "Without his [the slave's] aid the spindles and looms of Manchester, of Lowell and of all the large manufactories must in a great measure remain idle." For Bonner, enslaved African descendants represented the perfect engine for an Atlantic economy tied together by cotton. If slavery were somehow ended, it did not just spell the end of the cotton districts; the entire Atlantic economy would grind to a halt. In short, like Nott and other prominent racial theorists, students conceptualized the medical profession's aid as essential to the success of transnational capitalism. On a similar note, when it came to sugar and rice, MCSC student Peter L. Horn—the pupil who deliberately infected an enslaved man with measles—argued in 1860 that only African-descended laborers possessed bodies protected from malaria, the worst ailment of those laboring on rice and sugar plantations.[56] Thus, prospective physicians were required to understand Black people's health for their practice and to preserve the prosperity of the nation.

While students framed African descendants as ideally suited for the tropical aspects of the southern climate, in terms of disease environments, the South represented a liminal space between temperate and tropical. As a result, African descendants were protected from marsh fevers but particularly vulnerable to the nontropical ailments that plagued southern plantations. Specifically, most students perceived enslaved people to be more vulnerable to intestinal ailments such as dysentery, cholera, and typhoid fever. In contrast to their thinking about malaria and yellow fever, students were often unsure whether it was built environment or race that affected rates of contracting typhoid fever. In 1856, MCSC student Benjamin Fishburne explained,

"The negro has been observed to be especially liable to this disorder, but whether his proneness is attributable to some defect in primitive conformation, or whether it is the effect of locality and climate, or the result of mode of life, which he pursues, is a question which has never been satisfactorily solved."[57] In the three theses addressing racial susceptibility and cholera, students all agreed that the ailment disproportionately attacked the Black population. However, in contrast to the conclusions in theses on malaria and yellow fever, students avoided diagnosing the causes of the supposed demographic discrepancies.[58] Students writing on dysentery fit the general trend established by those writing on cholera and typhoid fever. While doctors believed that Black people on plantations had a greater likelihood of contracting dysentery, pupils were far more reluctant to attribute these higher rates of disease contraction to some sort of constitutional peculiarity.[59]

When comparing how students discussed questions of race and resistance/predisposition to tropical fevers versus intestinal diseases, no simple formula existed for discerning when students would attribute a race's perceived higher rate of contracting a certain ailment to inherited traits or inconclusive factors. If these students were simply proslavery theorists masquerading as scientists, they most likely would have declared that all demographic discrepancies were caused by inherent racial difference. Instead, students' diverse conclusions about the connections between race and disease painted antebellum racial medicine as far more theoretically diverse and complicated. While many prospective doctors had an interest in naturalizing slavery (or at least white supremacy generally), they did so when they believed the supposed facts supported a proslavery conclusion.

Students also applied these ideas to the relationship between Black people's physiology and the environment. Specifically, students were divided over whether Black girls menstruated earlier than whites, and if so, whether this was due to climate, culture, or innate physiology. In 1857, MCSC student Lewellyn E. Snow asserted, "When the female is thrown much or constantly in contact with the opposite sex [menstruation] appears sooner as is found by our black or slave population who are known to commence much younger than our white population." In contrast, another MCSC student, W. Weathersbee, claimed in 1855 that differential menstruation between each race was "mere conjecture having no foundation whatever."[60]

Through their discussion of menstruation, students grappled with the gendered meanings of race, potentially describing Black girls as overly sexualized, innately distinct, or, in some cases, as physiologically approximating their white counterparts. Likewise, since healthy menstruation was seen as essential to reproducing the enslaved population, physicians took the study of the relationship between menses, race, and climate seriously. The desire to understand menses also led to greater medical surveillance of Black girls' bodies. As with other medical and racial topics in this period, much of the importance of studying menstruation resided in turning the medical school into a space to discuss race, health, and the body, even though students often came to a diversity of conclusions. Moreover, student discourse over menstruation revealed the degree to which enslaved girls' reproductive organs were seen as a central battleground over the meaning of blackness and the future of slavery.[61]

Medical theory could also be bent toward making claims about the health risks of fugitivity and emancipation. Just as many students agreed with Nott that African descendants were best fit for the malarial climates of the South, they also argued that people of African descent were specifically unfit for the cold weather of the North and its attendant disease climate. In 1817, William Paxson, an MDUP student from Virginia, used Black people's supposed intolerance for cold weather as an explanation for their increased rates of contracting pneumonia. Paxson asserted, "Created to bask in the solar ray, the negro can only flourish, when he feels the genial influence of the tropic sun; remove him from it, like an exotic plant he droops and dies." Echoing the influence of polygenesis on physicians' approach to the health of African descendants, MCSC student McNeely Du Bose stated in 1854 that Black people were more liable to contracting pulmonary ailments because they were "constructed with a reference to . . . living in a hot, sultry [climate]." Through racial theories of the environment, deep political questions mingled with consideration of how to best approach medical practice. Students tacitly debated whether emancipation was medically sound, and whether it would be healthy for races to move to climates for which their bodies were not created. At best, students were divided over these questions, leaving serious doubts for Americans about the potential public health ramifications of racial migration and abolition.[62]

Just as some medical students believed that Black people faced serious physical health risks from cold weather and emancipation, others argued that freedom and cool climates endangered the psychological health of African descendants. In his 1852 thesis "On the Causes of Insanity in the United States," MCSC student Joseph Hinson Mellichamp set out "to account for the fact that the proportion of insane among the Blacks & Whites (especially the former) is much greater in the non-slaveholding than slaveholding states," and to demonstrate "that the negro [was] only insane in a state of Freedom."[63] For Mellichamp, the supposed increased levels of insanity among Black people in the North had two possible explanations, although both contained the underlying theme of biological determinism. First, Black people could be experiencing higher rates of insanity due to being put into social and intellectual situations that exceeded their intellectual potential. Second, in the North, Black people were exposed to far colder temperatures that went against their predisposition for tropical climes, thus causing mental collapse.

Mellichamp contrasted the high rates of mania among free Black people in the North with the seemingly sound mental health of Black people under southern slavery. He explained, "All the ills which he [the southern slave] may casually suffer from tyranny & injustice do not leave their impress upon him."[64] Building on this theme, another MCSC student in 1845 explained that Black people and Native Americans, as "savages," almost never contracted mania.[65] In these students' essays, insanity correlated to factors central to the doctrine of specificity. Black people were mentally healthiest in their proper environment and occupation, but once slaves grasped freedom and migrated north, their mental health suffered. Ironically, according to Mellichamp, whites experienced higher rates of insanity in the North as well, contradicting the notion that they were healthiest in temperate climates.[66]

Students' essays mirrored the larger holistic-racial worldview set out by authors such as Nott and Dickson. They imagined African descendants' bodies as something that reacted wholly differently to the environment compared with whites! Theoretically distinct, African descendants required alternative social and legal treatment. Mobility and freedom represented the largest public health threats to Black people in the antebellum era, according to polygenism. Fitting with polygenist logic, Black people would never be prepared for the mental stress of freedom. Perhaps more important, enslaved people faced serious health risks if they fled slavery to the cold climates of northern states.

According to students, since African descendants were created to exist in hot tropical climates, they were supposed to be protected from the most dangerous scourges such as yellow fever and malaria. Thus, the disease climate of the North represented significant dangers. Students also believed that plantation labor protected Black people from dyspepsia, or indigestion, a disease that was "the offspring of ease, luxury, and affluence." According to one student, the ailment was endemic to Scandinavia.[67] Protection from indigestion was further proof of the benefits of enslaved labor. One MCSC student explained in 1842, "The labouring negroes [are] a class that never has time to lead an inactive life; and we will find them strong, vigorous, and healthy, and enjoying richly all the pleasures that health can afford."[68] Through racial diagnostics, many pupils depicted Black people as both unaffected by many of the diseases of the plantation and, through their labor regime, protected from some of the illnesses of civilization. Disease resistance and susceptibility existed in the same set of binaries that shaped the social life of the United States—Black versus white and civilization versus savagery.

Just as students believed that the health of each environment was different for Black and white people, they also saw each race as requiring distinct therapeutics. As a result, aspiring doctors understood Black people as needing alternative treatments, within both medical practice and the U.S. social system.

In addition to their instruction on race and its relationship to disease environments, some professors also taught their students that Black people, unlike whites, were not strong enough to bear heroic medical treatments. Recalling his time as a medical student in Philadelphia, Josiah Nott explained that Professor Nathaniel Chapman told his students, "*The negro . . . rarely bears blood-letting, or depletion in any form.*"[69] Also while a student, Nott treated pulmonary diseases in Black patients at the Philadelphia Almshouse. The prescribed course of treatment for these cases focused on stimulants and quinine instead of bleeding, as would have been practiced on whites. From his earliest days of medical training in Philadelphia, Nott learned that beyond differential social treatments, physicians must also prescribe a different set of curatives to Black patients.[70]

Following Nott, in his 1850 thesis "Hints on the Medical Treatment of Negroes," MCSC student Moses McCloud wrote a detailed analysis of the peculiar problems facing a plantation physician. In addition to detecting whether an enslaved person was feigning illness, McCloud argued that plantation doctors needed to take a wholly different approach to medical therapeutics for the people under their care. While physicians must engage in heavy bleeding for white patients, McCloud asserted, "By attacking the disease of the negro by heroic treatment[,] the almost inevitable result will be extreme debility." According to McCloud, heroic treatments such as venesection and cathartics would only weaken enslaved patients. Instead, the plantation physician "must, therefore, sustain the strength of his patient from the commencement; if not by actual stimulation, he must by withholding all treatment which would necessarily weaken him." McCloud put the doctrine of specificity into a plan of action, highlighting the necessity of a racialized medicine for plantation practice. Students such as McCloud evidenced how practice was influenced by racial theorists like Nott. These students formulated African descendants as rhetorically unheroic and requiring treatments that stimulated their weaker constitutions.[71]

At the center of antebellum therapeutic skepticism was the practice of bleeding, or venesection. While many students, including Moses McCloud and the young Josiah Nott, showed a general skepticism toward the efficacy of heroic medicine on the enslaved, the notion that Black people could safely undertake little or no bleeding appeared to be a near-universal tenet of antebellum medicine. In 1852, MCSC student Benjamin F. Carter confirmed that Black patients felt "a more depressing influence" from cold than white patients did. Moreover, African-descended patients found their "recuperative powers . . . much more diminished" by bleeding than white patients did.[72] Of the ten students from MDUP, MCSC, and the University of Nashville that discussed venesection and race, all agreed that Black patients should be bled less because of their purportedly weak constitutions.[73] While white physicians in some ways envisioned Black people as particularly strong in their capacity for agricultural labor, their inability to withstand heroic treatments rhetorically positioned them as physically weaker than whites, or as not heroic enough to prosper from the brutal therapeutics of white medicine.

In addition to therapeutic questions, medical students discussed the need to control enslaved patients as a part of everyday practice. Wary of enslaved people feigning illness to avoid work, medical practitioners devised schemes to combat enslaved agency on the plantation. In 1843, writing in the margins of his notes on Professor Nathaniel Chapman's medical lectures, an unknown MDUP student highlighted how doctors took their cues from planters, relying on intimidation to manage the enslaved. The student wrote, "A Virginian was troubled vastly with his n—rs on account of intermittents, every n—r on his plantation shook 2 hrs. every day." In response, the student noted, "the Virginian had a grave dug and swore the first n—r got a chill should be buried alive. Not a chill was complained of again." Along similar lines, Moses McCloud explained that detecting enslaved people's false claims required physicians' total "discrimination and acuteness." Constantly on guard for deception, McCloud in one case ordered a slave to be whipped to "cure" his supposedly false claim of having a concussion. When working with enslaved patients, physicians relied on the same brutal norms as planters. Moreover, as a part of their education, medical students in the North and South grappled with the most effective ways to manage enslaved people, with terror being a legitimate medical practice.[74]

In their theses, students in the antebellum era articulated a new type of racial medical practice based on the theories of medical and racial authors such as Josiah Nott and Samuel Henry Dickson. Prospective doctors understood that keeping African descendants healthy required various treatments, some preventative and some active. Physicians saw Black people as both rhetorically and physically unfit for heroic medicine, requiring little or no use of the lancet when ill. More importantly, Black people had to be kept in or near the tropics, where they had supposedly natural resistance to the most dangerous diseases, such as yellow fever and malaria, along with a high tolerance for heat and sunlight, "it being the nature of all black bodies to absorb the rays of heat + light that fall upon them."[75] Through the act of writing, students shaped a racial practice that simultaneously naturalized African descendants as strong and weak. Black people were unfit for white heroic medicine or cold weather, but they were well suited to toil in rice swamps and cane fields. Moreover, students understood that to preserve the health of Black people, they must be confined to the only fit place in the United States, the subtropical plantations of the South.

Physicians used environmental concepts of health and race to fashion themselves as a managerial class whose expertise could be used not only to treat the diverse local population, but also to inform the United States' domestic and foreign policy. For example, in his 1852 thesis at MCSC, R. N. Cheves explained that monumental history proved that the races, in this case whites, had always been anatomically and visually distinguished. He asserted, "We [whites] have the same features exhibited in the paintings of Leonardo da Vinci, executed 300 years since. We have them in paintings from the Egyptian catacombs, 3000 years of age, where not only this race, but the native Egyptians, the negro, and the Persian can be distinguished by complexion and physiognomy." Building on the work of those like Morton, Cheves contended that the shape of the skull had always divided the world racially. By adopting Morton's model of using ancient Egyptian monuments as a route to understand the antebellum United States' racial present, Cheves further underscored the influence of racial science on medical students and the international nature of these discourses. With his focus on bodily features and assertions of whites' superior intelligence, he was employing the anatomical approach then dominating medicine. Evidencing this methodology, Cheves averred, "The mental characteristics of a race appear to be to the full as permanent, as those which mark the bodily structure."[76]

In his thesis, Cheves went beyond the borders of the United States not only in his evidence and methods but also in his vision of white superiority. "The great Caucasian race originating from one source, and now so widely disseminated," he pontificated, "have asserted their supremacy over all other divisions of mankind." While Cheves embodied the racism of the time in his work, he also captured its aggression as whites increasingly pushed into new territories around the globe, disrupting countless lives. He explained, "By the force of mental superiority, they [whites] are daily extending themselves through every portion of the earth's surface, exterminating or amalgamating all other races with which they come in contact."[77]

With no remorse, Cheves described whites and their "extensive encroachment upon Asia." He declared, "[Whites have] supplanted and almost exterminated the aborigines of North America. They are more or less diffused throughout South America, and the islands of the Pacific and Atlantic." They had even made considerable inroads into "Africa, the portion of the world least suited to the race, [where] the Caucasian Arabs possess[ed] one half. They [whites might] be called the great civilizers of the world." Almost five decades before Rudyard Kipling published his infamous poem "The White Man's Burden" during the height of Europeans' global empires, Cheves was triumphantly describing the violent spread of whites around the world through imperialism. Through the education of students like Cheves, antebellum medical schools disseminated a white supremacist ideology that not only undergirded enslavement but also justified violent white expansion on a global scale, presaging much of the imperial medical ideology of the turn of the twentieth century.[78]

Theses such as Cheves's underscore the increasingly international outlook of the clinical-racial gaze and the way in which this gaze was produced by medical professionals who regularly crossed borders to learn their trade. Thus, racial medicine was shaped in a country that was progressively more connected to neighboring countries and the rest of the world.

When Josiah Nott warned of the health repercussions of empire, he wrote for a white medical profession that had long been considering the notion that different races required separate medical treatments. By the end of the antebellum era, medical students like Cheves saw race as defining not only the nation's present but also its potential imperial future. In comparing the health of Black people in Africa and the Americas, students and professors created a medicine that served the South while speaking to an increasingly international version of white supremacy. Whereas Rush mostly presented all races as equally susceptible to diseases and characterized the influence of external stimuli as causing ill-health, antebellum students argued that the problem resided in not respecting the ingrained relationship between certain bodies and disease environments. Using the prevailing theories of specificity, medical regionalism, and polygenesis, pupils and professors framed Black people as naturally fit for labor in the hot weather of the tropics, where those of African descent maintained supposed resistance to dangerous ailments including yellow fever and malaria. In contrast, Black people faced serious physical and mental health dangers when they left the South for freedom and the cold climes of the North.

For students in the antebellum era, the southern subtropics represented a liminal space where both white enslavers and enslaved Black people could exist in relatively good health. Presaging the tropical health movement at the turn of the twentieth century, antebellum students and professors had begun to fashion a racial medicine suited to global imperialism. As much as polygenesis supported an internal gaze when diagnosing regional medical and political problems, physicians also used race to fix their vision outward. Formal medical training played a key role in inculcating doctors with this transnational orientation.

Finally, through the mutually constituted theories of polygenesis, medical regionalism, and the doctrine of specificity, medical students were able to reimagine African descendants as something medically "Other." Treating Black people through active therapeutics and disease prevention meant understanding each race's specific connection to its local environment. Through environmental theory, the physiological whole of African descendants' bodies was constructed as requiring unique treatments, both medically and socially. The health of the nation became about understanding the specific place of each race, particularly African descendants. White students believed that people of African descent would not be suited for social equality; instead, even if African descendants were nominally freed, many physicians saw them as built for toil and labor in the diseased lowlands of the South. Doctors believed it was their duty to incorporate racial medicine into their practice, protecting the health of their enslaved Black patients and the nation.

EPILOGUE

THE AFTERLIVES OF SLAVERY

AND RACIAL SCIENCE IN U.S. MEDICAL

EDUCATION

"I am the editor of the 'Dallas Herald' Newspaper and what you Philadelphians would call a fire-eater secessionist, but I still retain my partiality for the Profession of Medicine," wrote Dr. Charles R. Pryor to MDUP professor Joseph Leidy on March 12, 1861. An 1853 graduate of the University of Virginia's medical school, Pryor wrote to Leidy to request a copy of the professor's book after an 1860 fire destroyed Pryor's library. He also sought to assess his chances of studying medicine in Philadelphia the next winter. Pryor's letter to the northern professor captures a great deal about the nature of sectionalism, fraternalism, and nineteenth-century medicine. Ironically, Pryor, like many other southern doctors, saw little conflict between his allegiance to both the emerging Confederate States of America and the U.S. medical profession. The country's finest schools and centers of scientific knowledge production remained in the Northeast, and as war appeared imminent, southern doctors wrote letters to solidify their professional networks before the conflict erupted. Northern doctors, as the epilogue also reveals, shared the same fears with their southern counterparts, and they wrote consoling letters to their medical friends in the Confederacy, assuring them that political allegiances would not damage professional relationships. Furthermore, postwar correspondence reveals that these friendships survived, ensuring the endurance of a shared commitment to racial medicine across the national profession.

Like so many other young doctors, Pryor looked up to Leidy, who was not much older but already had risen to the top of the field. Pryor was indeed a secessionist, and, based on a cursory examination of the *Dallas Herald* in the spring of 1861, his self-description as a fire-eater appears apt, yet he did not seem to believe that the national division would also divide the medical profession. His loyalties to the emerging Confederacy did not seem to affect his affiliation with the United States' medical fraternity. He shared with many others of his time a naivety about the coming war, and he was already making plans to travel from the Confederacy to the United States for further medical study and networking, seemingly unaware of the imminent violence. Pryor's brief letter captures how sectionalism had divided the United States but not its physicians.[1]

In fact, Leidy's correspondence from the winter and spring of 1861 is filled with similar requests for favors and friendly entreaties from Confederate medical colleagues. On January 7, Professor Francis S. Holmes, a naturalist at the College of Charleston, described the city preparing for war and blamed the Republicans. Despite a sectional bias toward secession, he was not writing Leidy to debate politics, but to make sure that their friendship survived. He concluded, "Remember your promise Leidy, 'no matter what comes *we are friends forever.*" Around this same time, Leidy also wrote William A. B. Norcom, a Charleston physician and MDUP graduate, transmitting much the same message. Leidy's prewar sentiments are preserved in Norcom's first letter to the professor after the war. "The last letter I ever recd. from you ended thus," Norcom recalled in 1866: "If the Union goes to the devil we'll still be friends." Norcom wrote to assert that, indeed, the war had not changed their relationship, stating, "In a word, let me assure you that in me you have the same true & warm friend as in antebellum days." Adopting the descriptor that came to define the era before the Civil War, Norcom revealed the medical fraternity's strength in the face of the contentious politics of the era.[2]

Like Leidy, before the war, Josiah Nott wrote letters meant to ensure that political fractures did not mean enduring professional or personal collapse. On May 3, 1861, weeks after Confederates fired on Fort Sumter, Josiah Nott wrote the New York ethnologist E. G. Squier in an effort to protect their friendship. Nott believed that their commitment to science should overcome any differences over sectional politics or even war. Apparently it did, as Squier and Nott rekindled their friendship four years later. In May 1861, it seemed to be business as usual for Marylander William Stump Forwood. He wrote to the Louisiana physician and racial scientist Samuel Cartwright, asking him for advice on how to treat enslaved people who believed that they had been cursed.[3] As civil war loomed, elite physicians in the North and South wanted to ensure that political fracture would not break the bonds that they had forged through medical education, journalism, white male fraternity, and practice.

Another Charleston colleague even asked Leidy to help his nephew find a place to study medicine in the North and Europe. In February 1861, MCSC professor J. Edwards Holbrook asked Leidy's advice on the best course for his nephew's medical education. "It is our intention to send him to Europe next Spring and the first thing is to get him graduated," explained Holbrook. "I thought it might be best to send him to a friend of mine from Charleston now settled in N. York as a teacher, Dr. Thomas, there to learn midwifery and practice of medicine. Would this be advisable or have you a better plan for him in Philadelphia," he inquired. Not just interested in preserving his friendship, an elite faculty member like Holbrook wanted his nephew to enter into both national and transnational medical communities. For Holbrook, an impending civil war did not mean that his nephew should not receive the best medical education on the continent. For that, he must study in the Northeast before traveling to Europe.[4]

These letters to Joseph Leidy are just a sliver of the correspondence between northern and southern physicians and scientists in the months leading up to the Civil War's eruption. The professors, racial scientists, and students that had been building a white medical community for the last century were not willing to let this national institution die. That community did not perish, nor did medical schools' pension for teaching essentialist and embodied concepts of racial difference. Instead, medical education and racial science flourished in the decades following the Civil War. While the fighting caused a massive shift in the lives of enslaved people, medical professionals also saw their field gain authority during the war. The conflict over slavery did little to mitigate the influence of racial thinking on medicine.

If anything, racial thinking in medicine only grew in the period spanning from the U.S. Civil War and into the era of eugenics in the first half of the twentieth century. This period of U.S. medical education contained many titanic moments in the history of racism and Black people's health-care activism, but also in medical science more generally. Medical professionals—both white and Black—advocated for more rigorous medical education, building on the success of the first century of medical school founders. All of these changes increased the social and political power of American physicians, medical scientists, and medical schools. From many perspectives, this was a period of monumental and sometimes progressive shifts and discoveries: the founding of Black medical schools, the establishment of the National Medical Association, and so many other changes that made the American medical profession more equal. Yet this hundred-year period was also marked by extreme racial retrenchment with the founding of the Ku Klux Klan, the rise of Jim Crow laws, and the lynching of thousands.

Just like the first, the second century of U.S. medical schools and medical ideas was shaped by hotly contested racial politics. To an extent, medical science had changed, and Black people had more freedom to establish their own medical schools, journals, and hospitals. Yet U.S. medical education continued to reproduce many of the worst ideas and practices of its founding period. Correspondence between medical and scientific elites written immediately following the Civil War captures how the second century of racial science in U.S. medical schools would share ideologies and actors from the first.

It has been tempting to consider the Civil War as a cataclysmic rupture in U.S. culture from the perspective of medicine. To some extent, it was. However, the social networks created in the late antebellum period survived the war, even as some Americans built up deep resentments in the conflict's wake. Influential medical professors like Joseph Leidy and Oliver Wendell Holmes Sr. continued to hold their professional positions and preserve their southern networks of friends and influence long after the war. In December 1865, Francis Holmes, the College of Charleston naturalist, wrote to Leidy, explaining, "[With the war at an end,] my first thoughts are of you and my friends in Philadelphia." In addition, Holmes revealed that he needed help creating a new library since "the Negroes ha[d] burnt up" his books.[5] Letters to Leidy from southerners like this one show that any damage to friendships resulting from the conflict could be easily repaired.

In contrast to Francis Holmes's attempts to recreate his antebellum life in Charleston, Nott had trouble adjusting to the South after emancipation. In September 1866, he sought out Leidy for consolation, writing, "We got [the Medical College of Alabama] out of the hands of the negroes only a few weeks ago & we are trying to rake up the fragments & make a beginning again."[6] The school's restoration did not go as planned, though. Six months later, Nott moved to Baltimore, and after a year residing there, he moved farther North to New York City, where his friend and collaborator E. G. Squier already resided. Following decades of living in the South, Nott found professional invigoration in these scientifically minded cities in the mid-Atlantic and Northeast.[7] Correspondence between northern and southern medical friends before and after the Civil War highlights the strength of physicians' and racial scientists' professional identity, which was able to withstand the deadliest war in U.S. history. When the war ended, elite southern physicians and naturalists such as Francis Holmes and Josiah Nott found solace in the medical and scientific fraternity that previously had transcended regional and political boundaries.

Similarly, UVA professor James Lawrence Cabell wrote to Harvard's Jeffries Wyman on March 2, 1868, hoping to be consoled about Reconstruction's radical turn. The two were likely old friends from Wyman's days teaching at Hampden-Sydney in Virginia. Wyman had written to Cabell after the Civil War in hopes of news about the vitality of UVA's medical school. While the school had reopened in October 1865, incoming classes were not growing at the expected rate. The first year, 250 students enrolled, and 240 more joined the student body the next year. Afterward, though, enrollments stagnated. The faculty's outlook was "gloomy" about the next year, as some pupils already were unable to afford to board locally. However, more pressing was the perceived damage being wrought by the Radical Republicans, who intended to "Africanize the Southern States [which made the] future absolutely hopeless." Cabell's real question was about the stability of the national culture of white supremacy that he had enjoyed before the war. "Is it possible," he asked Wyman, "that the Northern people will suffer a political party to destroy every vestige of a constitutional government and bring ruin upon a whole country in order to perpetuate its own rule?" In short, while Cabell might have been skeptical of the Republican Party, he looked to an old northern colleague like Wyman for comfort that the racial order and its medical basis would remain intact.[8]

The professional bonds and racial ideas established in the antebellum era endured, and they shaped much of the future trajectory of racial science and medicine. During that first century of U.S. medical schools, racial scientists and physicians had made significant accomplishments. These experts had established medical schools as the primary route for medical education, a trend that would be codified into law during the second century of medical schools in the United States. They also used medical schools as a primary vessel for distributing racial science and essentialist ideas about racial difference.

In addition, the choice to teach racial science transcended whether faculty nominally supported monogenesis or polygenesis. No matter the causal narrative, most doctors were trained to believe that Black people possessed bodies that were differentiated indefinitely by their anatomy and relationships to different climates around the world. Most medical students would have witnessed or participated in the dissection of a stolen Black cadaver. This was even true of Samuel F. McGill, the first Black graduate of a U.S. medical school. Rare students also conducted life-threatening nontherapeutic experiments on enslaved patients that would not have been possible on whites. This most disturbing trend was hardly stymied by emancipation, as dangerous experiments on Black subjects increased in the second century of institutional medical education.[9] Finally, medical schools normalized the possession, measuring, and description of non-white remains to allegedly prove white supremacy as an anatomical fact. Students learned from textbooks, lectures, and collections of stolen skulls in medical museums the supposed fact that Black people had smaller crania, which was believed to correlate to lesser intelligence. While these ideas remained in medical education after the war, they also represented a critical foundation for professional anthropology, which eventually turned into the subfield of physical anthropology.[10]

When the Darwinian revolution arrived, it forced changes to the ideas of racial scientists and physicians, but there was continuity as well. Polygenists' causal explanation for human difference quickly disappeared from mainstream science after Charles Darwin first published his theory of natural selection. But even though polygenesis might have had a short life span in U.S. science and medicine as the dominant theory of human origins, many of medical polygenists' specific ideas about Black people's bodies survived. Leidy was an early convert to natural selection, but in the postbellum period, he still taught that Black people were anatomically distinct.[11]

In his 1874 thesis, MDUP student and Philadelphia native Hollingsworth Neill wrote about the anatomical peculiarities of Black people. While the nation had abolished slavery by this time, and Darwinists had mostly usurped polygenists in scientific circles, Neill created a work that closely resembled antebellum theses on racial anatomy. In familiar fashion, Neill argued that Black people had longer forearms, larger penises, and narrower pelvises.[12] Likewise, he pointed out Black people's supposedly longer heel bones, which were such common knowledge as to give "rise to the vulgar expression 'N—r Heels.'"[13] Neill cited his experience with dissecting Black people's bodies and measuring their skulls as a basis for his assertions of white superiority. He explained, "The frontal bones [of the skull], besides having a smaller cranial capacity and a receding direction, have also larger supra-orbital protuberances, very suggestive of the formation in the Gorilla."[14] While historians have treated the Civil War as a significant turning point in the history of medicine, Neill illustrated that, in terms of racial anatomy, little had changed.[15]

Oliver Wendell Holmes, too, continued to lecture about racial difference and craniometry well after the Civil War. Nearly every year that he kept notes after 1865, Holmes lectured on racial differences of crania. Differing descriptors were applied, but the broad strokes appeared to be the same. In 1872, he discussed "national diversities." In 1873, Holmes covered the "different Forms of the head," and a year later, he addressed the "crania of different races." In 1876 and 1877, he orated about "crania in different races." In 1879, his students learned about "ethnological crania, phrenological, d[itt]o." In 1880, Holmes taught about "orthognathous and prognathous" skulls, as well as "some hints on phrenology." Ensuring that further generations of physicians could learn to measure skulls, upon his retirement in 1882, Holmes donated his craniometer to the Warren Anatomical Museum, where it became object number 7806.[16]

Medical museums' skull collections remained relevant, and the practice of collecting human remains for science even grew in the postbellum period. According to many historians of science, the pre-Darwinian period of skull collecting was nascent and amateurish. Complementing this narrative was the fact that the study of race and human remains expanded during and after the Civil War. Historian Samuel Redman explains, "Medical officers working as agents for the Army Medical Museum (AMM) were among the first to systematically collect skeletons for a major medical museum collection in the United States." This trend continued, Redman observes, and new museums and collections were opened in major cities across the United States. Likewise, Leslie Schwalm has uncovered how Union army doctors were collecting anatomical measurements of Black and white soldiers during the war for scientific study.[17]

Moreover, the incorporation of the Boston Society for Medical Improvement's anatomical collection into the Warren Museum at Harvard was only completed in the postbellum period. The museum continued to add objects. In 1873, it cataloged the penis of a man of an unknown race whom students dissected at Harvard. Professor Jackson, though, clarified that the man was not Black, as his "hair [was] perfectly straight.—question between South Sea Islander and Japanese." As the collection grew, so did object numbers, and the aforementioned acquisition was number 7509. Likewise, as evidenced by the collection of racially ambiguous genitals of a man from the Pacific World, the international dimensions of this science had expanded rather than contracted. Again, then, the ideas and practices established in the antebellum era were hardly swept aside. Instead, antebellum medical educators had created a foundation for the profession to build on after the war.[18]

While racial science grew after the war, so did resistance to it. In 1879, Martin Delany, one of the three Black students admitted and then expelled from Harvard during 1850–51 session, published a refutation of polygenists' causal narrative, even if he was skeptical of white moral uplift. Delany opened the monograph on a cavalier note, explaining, "The theory of Chapollion, Nott, Gliddon and others, of the Three Creations of Man—one black, the second yellow, and the last white—we discard." Yet, like some other Black opponents to racial science, Delany had trouble transcending the problematic nature of this discourse more generally. Despite his distrust of polygenesis, in other respects, Delany's medical training may have manifested itself in his work. For example, he advocated strenuously against racial mixing, which he believed would destroy everyone. To Delany, Black people were the most religious race and the best redeemer for humanity. He also had a tendency toward fetishizing "pure," unmixed Africans, even noting that the racial groups of the 1870s were "indestructible."[19]

Few other Black thinkers were as racially essentialist as Delany in their refutation of racial thinking in the postbellum period. Nor did most embrace his advocacy for racial purity. As historian Mia Bay explains, "Even during the difficult days that followed Reconstruction, few Black thinkers were willing to make as much of racial distinctions as did Martin Delany, and fewer still shared his admiration of the African—'untrammeled in his native purity.'" While few Black thinkers embraced racial purity like Delany, his work hinted at the numerical growth of Black public academics and their critiques of racial science. Just a few decades later, in 1906, W. E. B. Du Bois would edit a collection of essays, proving that poverty, not Black inferiority, was the cause of racial inequality. Thus, just as the influence of racial science grew after the Civil War, so did its opponents.[20]

In the immediate aftermath of the Civil War and the Darwinian revolution, Joseph Leidy and Hollingsworth Neill still presented a narrative of racial difference as defined by anatomy. Neill, like his antebellum predecessors, wrote his thesis at a time when medical professionals' most famous cases of exploiting Black people's bodies were still well into the future. Medical and natural history museums increased in number and scope. While medical professionals continued to change the theories and language that they used to describe racial distinctions, many white twentieth-century physicians continued to view Black people as inferior and fit subjects for experimentation. Through forced sterilizations, the Tuskegee experiments, and numerous other actions, physicians continued to assert their right to exploit, control, and play master over Black people's bodies, and to define race medically.[21] The fact that racial medicine continued through the twentieth century further highlights the deep institutional relationship between medical knowledge and U.S. racism.

If the legacies of anatomical racism continued after the Civil War, the afterlives of environmental and transnational medical racism would be just as enduring. Not only did medical schools craft a racial pedagogy that spoke to domestic race relations, but they also created a racial medicine meant to bolster the United States' aspirations to become a global imperial power. During the antebellum period, this meant comparing the health of the enslaved to colonized peoples around the world. American physicians collected data on mortality from European empires, just like they purchased and received donations of stolen skulls of those slain in Europeans' colonial incursions. The emergence of an international racial health data set allowed white physicians to begin crafting arguments about the United States' larger role in the world as a white country. At the end of the first century of American medical schools, the United States had used its naval might to force open Japanese markets. Southerners had made various failed attempts to colonize parts of the Caribbean and Central America in the hopes of establishing further slave states. Therefore, it should be of little surprise that racial scientists were beginning to think about the health of U.S. imperialism in Africa, the Americas, and Asia in the 1850s. Still, the peak of the United States' role in overt global imperialism remained decades away. The country's true imperial heights awaited the second half of the twentieth century, with the adoption of soft-power corporate imperialism and the establishment of military bases in sovereign nations globally.

Medical practice, racial science, and troop deployments during the Spanish-American War perfectly captured how environmental racism and tropical medicine grew in influence after the Civil War. At the turn of the twentieth century, the U.S. military embraced environmental racism in its recruitment of Black women as fever nurses in Cuba, and in the types of work it relegated to Black men. More often than not, Black men in Cuba were assigned manual labor tasks, reproducing the notion that their bodies were built for hard exertion in the tropics. Black women, on the other hand, were selected as nurses because Black people were still seen as resistant to yellow fever. This also compounded racial stereotypes of Black female nursing rooted in the slave system. Ironically, Black men and women were attracted to military service because they hoped to prove their fitness for citizenship to whites. Instead, Jim Crow retrenchment began to strip them of the gains made during Radical Reconstruction, as evidenced by military medicine and their service roles.[22]

For white doctors, however, service in the United States' new Asian and Latin American colonies provided firsthand opportunities to study and racialize new populations. Military health officials made this dynamic clear during the U.S. occupation of the Philippines, which lasted until 1946. In the Philippines, U.S. public health officials established draconian hygiene regimes meant to control the local non-white population as much as illnesses. Similar to their participation in discourses on Black people, public health officials routinely vacillated between depicting Filipinos as immune to disease or as secret disease carriers.[23]

Private corporations, as well as governmental actors, embraced global models of medical racial essentialism. U.S. companies even invested in and endowed newly formed schools of tropical medicine. During this period, U.S. corporations' global footprint was growing rapidly. In the 1910s, Samuel "the Banana Man" Zemurray began to establish banana plantations in Honduras in collaboration with the United Fruit Company. Like working on a tropical sugar plantation, working on a banana plantation exposed local workers to dangerous illnesses such as yellow fever and malaria. Needing a cadre of physicians competent at treating the diseases of the tropics, Zemurray went on to fund the establishment of the United States' first school of tropical medicine at Tulane University. Stories like Zemurray's and Tulane's beg questions as to why there are no studies of universities' histories with corporate plantation medicine. Research on this subject would complement ongoing investigations of universities' historic ties to slavery, segregation, and eugenics.[24]

The introduction and production of racial ideas in medical education from the late colonial period through the antebellum era has had profound political, social, and material consequences. Ideas of race and health have lent weight to the notion that biological races are real, and that human bodies and genetic inheritance naturally divide humanity into simple categories. The adoption of racial ideas has led to a medical culture that takes advantage of and even sometimes harms the bodies of the most socially marginalized and disadvantaged people in global society. Rapid communication and transportation have encouraged these phenomena to globalize.[25] Moreover, the racialization of medicine allows doctors, societies, and individuals to blame the already marginalized and endangered for their health problems. Ideas that were once used to defend slavery are used to justify inequality on local, national, and global scales today.

In a study published in 2016 in the *Proceedings of the National Academy of Sciences of the United States of America*, four scholars from UVA seek to understand the relationship between pain, racial bias, and the treatment of Black patients. Their study is novel. The authors surveyed laypeople, but separately they also studied medical students at UVA. What they found astonished many and wrought considerable news coverage. The core of the investigation is a survey of whether participants held false biological beliefs about Black people. Scholars asked the participants whether they believed that Black people have thicker skin, are more susceptible to heart disease, are more fertile, and have "denser, stronger" bones and more sensitive nerve endings. This is just a sample of the questions asked, which seem plucked straight out of the history of the first century of medical schools in the United States. The study reveals that these future doctors harbored medical stereotypes of Black patients at alarming rates. Particularly appealing to medical students were notions like Black people possessing stronger bones and thicker skin, two false anatomical traits popularized during the nineteenth century. On the other hand, contemporary medical students were less likely to believe that

Black people had smaller brains, even as the notion had some appeal among lay participants.[26] Perhaps even more troubling than physicians holding biological essentialist beliefs about race was the fact that they also applied this to their practice. The authors find a direct correlation between medical students believing in biological racial traits "which are false and fantastical in nature" and the likelihood that they will pursue an incorrect treatment course for pain in Black patients. The study lays bare what many already know: racial medicine is not only unethical, but it leads to poorer outcomes for its victims. "Endorsing more false beliefs," the authors explain, "was associated with perceptions that blacks feel less pain and a 'commensurate' insufficient treatment recommendation for Black patients."[27]

The historical trajectory from the history related in the preceding pages to the present is clear and troubling, and it means that centuries of generally reforming medical education has not accomplished enough. Craniometry might have mostly moved out of medical schools, but many of the racial ideas that it supported have not. Far too many physicians and nurses—people working to preserve the bodies of others—are still trained to misunderstand human forms and the seemingly infinite diversities and similarities between them. The United States' medical system, like its politics, has found it convenient to divide patients into distinct groups that seem to rationalize the inequities in the system. Resolving these issues is an unclear, difficult process, and no matter what, it will mean dismantling an ideological system of racial essentialism that has been cultivated in U.S. medical education for centuries. To the extent that there is hope, it will come from those willing to do the work to change that system.

Masters of Health does not relate an optimistic story, and there may be little reason to assume that the future of racism and medical education will be very different or better than the past. However, taken at face value, this book does provide a potential blueprint for change. It relates the story of the creation of a new education system that would have profound influence on the future trajectory of the United States. Doctors, professors, and medical students created locally novel, influential, and enduring institutions. These medical professionals shaped the discourse of their era. They framed many of the most profound political questions of their period in terms of health, race, and bodily control. They used their profession to gain greater influence and respect in their society by making their work speak to the politics of the moment. They executed this aim effectively and built a new set of institutions that shaped many future generations. They did so to terrifying and destructive ends. They set medicine on the path to exploit the bodies of those the world over for profit. They normalized the lower life expectancies and higher infant mortality rates of Black and other marginalized peoples in the United States and abroad. They revealed the profound power of medicine and education to influence social, cultural, and material life over long periods of time.

While this history reveals the destructive power of these institutions, contemporary and future Americans and medical professionals must seize such power for themselves to dismantle racism and the inequality it supports. They must imagine and work to enact an alternative future without race in medical education. Just like those who introduced race into medical education, others can reform old institutions or build new ones that do not divide humanity along false biological lines but instead support the fundamental equality of all people and treat health care as a human right.

ACKNOWLEDGMENTS

Writing this book has been a collaborative process. It has been improved by countless conversations with fellow scholars, archivists, friends, family, and audience members. The volume of unofficial collaborators means that I should quickly proceed with the thank-yous, or else front matter may threaten to consume the book.

Like most writers and scholars, I find that my best habits are the result of listening closely to those willing to teach me. At Tulane University, Randy Sparks was a fantastic PhD adviser who embraced both the human and academic sides of mentorship. He and his work continue to teach me that good scholarship and human storytelling work in tandem and make for the most powerful histories. Since we met early in my career as a graduate student, Deirdre Cooper Owens has been a keen mentor, and she continues to be a model of an ethical scholar. Her advice remains gospel for me, and I aspire to scholarship like hers that can center everyday actors in a world controlled by forces far larger than individuals.

As well as having been given helpful guidance on this work, I have been lucky to have had a number of friends, colleagues, and mentors who have guided my development as a historian and a writer since I began studying history in college. They have not only given incisive and helpful feedback but also spent hours on the phone or elsewhere providing emotional and intellectual support to me as I completed this project. A special thanks, then, is owed to Peyton Jones, Beau Gaitors, Peter McCandless, Jim Downs, Alix Riviere, Rana Hogarth, Stephen Kenny, and Sean Smith. Likewise, I accrued intellectual debts from many of my past teachers, including Thomas Adams, Laura Rosanne Adderley, Kathleen Béres-Rogers, Emily Clark, Jason Coy, the late Lee Drago, Michael Duvall, Guadalupe García, David Gleason, Carole Haber, Scott Peeples, the late Judith Schafer, Myra Seaman, and Justin Wolfe.

I am grateful to the colleagues and friends who were willing to read this entire manuscript. First, while at the Center for Humanities and Information at Penn State, I was lucky to have the opportunity to invite Pablo Gomez to undertake the herculean task of pre–peer reviewing my manuscript. Pablo's comments and our conversations about the scope and structure of the book were transformative, and I owe him a great debt. Likewise, from submitting my partial manuscript in 2018 for peer review to receiving review of the full manuscript in the summer of 2021, I have been lucky to be in conversation through writing with my two anonymous peer reviewers. Their comments fundamentally shaped the book, in particular its transnational scope. They were models of generative colleagues. They gave engaged and supportive feedback to this junior scholar, and it's a much better and different book because of these anonymous individuals.

I also owe a great debt to UNC Press for publishing this book and to my fantastic editor, Brandon Proia. I had the pleasure of meeting Brandon as we chatted at the Press's booth at the 2018 meeting of the American Society for Environmental History. After a meeting the next day, I finally understood the advice that finding a good editor and press is about fit. Brandon immediately got the project and encouraged its development over the last four years, and he has been a helpful and insightful editor of my writing. I am truly lucky for the experience of getting to work with him. Since I first signed an advance contract, I have had the pleasure of getting help and encouragement from other editors and staff at the Press, and for that I need to thank Dino Battista, Sonya Bonczek, Mary Carley Caviness, Elizabeth Crowder, Chuck Grench, Catherine Robin Hodorowicz, Iris Levesque, Elizabeth Orange, Dylan White, and Andrew Winters.

Other friends and colleagues read earlier drafts of parts of this book or provided feedback on conference presentations. Still other colleagues were generous in providing advice, helping with sources, and organizing opportunities for me to workshop parts of this book. I must thank Mohamed Adhikari, Sari Altschuler, Seth Archer, Babak Ashrafi, Mario Barbosa, Jenifer Barclay, David Barnes, Daina Ramey Berry, Lundy Braun, Kellie Carter Jackson, Lauren (Robin) Derby, Lucas Desmond, Sharla Fett, Elodie Edwards-Grossi, Glenn Ellis, Mariola Espinosa, Sharla Fett, Joseph Gabriel, Vanessa Northington Gamble, Evelynn Hammonds, Leslie Harris, Elizabeth Herbin-Triant, Eric Herschthal, Mary L. Hicks, Margaret Humphreys, Tera Hunter, Jonathan Jones, Terence Keel, Elaine LaFay, Jonathan Lande, Mia Levenson, Beth Linker, Elise Mitchell, Paul Wolff Mitchell, Jon Moore, Wangui Mugai, Sowande'Mustakeem, Sarah Naramore, Molly Nebiolo, Ayah Nuriddin, Kathryn Olivarius, Chris Parsons, Nigel Penn, Scott Podolsky, James Poskett, Richard Price, Ian Read, Adolph Reed Jr., Jonathan Reynolds, Carolyn Roberts, Dorothy Roberts, Naomi Rogers, Joshua Rothman, Ezelle Sanford III, Michael Sappol, Sarah Senette, Todd Savitt, James Schafer, Leslie Schwalm, Suman Seth, Kylie Smith, Peter Stallybrass, Jacob Steere-Williams, Melissa Stein, Cameron Strang, Ula Y. Taylor, Michael Thompson, Nancy Tomes, Sasha Turner, Joel Vargas-Dominguez, Keith Wailoo, Kerry Ward, John Harley Warner, Craig Steven Wilder, Savanah Williamson, and Kanisorn Wongsrichanalai.

This project has also been a collaboration with many archivists. They have guided me to sources like medical theses, asked critical questions, and helped me navigate yet-to-be-cataloged collections. Some even bought me coffee or lunch when I was a graduate student. I have been lucky to have the help of Susan Hoffius, since retired from the Waring Historical Library at the Medical University of South Carolina. Likewise, John Pollock, Mitch Fraas, and Lynne Farrington at the University of Pennsylvania's Kislak Center for Special Collections, Rare Books and Manuscripts have been infinitely helpful and supportive of this project since its inception. Likewise, I found an enthusiastic friend and archivist in Beth Lander when she was the librarian at the College of Physicians of Philadelphia, and she is now the managing director at the Philadelphia Area Consortium of Special Collections Libraries. Dominic Hall, the curator of the Warren Anatomical Museum, made my work on Harvard's skull collection possible. He, Scott Podolsky, and Jessica Murphy at the Center for the History of Medicine at Harvard were always ready to supply suggestions and resources for this book. Finally, BJ Gooch and Jamie Day were invaluable in navigating Transylvania University's archives, and they helped make Lexington a welcoming place to conduct research.

I have been lucky to complete this book as a residential fellow at multiple institutions. During the 2017–18 academic year, Emory University's Bill and Carol Fox Center for Humanistic Inquiry provided a fantastic place to begin work on revising my manuscript and putting together a book proposal. All of the fellows were phenomenal to be in conversation with, and the Fox Center provided a supportive and genial intellectual environment for academic work. Walter Melion, the director of the Fox Center, was a model academic and supervisor, and his warmth made my first position in academia unforgettable. During my time at Emory, I accrued many social and intellectual debts, and I owe special thanks to Kiera Allison, Keith Anthony, Jennifer Ayres, Colette Barlow, Clifton Crais, Amy Erbil, William Fogarty, Kelsey Klotz, Mark Ravina, Benjamin Reiss, Thomas Rogers, and Dianne Marie Stewart.

My time during the 2018–19 academic year at the Lapidus Center for the Historical Analysis of Transatlantic Slavery at the Schomburg Center for Research in Black Culture was simply transformative for me. Michelle Commander and Brent Hayes Edwards were amazing mentors, and their advice and feedback continue to shape my work. I first presented chapter 5 of this book in the scholars' center colloquium at the Schomburg, and my colleagues' responses greatly improved my writing and gave me the confidence to write a bottom-up history of the Warren Anatomical Museum's racial skull collection. I wish to thank my cohort and others at the Schomburg Center for their advice and encouragement on this project, including Sister Aisha al-Adawiya, Denisse Andrade, Abena Asare, Gaiutra Bahadur, Dan Berger, Garrett Felber, Kelly Josephs, Jasmine Johnson, Brian Jones, Sid Lapidus, and Hasna Muhammad.

From the fall of 2019 through the spring of 2021, I had the pleasure of being a visiting fellow at the Center for Humanities and Information at The Pennsylvania State University. During this time, the center's leadership, Eric Hayot, John Russell, and Pamela VanHaitsma, made CHI a welcoming and stimulating intellectual home. The center's generosity and genial academic culture made it an ideal place to prepare this book for peer review. My fellow postdocs Jeffrey Binder, Georgia Ennis, Josh Shepperd, and Jennifer Shook were and continue to be fantastic comrades. At Penn State, I was also lucky to work with great scholars including Jim Casey, Richard Daily, Heidi Dodson, J. Marlena Edwards, Christopher Heaney, Shirley Moody-Turner, Rachel Shelden, and Leigh Soares.

I have had the pleasure of making the final changes to my manuscript while a fellow at the Huntington Library and Harvard University's Charles Warren Center for Studies in American History. At the Huntington, I must thank Steve Hindle, the director of research, for making the library such an intellectually vibrant work environment. At Harvard, Charles Warren Center director Walter Johnson, along with Sven Beckert and Evelynn Hammonds, the faculty in charge of this year's program, have likewise been a pleasure to work with as I complete this project. Additionally, I am glad for the opportunity to thank both institutions' administrative staff, including Juan Gomez, Monnikue McCall, Natalie Serrano, and Catherine Wehrey-Miller, for making this type of work possible.

In addition, I am grateful to have received numerous other research grants and fellowships in support of this project, including a Dissertation Research Improvement Grant from the National Science Foundation's Division in Science, Technology, and Society (grant number 1353086), a Countway Fellowship in the History of Medicine from the Center for the History of Medicine at Harvard University, a Wood Institute Travel Grant from the College of Physicians of Philadelphia, a Consortium for the History of Science, Technology, and Medicine Research Fellowship, a Mellon Research Fellowship from the Virginia Historical Society, a dissertation fellowship from Tulane University's Murphy Institute's Center for Ethics and Public Affairs, and multiple Summer Merit Fellowships from Tulane's School of Liberal Arts. To say the least, these funding resources have been indispensable to completing this book.

Over the years, I have also had the privilege of being invited to several colloquia and speakers series to workshop parts of this project. These opportunities allowed me to test my ideas, sharpen my analysis, and improve my prose. I must thank the audiences and organizers who have invited me to speak, including those at the History of Material Texts Workshop at the University of Pennsylvania, the Emerging Scholar Series at Brown University's Center for the Study of Slavery and Justice, the Early Modern Empires Workshop at Yale University, the National Autonomous University of Mexico's Center of Interdisciplinary Research in Sciences and Humanities, the Massachusetts Historical Society's Seminar on African American History, the University of Pennsylvania's Penn & Slavery Project Symposium, Soka University of America, and the University of California, Los Angeles's History of Science Colloquium and Atlantic Forum. Like everyone thanked here, these generous hosts are responsible only for the book's strengths and none of its weaknesses.

I also need to thank my family. My siblings, Andrew and Susanne, have been true sources of love and strength since I was born. Their spouses and children, Eli, Henry, Josh, Laura, Mac, Rollins, and Wade, have all brightened up my life. I owe too many thanks to my parents, Mike and Ruth Willoughby. They have been supportive of this long process, even when they could not understand why I was doing it. I love them very much, and I am glad to have dedicated this book to them and my partner.

Finally, I owe a huge intellectual and personal thanks to my partner, Dr. Urmi Engineer Willoughby. Since we met, I have known I was in the presence of my intellectual superior, and I have become a much smarter and better historian while at her side. Our nightly conversations (while occasionally exhausting, which is purely my fault!) continue to complicate my understanding and analysis of human existence and history. Writing a book is difficult and takes a long time. For seven years, she has heard countless diatribes and repetitive points about the history of medical education. Her mental endurance is stunning. In addition to being an intellectual companion, Urmi has been my most sturdy pillar of emotional support. Having met her makes me thankful to be a historian. So to my brilliant and loving partner, I give my last thank-you.

NOTES

ABBREVIATIONS

CHM   Center for the History of Medicine, Francis A. Countway Library of
        Medicine, Harvard Medical School, Boston

HLA   Holmes Lectures on Anatomy, 1850-1882, Center for the History of
        Medicine, Countway Library of Medicine, Harvard Medical School,
        Boston

JLC   Joseph Leidy Correspondence, Academy of Natural Sciences of Drexel
        University, Philadelphia

JLP   Joseph Leidy Papers, College of Physicians of Philadelphia

JWP   Jeffries Wyman Papers, Center for the History of Medicine, Countway
        Library of Medicine, Harvard Medical School, Boston

MDUPST Medical Department of the University of Pennsylvania Senior Theses,
        Kislak Center for Special Collections, Rare Books and Manuscripts,
        University of Pennsylvania, Philadelphia

SGMP   Samuel George Morton Papers, American Philosophical Society,
        Philadelphia

WAMR   Warren Anatomical Museum Records, Center for the History of
        Medicine, Countway Library of Medicine, Harvard Medical School,
        Boston

WHL   Waring Historical Library, Medical University of South Carolina,
        Charleston

WSFP   William Stump Forwood Papers, Southern Historical Collection, Louis
        Round Wilson Library, University of North Carolina at Chapel Hill

INTRODUCTION

1. This conflict between elite scientists supporting polygenesis against lay opposition also typifies some scholars' depictions of antebellum racial science. Rather than concentrating on a discredited medical and scientific theory, many U.S. historians have focused on the conflict's religious and political dimensions. Samuel Forwood to William Stump Forwood, July 1, 1857, WSFP; Stanton, *Leopard's Spots*, 194-96.

2. Samuel Forwood to William Stump Forwood, July 1, 1857, WSFP; Forwood, "Negro—a Distinct Species," 225-34; Senex, "Negro Not a Distinct Species," 300-301; Senex, "Is the Negro a Distinct Species?," 375-86; Charles F. J. Lehlbach, "Is the Negro a Distinct Species?," 532-41; Thornton, "Ethnological Question," 541-46; Ewcorstart, "Negro Not a Distinct Species," 577-82; Coles, "Unity of the Origin of Mankind," 582-99; Baldwin, "Unity of the Human Race," 141-51.

3. Senex, "Negro Not a Distinct Species," 300-301.

4. Rush, *Syllabus of a Course of Lectures*, 19; Benjamin Smith Barton, "Notes from Dr. Barton's Lectures on Natural History, or Zoology, 1809-1810," Medical Heritage

Library, College of Physicians of Philadelphia; Wood, *Treatise on the Practice of Medicine*, 1:270, 289.

5. Wilder, *Ebony & Ivy*, 196–97.

6. Warner, *Against the Spirit of System*, 34–39.

7. William Stump Forwood, "Ethnology Notes," WSFP. For more on the rise of tropical medicine, see Anderson, *Colonial Pathologies*; Sutter, "Nature's Agents or Agents of Empire?," 724–54; Espinosa, *Epidemic Invasions*; Willoughby, *Yellow Fever, Race, and Ecology*; and Polk, *Contagions of Empire*.

8. Forwood, "Ethnology Notes."

9. Kilbride, *American Aristocracy*, 85.

10. Here, I am building off three recent works in the history of science and medicine. In Cameron Strang's *Frontiers of Science*, he illustrates the centrality of colonial violence to the production of scientific knowledge in the Gulf South. Likewise, in *Materials of the Mind*, James Poskett unpacks the diverse intellectual and material networks of exchange that were foundational to the construction of phrenology. Both works reveal that science (and medicine) cannot just be studied at the point of knowledge production, and instead reveal the centrality of political and social factors to the construction of science. Finally, Deirdre Cooper Owens's *Medical Bondage* works diligently to center the intellectual contributions and lives of the enslaved subjects on whom American gynecologists pioneered their trade.

11. Stanton, *Leopard's Spots*, 194–96.

12. Fredrickson, *Black Image in the White Mind*, 84–96; Smedley, *Race in North America*, 239–43; Dain, *Hideous Monster of the Mind*, 224–26; Freehling, *Road to Disunion*, 2:41; and Johnson, *River of Dark Dreams*, 200–203.

13. Fredrickson, *Black Image in the White Mind*, 84–96.

14. Keel, "Religion, Polygenism, and the Early Science of Human Origins," 10; Stein, *Measuring Manhood*, 10–11; and Stanton, *Leopard's Spots*, 196. Nancy Stepan makes a similar point in her pathbreaking work on British racial scientists, *Idea of Race in Science*, xvi. Likewise, Reginald Horsman depicts Josiah Nott as a complicated figure committed to both science and slavery, describing him as "an impassioned racist who firmly believed in the integrity of what he was doing." Horsman, *Josiah Nott of Mobile*, 3. It is also worth noting that several scholars have assessed how Black people depicted white bodies in relation to racial science. See Dain, *Hideous Monster of the Mind*; and Bay, *White Image in the Black Mind*.

15. Desmond, *Politics of Evolution*, 4–7; and Kidd, *Forging of Races*, 121–22. Terence Keel also shows that while polygenists were critical of the Christian account of creation, they were many respects still indebted to a Christian worldview. He explains, "Christian ideas about time, the order of nature, and human descent played a key role in the scientific theories of American polygenists." Keel, "Religion, Polygenism, and the Early Science of Human Origins," 5.

16. As a recent example, scholars at Mount Sinai Hospital used eighteenth-century racial categories to argue that Black people have higher TMPRSS2 nasal gene expression than other races. Bunyavanich, Grant, and Vicencio, "Racial/Ethnic Variation in Nasal Gene Expression."

17. Savitt, *Medicine and Slavery*; Sheridan, *Doctors and Slaves*. See also Haller, "Negro and the Southern Physician"; Kiple, *Caribbean Slave*; and Jensen, *For the Health of the Enslaved*.

18. Fett, *Working Cures*; Morgan, *Laboring Women*. Katherine Bankole-Medina has also done important research on slavery and medicine in antebellum Louisiana. See her *Slavery and Medicine*. More recent scholars have taken this further, examining power relations on slave ships, the role of abolitionists in these dynamics, and the dynamic multicultural world of enslaved healers and European physicians in early modern slave societies. See Mustakeem, *Slavery at Sea*; Gómez, *Experiential Caribbean*; Paugh, *Politics of Reproduction*; and Turner, *Contested Bodies*.

19. Gómez, *Experiential Caribbean*, 1–15. For more on Black healing in the Atlantic World, see Weaver, *Medical Revolutionaries*; Sweet, *Domingos Álvares*; Schiebinger, *Secret Cures of Slaves*; and Smith and Willoughby, *Medicine and Healing in the Age of Slavery*.

20. Downs, *Sick from Freedom*; Kenny, "Medical Museums in the Antebellum American South"; Cooper Owens, *Medical Bondage*; Hogarth, *Medicalizing Blackness*.

21. Beckert, *Empire of Cotton*; Beckert and Rockman, *Slavery's Capitalism*; Berry, *Price for Their Pound of Flesh*; Johnson, *Soul by Soul*; Johnson, *River of Dark Dreams*; Mintz, *Sweetness and Power*; Williams, *Capitalism & Slavery*.

22. Fields and Fields, *Racecraft*, 16–19, quote on 18–19. See also Duster, *Backdoor to Eugenics*; Roberts, *Fatal Invention*; Yudell, *Race Unmasked*; and Washington, *Medical Apartheid*.

23. Hayley, "Essay on Thesis," 5, MDUPST. See also Stowe, *Doctoring the South*, 69–74; Corgan, "Some Medical Dissertations"; and Forrest, "Introduction: The Medical Student Thesis at Yale."

24. Despite the term's potential to reinforce enslavers' own perception of themselves, I use "master" because of its dual meaning in medicine and slavery. That being said, I use the term tactfully and intentionally, and I never uncritically refer to an enslaver as a master. Mastery of medicine and race is about the possessors' self-perception of authority over others' bodies. Describing students' engagement with dead bodies, historian of anatomy Michael Sappol explains, "In the anatomical encounter, then, the medical student acquired and demonstrated a powerful mastery of both the subject and himself." Thus, as both purveyors of racial science and medical practitioners, students sought mastery. They hoped to master ideas, diseases, and people. Sappol, *Traffic of Dead Bodies*, 80.

CHAPTER 1

1. Sweet, *Bodies Politic*, 280–81.

2. Barton, "Account of Henry Moss," 4. Parts of this description are also quoted in Sweet, *Bodies Politic*, 282.

3. Barton, "Account of Henry Moss," 15.

4. Jordan, *White Over Black*, 218–21.

5. Caldwell, *Autobiography of Charles Caldwell*, 163–64, 268–69; Sweet, *Bodies Politic*, 283–84.

6. Cassedy, *Medicine and American Growth*; Rothstein, *American Physicians in the 19th Century*; Rothstein, *American Medical Schools*; Stowe, *Doctoring the South*.

7. Stepan, *Idea of Race in Science*; Keel, "Religion, Polygenism, and the Early Science of Human Origins"; Stein, *Measuring Manhood*; Poskett, *Materials of the Mind*; Keel, *Divine Variations*.

8. Wilder, *Ebony & Ivy*; Oast, *Institutional Slavery*; Brophy, *University, Court, & Slave*; Harris, Campbell, and Brophy, *Slavery and the University*.

9. Since at least the 1960s, scholars have cited and discussed early medical professors' racial beliefs, but they rarely analyze these individuals' roles as instructors as well as racial theorists. Many scholars also have discussed how medical schools used enslaved people's bodies (living and dead) to train students. Stanton, *Leopard's Spots*; Jordan, *White Over Black*; Sappol, *Traffic of Dead Bodies*; Berry, *Price for Their Pound of Flesh*; and Hogarth, *Medicalizing Blackness*.

10. As one example of a subject related to race discussed in early medical journals, editors published numerous articles just concerning racial transformation. Catlin, "Ethiopian Turning to a White Man"; Hutchison, "Remarkable Case of Change of Complexion"; Hood, "Another White African"; Cassedy, *Medicine and American Growth*, 66–67.

11. "Review of Cartwright," 93; Kilbride, *American Aristocracy*, 80–85.

12. Seth, *Difference and Disease*, 18.

13. Jordan, *White Over Black*, 95–96. See also Fredrickson, *Racism*; Braude, "Sons of Noah and the Construction of Ethnic and Geographical Identities"; Hannaford, *Race*; Goldberg, *Racist Culture*; Smedley, *Race in North America*; and Horsman, *Race and Manifest Destiny*. On the other hand, James H. Sweet contends that race came out of the fifteenth-century North African Muslim slave trade of sub-Saharan Africans and survived in Spain through the Reconquista. Likewise, Thomas Gossett avers that there is evidence of racial thinking dating back to the ancient world. Sweet, "Iberian Roots of American Racist Thought," 145; Gossett, *Race*, 3.

14. DiPiero, "Missing Links," 161. On a similar note, Joyce Chaplin argues that seventeenth-century English colonists saw the muscularity of Native American bodies as a product of custom, not essential difference. She explains that colonists believed "Indian men had been subjected, since their infancy, to a regimen that artificially strengthened their bodies." *Subject Matter*, 255.

15. Livingstone, *Adam's Ancestors*, 19–20. For more on this and other similar controversies in the sixteenth and seventeenth centuries, see chapter 1 of Livingstone.

16. Seth, *Difference and Disease*, 18–20.

17. Chaplin, *Subject Matter*, 172–98, quote on 192. Recent scholarship has corrected narratives that focus exclusively on virgin soil epidemics as the cause of Native deaths. These narratives made Europeans appear more as passive, if jeering, observers, rather than active participants in genocide. In the past twenty years, new scholarship has emphasized the combination of disease and warfare in the high rates of mortality among Native American groups. See Jones, *Rationalizing Epidemics*; Kelton, *Epidemics and Enslavement*; and Kelton, *Cherokee Medicine, Colonial Germs*. For more on the rise of the African slave trade, see Thornton, *Africa and Africans in the Making of the Atlantic World*.

18. The extreme violence and health risks of enslaved labor and the Atlantic slave trade have been well documented by scholars for decades. See Curtin, *Atlantic Slave Trade*; Brown, *Reaper's Garden*; and Browne, *Surviving Slavery in the British Caribbean*.

19. Seth, *Difference and Disease*, 170–73.

20. Seth, *Difference and Disease*, 188–96.

21. Linnaeus, *General System of Nature*, 1:9. The first edition was published in Latin in 1735. Dain, *Hideous Monster of the Mind*, 13.

22. DiPiero, "Missing Links," 155. Environmental factors included both the social and physical environment. More specifically, these factors included a variety of influences such as diet, climate, and even intellectual stimulation.

23. Peabody, *"There Are No Slaves in France,"* 96–97; Curran, *Anatomy of Blackness*, 140–41; Kidd, *Forging of Races*, 93–95. Historian David Livingstone even argues that the general concept of polygenesis dates at least back to fourth-century Rome with Emperor Julian the Apostate. Livingstone, *Adam's Ancestors*, 6.

24. Dain, *Hideous Monster of the Mind*, 30–36; Curran, *Anatomy of Blackness*, 141–42.

25. Jefferson, *Notes on the State of Virginia*, 146–54.

26. Home, *Six Sketches*, 26; Valenčius, *Health of the Country*, 236.

27. Home, *Six Sketches*, 37–38. This did not mean that Home opposed slavery, but he did not believe that polygenesis inherently argued for slavery.

28. Hogarth, *Medicalizing Blackness*, 21–25.

29. Rather than focus on the shifting titles and language to describe racial scientists in the eighteenth and nineteenth centuries—such as "naturalist," "natural philosopher," "natural historian," "ethnologist," and, occasionally in this period, "anthropologist"—I have elected to mostly refer to them as racial scientists, even if this term was not common until the middle of the nineteenth century. Using "scientist" creates a clearer continuity between the nineteenth and twentieth centuries, even as the term is slightly anachronistic for the eighteenth century.

30. Benjamin Rush to John Morgan, 1768, in Joseph Carson, History of the Medical Department of the University of Pennsylvania Scrapbooks, vol. 2, p. 23, College of Physicians of Philadelphia.

31. Rothstein, *American Physicians in the 19th Century*, 86–87.

32. "By the Election of Dr. Rush," *Pennsylvania Chronicle, and Universal Advertiser*, August 14, 1769; Sweet, *Bodies Politic*, 290–91.

33. "By the Election of Dr. Rush."

34. Rothstein, *American Medical Schools*, 32–33.

35. Nash, *Forging Freedom*, 62–63; Sweet, *Bodies Politic*, 251–63.

36. Nash, *Forging Freedom*, 2–3.

37. "Letter II. From Dr. R—, to Mr. H—l—n, New York," *Newport (R.I.) Mercury*, March 24, 1788.

38. Nash, *Forging Freedom*, 104–5; Long, *Doctoring Freedom*, 154–55.

39. Rothstein, *American Medical Schools*, 34–35.

40. Rothstein, *American Medical Schools*, 31.

41. Rothstein, *American Medical Schools*, 48–49.

42. Cassedy, *Medicine and American Growth*, 67–72.

43. Rothstein, *American Physicians in the 19th Century*, 74–80.

44. Long, *Doctoring Freedom*, 137.

45. January 1 and 6, 1831, Minutes of the Medical Society of South Carolina, WHL; Force and Hoffius, "Negotiating Race and Status."

46. *Evening Bulletin*, May 13, 1854. This article was cut out and put in a scrapbook on the history of MDUP. While it is likely that this was a Philadelphia newspaper, it is unclear from the clipping. In Joseph Carson, History of the Medical Department of the University of Pennsylvania Scrapbooks, 6:69, College of Physicians of Philadelphia.

47. Kilbride, *American Aristocracy*, 80–85.

48. David Pusey, diary entry, November 28, 1853, David Pusey Papers, History Collections, Kornhauser Health Sciences Library, University of Louisville, Louisville, Ky.

49. Stowe, *Doctoring the South*, 80–83.

50. Cassedy, "Early American Medical Journalism," 139–45.

51. Cassedy, "Early American Medical Journalism," 138.

52. Cassedy, "Early American Medical Journalism," 145–47.

53. Receipts, WSFP; Forwood, "Ethnological Papers," 123; Forwood, "Negro—a Distinct Species," 228.

54. Barton, "Account of Henry Moss," 4; Catlin, "Ethiopian Turning to a White Man," 83–84; Hutchison, "Remarkable Case of Change of Complexion," 146–48; Cartwright, "Diseases and Physical Peculiarities of the Negro Race," 691; "Review of Cartwright," 93.

55. "Mr. Printer," *Daily Advertiser* (New York, N.Y.), April 23, 1788. See also Wilf, "Anatomy and Punishment," 509–13; Wilder, *Ebony & Ivy*, 196–97.

56. *"Commissioners of the Alms-House vs. Alexander Whistelo,"* 10–13.

57. *"Commissioners of the Alms-House vs. Alexander Whistelo,"* 14–16.

58. *"Commissioners of the Alms-House vs. Alexander Whistelo,"* 16–31. Quote on 20.

59. *"Commissioners of the Alms-House vs. Alexander Whistelo,"* 16–31. Quote on 23. Sari Altschuler has illustrated how imagination and even fiction writing were important methods for producing medical knowledge during this period. *Medical Imagination*, 8–13. Likewise, historian Stefanie Hunt-Kennedy has argued convincingly that ideas of monstrous births as shaped by maternal imagination influenced notions of racial difference and its inheritance dating back to the sixteenth and seventeenth centuries. Hunt-Kennedy, *Between Fitness and Death*, 13–38.

60. Elijah Griffiths, Notes from Dr. Rush's Lectures, 1797–1798 Session, vol. 2, no page numbers, College of Physicians of Philadelphia. I owe a special thanks to Sarah Naramore for first sharing with me transcriptions of Griffiths's lecture notes. See also Rush, "Black Color (as It Is Called) of the Negroes." For the best comprehensive analysis of Rush, see Naramore, "I Sing the Body Republic."

61. Elijah Griffiths, Notes from Dr. Rush's Lectures, 1797–1798 Session, vol. 2, no page numbers, College of Physicians of Philadelphia.

62. Jordan, *White Over Black*, 225–30; Benjamin Waterhouse, "Lecture: Recapitulation of Scale of Beings, Gradations of Man & Conclusion of the Last Lecture on, Comparison between Things Mater & Intellectual & . . . Jun. 30, 1805," Box 2, Benjamin Waterhouse Papers, CHM.

63. White, *Account of the Regular Gradation in Man*, 61–66; Jordan, *White Over Black*, 500–501. See also *Catalogue of Anatomical Preparations*.

64. White, *Account of the Regular Gradation in Man*, 67.

65. John Taulman, Lecture Notes, 1812–1813 Session, Archives and Special Collections, August C. Long Health Sciences Library, Columbia University, New York, N.Y.;

Charles Drake, Notes on Smith's Anatomy Lectures, 1812–1813, 233–38, Archives and Special Collections, August C. Long Health Sciences Library, Columbia University, New York, N.Y.

66. Caldwell, *Original Unity of the Race*, 16. This view of the Scriptures was common among antebellum polygenists, even though in many respects they still worked from a worldview informed by Christianity. Keel, "Religion, Polygenism, and the Early Science of Human Origins," 6–7.

67. Caldwell, *Original Unity of the Race*, 88.

68. Caldwell, *Original Unity of the Race*, 48. For more on Long, see Seth, *Difference and Disease*, 208–40; Jefferson, *Notes on the State of Virginia*, 146–54.

69. Augstein, *James Cowles Prichard's Anthropology*, xii; Prichard, *Natural History of Man*, 1:7. For more on Blumenbach, see Keel, *Divine Variations*, 23–53.

70. Prichard, *Natural History of Man*, 1:10, 2:714, quote on 1:10.

71. Prichard, *Natural History of Man*, 1:115–17, 339.

72. Gibson, *Rambles in Europe in 1839*, 274–76.

73. McCandless, *Slavery, Disease, and Suffering*, 143–44; McCandless, "Political Evolution of John Bachman," 17. See also Stephens, *Science, Race, and Religion*.

74. Bachman, *Unity of the Human Race*, 115. See also Bachman, "Reply to the Letter of Samuel George Morton"; and Bachman, "Second Letter to Samuel G. Morton."

75. John Bachman, excerpt from *The Doctrine of the Unity of the Human Race Examined on the Principles of Science*, in *John Bachman: Selected Writings*, 259–60, quote on 259.

76. Fabian, *Skull Collectors*, 17–27.

77. S. Henry Dickson to Samuel George Morton, March 20, 1837, SGMP. Dickson explained, "The profession everywhere [is] deeply indebted to you for your useful and beautiful illustrations of phthisis." Morton even corresponded about race with South Carolina senator John C. Calhoun, providing him with copies of Crania Aegyptiaca; *or, Observations on Egyptian Ethnography, Derived from Anatomy, History and the Monuments* and Crania Americana; *or, a Comparative View of the Skulls of Various Aboriginal Nations of North and South America*. Morton overall classified humanity into "*twenty-two* families." However, the groups fit into larger overarching racial categories. In Crania Aegyptiaca; *or, Observations on Egyptian Ethnography*, Morton identifies five overarching groups. Nott and Gliddon, *Types of Mankind*, 51, 83, 423, quote on 83.

78. "Proceedings of the Phrenological Association Held at Glasgow in September, 1840," Samuel George Morton Letters, Microfilm, American Philosophical Society, Philadelphia.

79. Fabian, *Skull Collectors*, 10.

80. Jeffries Wyman to Elizabeth A. Wyman, November 24, 1844; and Jeffries Wyman to Elizabeth A. Wyman, January 9, 1847, JWP.

81. Morton, Crania Aegyptiaca; *or, Observations on Egyptian Ethnography*, 21. On the Negro versus Negroid crania, Morton explains that "Negro" refers to skulls with pure negro features, but "negroid crania . . . [are] heads with decidedly mixed characters, in which those of the Negro predominate." It is also worth noting that Morton's sample size was quite small for ancient Egyptian skulls, only possessing one "Negro" crania and a handful of "Negroid" skulls.

82. Italics for emphasis in original. George Gliddon to Samuel George Morton, February 7, 1842, Samuel George Morton Letters, Microfilm, American Philosophical Society, Philadelphia.

83. Morton, *Crania Aegyptiaca; or, Observations on Egyptian Ethnography*, 66.

84. Nott and Gliddon were even given carte blanche access to Morton's papers by his wife, and they used them as a blueprint for organizing *Types of Mankind*. The volume was also dedicated to "the memory of Morton," and it contains a biographical sketch of him. Finally, Nott and Gliddon elected to place Morton's picture opposite the title page instead of their own, hinting that they saw Morton as the true author of the work. Nott and Gliddon, *Types of Mankind*, ix–xiv.

85. Douglass, *Claims of the Negro*, 16–18.

86. Douglass, *Claims of the Negro*, 16–18.

87. "CALVINISM *vs.* 'TYPES OF MANKIND'; or, DAVID and GOLIAH. A Covenanter's Snuffle. Old Scotch Air—'There Was a Little Man.' DEDICATED (SINE LICENTIA) to THE GENERAL ASSEMBLY." A printed source of unknown origin dated May 27, 1854, this song was glued into the cover of the racial scientist and medical professor James Aitken Meigs's copy of *Types of Mankind* held at the library of the Academy of Natural Sciences of Drexel University, Philadelphia.

88. Johnson, *River of Dark Dreams*, 200–203; Freehling, *Road to Disunion*, 2:41–44; Kidd, *Forging of Races*, 144–47; Dain, *Hideous Monster of the Mind*, 197–99.

89. "Treason against Adam and Noah," *Boston Investigator*, June 14, 1854; "New Publications," *Boston Daily Atlas*, May 22, 1854; "Types of Mankind," *Daily National Intelligencer* (Washington, D.C.), April 21, 1854; "A Man before Adam," *Daily National Intelligencer* (Washington, D.C.), April 27, 1854.

90. Subscribers were those who bought their copy before publication.

91. Nott and Gliddon, *Types of Mankind*, 733–38.

92. Keel, "Religion, Polygenism, and the Early Science of Human Origins," 10.

93. D. A. W., "Types of Mankind," *Liberator* (Boston), June 2, 1854.

94. Cartwright, "Diseases and Physical Peculiarities of the Negro Race," 691. For more on Cartwright, see Willoughby, "Running Away from Drapetomania," 579–614.

95. Cartwright, "Diseases and Physical Peculiarities of the Negro Race (Continued)," 194.

96. "Review of Cartwright," 93.

97. Dickson, *Syllabus*, 8.

98. Cabell, *Syllabus*, 58–59. Cabell also wrote a monograph in favor of monogenesis in 1859. Cabell, *Modern Testimony*; Charles M. Ellis to Joseph Leidy, March 21, 1861, JLC; vol. 1: notes 1850–1851, HLA.

99. Cooke, "Inaugural Dissertation," 29, MDUPST.

100. Cooke, "Inaugural Dissertation," 33.

101. Ball, "Origin of the Different Human Species," no page numbers, WHL.

102. About medical student theses, historian Stephen Stowe explains, "Mentors' voices can be heard just beneath the surface of theses, of course, and that is one reason theses are so valuable as historical sources. And although many theses are technical and closely focused, something of the expressive style of mid-nineteenth century American intellectual life resided in them, too: Romantic apostrophes to Nature; warnings about (or paeans to) the bustling, modernizing world; scenes from

the medical past; an empirical toting up of objects seen and categorized." Stowe, *Doctoring the South*, 69-74, quote on 69. One of the more interesting primary sources on theses was written by MDUP medical student L. B. Hayley. In his senior thesis, Hayley actually argued against the practice of thesis writing due to rampant plagiarism by students. Hayley, "Essay on Thesis," MDUPST.

103. Gibson, "Essay on Plurality," 13, MDUPST; McDow, "Essay on the Negro," no page numbers, MDUPST.

104. Gibson, "Essay on Plurality," 5.

105. Louis Agassiz, "Sketch of the Natural Provinces of the Animal World and their Relation to the Different Types of Man," in Nott and Gliddon, *Types of Mankind*, lviii-xxvi. Evidence of the commonly held belief that African Americans were best fit for southern labor can be seen in this passage from Mississippi's justification of secession: "By an imperious law of nature, none but the Black race can bear exposure to the tropical sun." "Declaration of the Immediate Causes."

106. McDow, "Essay on the Negro," no page numbers.

107. Polygenesis declined in the 1860s in scientific circles, but the theory had a much longer life in popular circles, most clearly shown in Charles Carroll's *"The Negro a Beast,"* published in 1900.

108. Duffy, *Tulane University Medical Center*, 40-41.

109. Kilbride, *American Aristocracy*, 92-93.

110. MDUPST.

111. Long, *Doctoring Freedom*, 124-28.

CHAPTER 2

1. Josiah Nott to Joseph Leidy, April 12, 1859, JLC.

2. Horsman, *Josiah Nott of Mobile*, 10-15, 42-45.

3. Richerand, *Elements of Physiology*, 606-7; Altschuler, *Medical Imagination*, 128, 240n30; Crais and Scully, *Sara Baartman and the Hottentot Venus*, 130-49; Poskett, *Materials of the Mind*, 58-62.

4. Warner, *Against the Spirit of System*, 34-39.

5. Warner, *Against the Spirit of System*, 175-76.

6. Warner, *Against the Spirit of System*; Curran, *Anatomy of Blackness*; and Cassedy, *American Medicine and Statistical Thinking*.

7. Bates, *Anatomy of Robert Knox*, 6.

8. Ackerknecht, *Medicine at the Paris Hospital*, 15. This universality would have been limited to the types of bodies and diseases local to French physicians.

9. Ackerknecht, *Medicine at the Paris Hospital*, 51, 87, 102. See also Sappol, *Traffic of Dead Bodies*, 52-53.

10. Ackerknecht, *Medicine at the Paris Hospital*, 87.

11. Bartlett, *Essay on the Philosophy of Medical Science*, 225.

12. Warner, *Against the Spirit of System*, 127; Ackerknecht, *Medicine at the Paris Hospital*, 193.

13. Italics for emphasis added. Louis, *Essay on Clinical Instruction*, 1.

14. Ackerknecht, *Medicine at the Paris Hospital*, 9.

15. Louis, *Essay on Clinical Instruction*, 9-10.

16. Caffey, "Thesis on Calomel in Southern Fevers," 11, WHL.

17. Foucault, *Birth of the Clinic*, 129.

18. Foucault, *Birth of the Clinic*, 164. Foucault was undoubtedly a poor historian, and these comments are certainly oversimplified. Yet he coined this essential term that continues to resonate and capture how clinicians saw the body. There were, however, important seventeenth- and eighteenth-century precedents for this type of gaze, like the approach of Herman Boerhaave at the University of Leiden. French clinicians popularized the clinical gaze again in the nineteenth century in response to symptomatic universalists of the University of Edinburgh like Benjamin Rush, who had dominated late Enlightenment U.S. medicine.

19. Cassedy, *American Medicine and Statistical Thinking*, 69–80.

20. Rosenthal, "Slavery's Scientific Management," 86.

21. Cassedy, *American Medicine and Statistical Thinking*, 63.

22. Heck, *Iconographic Encyclopædia*, 2:707–14, 853. Volume 3 also contains a section entitled "Ethnology of the Present Day." Willoughby, "Running Away from Drapetomania," 595–96. Likewise, historians of polygenesis and racial theory have shown that these ideas had deep roots in the Atlantic history of science and religion that merely culminated in the mid-nineteenth century. Curran, *Anatomy of Blackness*, and Livingstone, *Adam's Ancestors*.

23. Johnson, *Soul by Soul*, 161. This racial gaze affected nonsouthern physicians through readings and lectures, but the practical experience of southern physicians gave this racial gaze added weight in their analysis of race.

24. Horsman, *Josiah Nott of Mobile*, 12, 130.

25. Johnson, *Soul by Soul*, 149.

26. Johnson, *Soul by Soul*, 146.

27. Fett, *Working Cures*, 20–21; Johnson, *Soul by Soul*, 137. Historian Stephen Kenny argues that the chattel principle shaped southern medical approaches to Black people's bodies in terms of how their bodies were sourced for dissection materials. Kenny, "Medical Museums in the Antebellum American South," 37.

28. Bruce Dain has pointed out, however, that Morton's antislavery stance was suspect by the late 1840s, as evidenced by his offering John C. Calhoun permission to cite his work. Dain, *Hideous Monster of the Mind*, 217–18.

29. Samuel Morton, Journal, 1833–ca. 1837, SGMP; Cartwright, "Diseases and Physical Peculiarities of the Negro Race," 701–14; Caldwell, *Original Unity of the Race*, 48. Bruce Dain also gives an account of Morton's trip. Dain, *Hideous Monster of the Mind*, 202–3.

30. Morton, Journal, 1833–ca. 1837, SGMP.

31. Home, *Lectures on Comparative Anatomy*, 3:317. This account also encapsulated historian Suman Seth's contention that, when it came to race, metropolitan scientists relied on knowledge produced in the colonies. See Seth, *Difference and Disease*, 6–14. See also Poskett, *Materials of the Mind*, 115–49.

32. Home, *Lectures on Comparative Anatomy*, 3:317; Cooper Owens, *Medical Bondage*, 79.

33. Home, *Lectures on Comparative Anatomy*, 3:317; Cooper Owens, *Medical Bondage*, 79.

34. George Gliddon to Samuel Morton, March 31, 1839, SGMP; Morton, *Skulls of Man and the Inferior Animals*, 91, 95–96, 98–100. I owe a special thanks to Paul Wolff Mitchell for help with this note.

35. Nott and Gliddon, *Types of Mankind*, xxxv; Headrick, *Tools of Empire*, 150–56; Streets-Salter and Getz, *Empires and Colonies*, 248–50.

36. Nott and Gliddon, *Types of Mankind*, xxxv; George Gliddon to Samuel Morton, March 31, 1839, SGMP; Morton, *Skulls of Man and the Inferior Animals*, 91, 95–96, 98–100.

37. John Collins Warren to Samuel Morton, February 3, 1837, SGMP; Daniel Drake to Samuel Morton, September 28, 1833, SGMP; James Cowles Prichard to Samuel Morton, December 11, 1839, SGMP. See also Lindquist, "Stealing from the Dead."

38. Other historians have discussed how empires allowed for the emergence of modern racial science. See Sera-Shriar, "Ethnology in the Metropole" and MacDonald, *Human Remains*.

39. Samuel George Morton to John Collins Warren, April 13, 1849, John Collins Warren Papers, Massachusetts Historical Society, Boston.

40. Morton, *Crania Americana; or, a Comparative View of the Skulls of Various Aboriginal Nations*, 252–54.

41. Morton, *Crania Americana*, v.

42. Historian Michael Worboys explains, "The nineteenth century saw the medical profession develop a near monopoly in the labeling and management of disease." "Medical Perspectives on Health and Disease," 5:65–66.

43. Samuel George Morton to John Collins Warren, March 25, 1837; and Samuel George Morton to John Collins Warren, December 15, 1839, John Collins Warren Papers.

44. Augustus Addison Gould to Jeffries Wyman, January 16, 1845, Jeffries Wyman Papers, University Archives, Harvard University, Cambridge, Mass.; Jeffries Wyman to Elizabeth A. Wyman, November 24, 1844, and January 9, 1847, JWP; McDow, "Essay on the Negro," no page numbers, MDUPST; Gambel, "Essay on Organic Forms or Species," 12, MDUPST. Gambel also apprenticed for Morton.

45. Leidy, *Elementary Treatise on Human Anatomy*, 637. Leidy's personal copy is held today at the College of Physician of Philadelphia. "Descriptive Catalogue of the Museum of the Mass. Medical College, August 1850," Box 17, 232, WAMR.

46. P. A. Browne Hair Albums, Academy of Natural Sciences of Drexel University, Philadelphia.

47. Browne, *Classification of Mankind*, 20.

48. Volumes 1–9, P. A. Browne Hair Albums; Samuel G. Morton to Peter Arrell Browne, Correspondence File, P. A. Browne Hair Albums.

49. Nott and Gliddon, *Types of Mankind*, 452–53.

50. Josiah Nott to Jeffries Wyman, February 13, 1845, Wyman Family Papers, University Archives, Harvard University, Cambridge, Mass. In many ways, Nott's belief in the need for the greater collection of human remains would be realized in the postbellum era. Postbellum collections of human remains dwarfed their antebellum predecessors. For more, see Redman, *Bone Rooms*.

CHAPTER 3

1. Addams, "Inaugural Dissertation on the Internal Changes Produced by the Operation of the Remote Causes of Fever," Special Collections Department, J. Douglas Gay Jr./Francis Carrick Thomas Library, Transylvania University, Lexington, Ky.

2. Addams, "Inaugural Dissertation on the Internal Changes," 22–23.

3. Morrill, "Essay on the Formation of Medical Character," 28, MDUPST.

4. Sappol, *Traffic of Dead Bodies*, 1–7; Richardson, *Death, Dissection, and the Destitute*, 61–62. See also Kenny, "Medical Museums in the Antebellum American South," 32–62; Stowe, *Doctoring the South*; Wilf, "Anatomy and Punishment"; Breeden, "Body Snatchers and Anatomy Professors"; and Humphrey, "Dissection and Discrimination."

5. Richardson, *Death, Dissection, and the Destitute*, 30.

6. Savitt, "Use of Blacks," 342–48; Kenny, "Power, Opportunism, Racism." See also Schiebinger, "Medical Experimentation and Race."

7. "Nat Turner's Insurrection," *Liberator* (Boston), August 9, 1861.

8. Jackson, *Descriptive Catalogue of the Warren Anatomical Museum*, 74–75.

9. Wilf, "Anatomy and Punishment," 509.

10. In 1788, New York was still a slave state, and it would not pass a law providing for the gradual emancipation of the enslaved for eleven more years. Wilf, "Anatomy and Punishment," 510–13.

11. Hogarth, "Comparing Anatomies, Constructing Races," 218. See also Kenny, "Medical Museums in the Antebellum American South"; Savitt, "Use of Blacks"; Humphrey, "Dissection and Discrimination," 819–27; and Breeden, "Body Snatchers and Anatomy Professors," 321–45.

12. "Ourang Outang," *Raleigh Register, and North-Carolina State Gazette*, September 23, 1825; "Dissection of an Ouran Outang," *United States Telegraph* (Washington, D.C.), September 15, 1826; "Dissection of an Ouran Outang," *Daily National Journal* (Washington, D.C.), September 16, 1826; "Dissection of an Ouran Outang," *Louisiana Advertiser*, October 16, 1826; "The Dissection of the Ourang Outang," *Southern Patriot* (Charleston, S.C.), October 7, 1835; and "The Dissection of the Ourang Outang," *Virginia Free Press*, October 15, 1835.

13. "Dissection of the Ourang Outang," *Southern Patriot* (Charleston, S.C.), October 7, 1835.

14. "Object 763," in "Descriptive Catalogue of the Cabinet, Volume II, Wyman Collection, ca. 1837–1847," Folder 11, Box 10, Collection Registration Records, WAMR.

15. Quoted in Nott and Gliddon, *Types of Mankind*, 457.

16. Joseph Leidy to Josiah Nott, April 18, 1855, quoted in the appendix to Gobineau, *Moral and Intellectual Diversity of Races*, 480.

17. Quoted in E. J. Nolan, Report of a Conversation with Dr. Leidy, October 29, 1867, vol. 1, p. 10. Joseph Leidy Memorial Albums, Academy of Natural Sciences of Drexel University, Philadelphia, Pa.

18. Titus M. Coan to his parents, July 9, 1860, Titus Munson Coan Papers, New York Historical Society, New York, N.Y.

19. Sappol, *Traffic of Dead Bodies*, 79, 84.

20. William E. Horner, entry for May 10, 1821, Travel Journals, vol. 4, William Edmonds Horner Papers, University Archives and Records Center, University of Pennsylvania, Philadelphia, Pa.

21. Italics for emphasis in original. Francis Bowen to Jeffries Wyman, November 25, 1845, JWP. Daina Ramey Berry's monograph has a slight transcription error when describing this letter, quoting Bowen as saying "taboo crops" rather than "tobacco crops." Likewise, Berry reads Bowen as seriously asking Wyman about purchasing cadavers from Virginia for Harvard. While this agenda was not impossible, as Black people's bodies were certainly shipped from the South to New England, Bowen spends three out of four pages of the letter relating Boston gossip. His inquiry comes at the end, when he might ask about his friend's life in slave country. This is how I read the letter. Likewise, in my analysis of the papers of John Collins Warren, a Harvard professor of anatomy and colleague of Wyman's, I found no evidence of Warren requesting Bowen to act as an intermediary, and to my knowledge Bowen was never employed by the anatomy department. I did find evidence of Warren using his network to try to obtain bodies from Baltimore, Maine, Montreal, and New York City during the antebellum period. In an 1839 diary entry, he even noted that he purchased a body from New York City. Thus, while Berry's reading is possible, I have not found enough clear evidence to corroborate her account. Berry, *Price for Their Pound of Flesh*, 159–61; J. Revere to J. C. Warren, December 14, 1827; James Hederson to J. C. Warren, December 23, 1828; Moses Shaw to John Collins Warren, November 11, 1839; and diary entry, November 26, 1839, John Collins Warren Papers, Massachusetts Historical Society, Boston.

22. Jeffries Wyman to Elizabeth A. Wyman, November 9, 1844; and October 19, 1844, JWP.

23. Quoted in Warner and Edmondson, *Dissection*, 26, caption to photo.

24. Quoted in Warner and Edmondson, *Dissection*, 25.

25. Hogarth, "Comparing Anatomies, Constructing Races"; and Hogarth, "Charity and Terror in Eighteenth-Century Jamaica"; Nash, *Forging Freedom*, 2.

26. Much of the literature that has addressed body snatching of Black cadavers in the Northeast has focused on the 1788 anatomy riots in New York. This event-driven narrative loses sight of the systematic and often uncontested appropriation of Black bodies in northeastern cities with large free Black populations. See Wilf, "Anatomy and Punishment"; and Swan, "Doctors' Riot of 1788." David Humphrey's 1973 article on the social origins of cadavers provides a notable exception to this trend. Humphrey explains that for New York physicians, "obviously, dissecting a white was risky business. Dissecting a black was largely a matter of finding a body." Humphrey, "Dissection and Discrimination," 820.

27. In an 1844 census of the Philadelphia and Blockley Almshouses (Blockley was a town later incorporated into Philadelphia), Black people represented 12 percent of the population compared to occupying only 9 percent of the city's total population in 1830. This number continuously diminished throughout the antebellum era as waves of European immigrants entered the city. In 1860, Black people only represented 4 percent of the city's population. "Census of the Blockley Alms House and Philadelphia Hospital," 61; Warner, *Private City*, 55, 127; Nash, *Forging Freedom*, 154–57.

28. In Bettner's thesis, he gives the ward where each patient was admitted. Bettner, "Inaugural Essay on Ulceration," 7, 13, MDUPST.

29. Bettner, "Inaugural Essay on Ulceration," 7, 13.

30. Gwathmey, "Cholera Infantum, An Essay," 21–23, MDUPST.

31. Savitt, "Use of Blacks," 338–40.

32. Gorham, "Collections in Morbid Anatomy," 34–36; Gorham, "Cases in Morbid Anatomy," 349.

33. Receipt, L. L. Tarbell, Funeral Undertaker, May 9, 1860, Records of the Warren Anatomical Museum, 1828–1892, CHM.

34. Horner, *United States Dissector*, 192.

35. Augustus Addison Gould to Jeffries Wyman, January 10, 1847, JWP.

36. "Death of Joice Heth," *Herald* (New York, N.Y.), February 24, 1836. Benjamin Reiss relates the story of Barnum and Heth in detail in his monograph, *The Showman and the Slave*.

37. "Physical; Joice Heth's; Dr. D. L. Rogers," *Daily National Intelligencer* (Washington, D.C.), March 7, 1836.

38. "Another Hoax," *Herald* (New York, N.Y.), February 27, 1836; Reiss, *Showman and the Slave*, 134–37.

39. "Physical; Joice Heth's; Dr. D. L. Rogers"; Reiss, *Showman and the Slave*, 135; Sappol, *Traffic of Dead Bodies*, 137.

40. Perry, Howson, and Bianco, *Archaeology of the African Burial Ground*, 1:192–93, 209–10. Quote on 210.

41. Perry, Howson, and Bianco, *Archaeology of the African Burial Ground*, 1:192–93, 209–10. Quote on 210.

42. Medford et al., "'By the Visitations of God,'" 88–90.

43. McKnight, *Pioneer Outline of Northwestern Pennsylvania*, 294.

44. McKnight, *Pioneer Outline of Northwestern Pennsylvania*, 296–300.

45. John D. Godman to John Collins Warren, January 1, 1829, John Collins Warren Papers, Massachusetts Historical Society, Boston; Sappol, *Traffic of Dead Bodies*, 114–16.

46. Webster, *Anatomical Instruction in Philadelphia*, 6–17.

47. John D. Godman to John Collins Warren, January 1, 1829.

48. I need to thank Robert Murray for sharing his article on McGill's story with me prior to its publication. Murray, "Bodies in Motion," 639–43.

49. Murray, "Bodies in Motion," 639–43.

50. *Annual Announcement of the Trustees and Faculty*, 4. Stephen Kenny has shown a dimension of how physicians employed the chattel principle (although he does not employ this term). Southern physicians engaged in the chattel-making process through procuring slaves for experimentation. Kenny explains, "As slaves were legally considered as commodities and were framed as an inferior race by white slaveholding ideology, the southern medical profession faced few obstacles appropriating and utilizing slave bodies for teaching and research." Kenny, "'Dictate of Both Interest and Mercy'?," 17.

51. "Recent Southern Atrocities," *Liberator* (Boston), August 10, 1849. Other examples included "Charleston; Negro Joe; Convicted; Assault; Conformably; Delivered; Understand; Surgeons," *Evening Post* (New York, N.Y.), October 5, 1831; and

"Mr. Ford; Frequent; Pursuers; Negro Jack," *Daily Advertiser* (New York, N.Y.), June 20, 1821.

52. Jeffries Wyman to Morrill Wyman, December 12, 1847, JWP.

53. "Petersburg; Southampton; Nat Turner; Friday; Jerusalem," *Liberator* (Boston), November 26, 1831; Reiss, *Showman and the Slave*, 134; Greenberg, "Introduction, *The Confessions of Nat Turner*," 19–20.

54. Wilf, "Anatomy and Punishment," 512.

55. Fett, *Working Cures*, 152–53; Savitt, "Use of Blacks," 340. Fett and Savitt explain that enslaved people knew to fear dissection and medical schools generally. Moreover, scholarship on the networks of intelligence shared among the enslaved, especially regarding rebellion and politics, lends strong support to the idea that many enslaved people would have known about the dissection of rebels. Hahn, *Nation under Our Feet*, 7–8. See also Troutman, "Grapevine in the Slave Market."

56. "John Brown's Invasion," *New York Tribune*, November 28, 1859.

57. Fett, *Working Cures*, 152–53; Savitt, "Use of Blacks," 340.

58. Hogarth, "Comparing Anatomies, Constructing Races," 5–6.

59. "Mr. Printer," *Daily Advertiser* (New York, N.Y.), April 23, 1788; Wilf, 511. See also Richardson, *Death, Dissection, and the Destitute*, 90–93; and Sappol, *Traffic of Dead Bodies*, 136–37.

60. Brown, *Slave Life in Georgia*, 45. Sharla Fett and Todd Savitt also give accounts of Hamilton's experiments. Fett, *Working Cures*, 152; Savitt, "Use of Blacks," 344; *Catalogue of the Alumni*, 75.

61. Brown, *Slave Life in Georgia*, 46–47.

62. Brown, *Slave Life in Georgia*, 47–48.

63. Brown, *Slave Life in Georgia*, 48.

64. Brown, *Slave Life in Georgia*, 48–49.

65. Vesicovaginal fistula is defined by a tear in the vaginal wall causing general incontinence. Cooper Owens, "Manifesting Power," 176–81; Schwartz, *Birthing a Slave*; McGregor, *From Midwives to Medicine*.

66. Kenny, "Power, Opportunism, Racism," 11.

67. Schwartz, *Birthing a Slave*, 237–40.

68. Lesch, *Science and Medicine in France*, 99.

69. Lesch, *Science and Medicine*, 112.

70. Schaffer, "Essay on Experiments on the Heart's Action," no page numbers, MDUPST.

71. Lesch, *Science and Medicine in France*, 112.

72. Caruthers, "Essay on Emetics," 27, MDUPST. This experiment was also described by MCSC student James Cleckley in his thesis, "Dissertation on the Modus Operandi of Emetics," 8, WHL. Other students described experiments by Magendie that were fatal to numerous dogs and other animals. Compton, "Inaugural Treatise on Iodine," 6–7, WHL; Thornton, "Inaugural Dissertation upon Iodine," 4–5, WHL; Leak, "Thesis on the Modus Operandi of Medicines," 5, WHL; and Raysor, "Inaugural Dissertation on the Modus Operandi of Cathartics," 9, WHL. For more on Magendie's experiments, see Lesch, *Science and Medicine in France*, 99–124, 149; Fye, *Development of American Physiology*, 4–5.

73. Caruthers, "Essay on Emetics," 27.

74. Schaffer, "Essay on Experiments on the Heart's Action," no page numbers, MDUPST; Carrington, "Inaugural Essay on Hydrophobia," 16, MDUPST; Phillips, "Inaugural Dissertation on the Modus Operandi of Opium," 5, WHL.

75. *Code of Ethics*, 7–10. Quote on 8.

76. Lederer, *Subjected to Science*, 97–100.

77. Gross, *Double Character*, 65–66.

78. Lederer, *Subjected to Science*, 115.

79. Bylebyl, "William Beaumont, Robley Dunglison, and the 'Philadelphia Physiologists,'" 9–11. See also Pitcock, "William Beaumont, M.D. and Malpractice"; and Numbers and Orr, "William Beaumont's Reception at Home and Abroad."

80. Beaumont, *Experiments and Observations*, 18–19.

81. Dracobly, "Ethics and Experimentation," 332–33.

82. Dracobly, "Ethics and Experimentation," 360–61.

83. Dracobly, "Ethics and Experimentation," 356.

84. Kenny, "Power, Opportunism, Racism," 15.

85. Cooper Owens, "Manifesting Power," 176–81.

86. Home, *Lectures on Comparative Anatomy*, 3:216–20; Curran, *Anatomy of Blackness*, 120–21.

87. Horn, "Inaugural Dissertation on the Subject Is Yellow Fever Contagious," no page numbers, WHL.

88. DeLancey, "Vaccinating Freedom," 300–302; Colman, *New Method of Receiving the Small-Pox*, 15–16.

89. Horn, "Inaugural Dissertation," no page number.

90. Horn, "Inaugural Dissertation," no page number.

91. Higgins, "Inaugural Dissertation on Cutaneous Absorption," 14–16, WHL.

92. Higgins, "Inaugural Dissertation," 14–16.

93. Higgins, "Inaugural Dissertation," 14–16.

94. Higgins, "Inaugural Dissertation," 14–16. Higgins's process of stripping, coating, and cleaning the enslaved woman resembled many of the common features of white physicians' interactions with their female enslaved patients. Historian Deirdre Cooper Owens explains, "A major part of female slave care was the physical manipulation of the female body. Doctors examined, prodded, and displayed slave women's bodies with regularity. Black women like Nanny, were assumed by most whites to be oblivious to the invasive handling of their bodies." Cooper Owens, "Manifesting Power," 181.

CHAPTER 4

1. Charles M. Ellis to Joseph Leidy, March 29, 1861, JLP.

2. Charles M. Ellis to Joseph Leidy, March 29, 1861, JLP.

3. Charles M. Ellis to Joseph Leidy, March 29, 1861, JLP.

4. Charles M. Ellis to Joseph Leidy, March 29, 1861, JLP.

5. Sappol, *Traffic of Dead Bodies*, 44.

6. Rothstein, *American Medical Schools*, 48–49.

7. Berkowitz, *Charles Bell and the Anatomy of Reform*, 49.

8. Morton, *Illustrated System of Human Anatomy*, iii.

9. Morton, *Illustrated System of Human Anatomy*, 69–76. Quote on 69–70. Reflecting racial scientists' interests in other parts of the body, Morton demarcated a few other supposed anatomical differences that separated the races, ranging from the shape and pigmentation of women's nipples to the supposedly rounder pigment cells of whites. He depicted these ostensible anatomical distinctions as spread across the body, enduring, and inherited, and they were neither cultural nor created by variances in climate. Morton, *Illustrated System of Human Anatomy*, 151–54, 362.

10. Carson, *History of the Medical Department*, 134–44. As evidence of the wide influence of the textbook authors selected for this chapter, in his *History of American Medical Literature, from 1776 to the Present Time*, Jefferson Medical College professor Samuel D. Gross explained in 1876, "After Wistar's treatise appeared, in 1826, that of Dr. William E. Horner, then adjunct and subsequently sole professor of anatomy in the University of Pennsylvania, a work in two volumes, entitled 'Special Anatomy and Histology'; and then the elementary treatises of Morton, of Handy, of Richardson, and of Leidy, productions extensively employed as text-books, and composed, for the most part, by men of great reputation." Gross, *History of American Medical Literature*, 9. Likewise, in the 1840–41 circular for MCSC, the anatomy professor J. Edwards Holbrook put Horner's textbook first in his list of reference works. *Annual Announcement of the Trustees and Faculty*, 7.

11. Wistar, *System of Human Anatomy*, 1:407–12. See discussion of Barton and Rush in the introduction and chapter 1. Wistar's only protracted consideration of race and Blackness in his textbook was on the subject of skin, a matter of medical and scientific inquiry since the seventeenth century. Physicians and theorists saw skin color as a remarkably malleable anatomical difference.

12. Wistar, *System of Human Anatomy*, 1:66, 338. For more on phrenology, see Poskett, *Materials of the Mind*, and Thompson, *Organ of Murder*.

13. Rush, *Medical Inquiries and Observations*, 2:372; Sappol, *Traffic of Dead Bodies*, 53.

14. For more on the history of the politics of the sectional crisis, see Freehling, *Road to Disunion*, vol. 1, *Secessionists at Bay*; Freehling, *Road to Disunion*, vol. 2, *Secessionists Triumphant*; Ford, *Deliver Us from Evil*; and Blackett, *Captive's Quest for Freedom*.

15. Horner, *Treatise on Special and General Anatomy*, 1:208–16, 283, 291, 347. Quote on 211.

16. Horner even cited the famous French clinician Xavier Bichat's idea that greater aptitude for taste and smell corresponded to smaller brain size and lesser intelligence. Thus, he endorsed for students the idea that African descendants possessed heightened senses. Horner, *Treatise on Special and General Anatomy*, 1:211.

17. Horner, 1:212–15. Quote on 213.

18. Leidy, *Elementary Treatise on Human Anatomy*, 65–92. First quote on 65. Second quote on 76.

19. Leidy, 87–88. In addition to skull bones, Leidy analyzed other supposed differences on the head. He claimed that the nose, eyelids, and hair shape varied by race. The only substantial passage that Leidy included about racial traits below the neck was on the "*odifer'erous glands* of the *axilla*." Leidy, *Elementary Treatise on Human Anatomy*, 588, 595, 634, and 636–37. For more on slavery, race, and scent, see Smith, *How Race Is Made*; and Smith, "Transcending, Othering, Detecting."

20. Leidy, *Elementary Treatise on Human Anatomy*, 514. For more on how gender complicated ideas of race and intelligence, see Schiebinger, "Anatomy of Difference"; Stein, *Measuring Manhood*; and Gonaver, *Peculiar Institution*, 54–55.

21. Todd, *Descriptive and Physiological Anatomy*, 123–26. This had some precedent in France as well, dating back to the turn of the nineteenth century. Richerand, *Elements of Physiology*, 606–7.

22. Knox, *Manual of Artistic Anatomy*, 71.

23. Richardson, *Elements of Human Anatomy*, 165–68. Richardson's text was adopted by the University of Louisiana at the end of this period. *Annual Circular*, 10.

24. Lee, *Human Physiology*, 36, 75, 92; Comings, *Class-Book of Physiology*, 149. Usher Parsons also discussed facial angles and race in his introductory lecture to Brown University undergraduates in 1826, placing whites in a superior position to African Americans, whose facial angles more closely approximated those of orang-utans. Parsons, *Sciences of Anatomy and Physiology*, 27.

25. Rollin, *Martin R. Delany*, 68–69; Abraham R. Thompson and Joseph Fray [managers of the Massachusetts Colonization Society] to the Medical Faculty of Harvard College, November 1, 1850; and the Medical Faculty of Harvard College to Abraham R. Thompson, December 26, 1850, Petitions and Correspondence, Re Admission of Colored Students, CHM; Wilkinson, "1850 Harvard Medical School Dispute," 13–27; Cash, "Pride, Prejudice, and Politics," 22–24. It is not clear whether Delany made a similar agreement to leave for Liberia, but it seems likely. The school was reluctant to train Black doctors, and Delany at times showed serious interest in emigration.

26. Also worth noting, for the previous lecture, Holmes had cited Morton as the central authority. Vol. 1: notes 1850–1851, HLA. Robert Bogdan has written a helpful account of Maximo and Bartola, especially their cultural impact. That being said, much of the language he uses to describe these people reads as outdated, to say the least. Bogdan, *Freak Show*, 127–34.

27. Joseph Leidy, Envelopes 8 and 10, Notes to his Courses on Anatomy at the University of Pennsylvania, undated, College of Physicians of Philadelphia. Leidy's notes are highly disorganized and mostly undated, making it difficult to say with certainty that these are from the antebellum era. There are also multiple similar sets of notes, presumably updated every few years, making it likely that this material was representative. These facts, combined with Ellis's letter, Leidy's textbook, and William Stump Forwood's article based on education from Leidy at MDUP in the 1850s, make it clear that Leidy had a well-developed racial anatomy curriculum.

28. In the first installment of his 1857 "The Negro—a Distinct Species," published in the *Medical and Surgical Reporter*, Marylander, MDUP graduate, and former Leidy student William Stump Forwood used six of the article's ten pages to set out the perceived anatomical differences between Black and white people. In his article, Forwood called on Leidy's lectures at MDUP more than on any other authority. Forwood, "Negro—a Distinct Species," 228–31. Professors at MCSC, among other schools that have already been enumerated, also lectured on racial difference. *Annual Announcement of the Trustees and Faculty*, 11.

29. Joseph Leidy to Josiah Nott, April 18, 1855, quoted in Gobineau, *Moral and Intellectual Diversity of Races*, 480–81.

30. Thomas Dwight, typed "Reminiscences of Dr. Oliver Wendell Holmes as Professor of Anatomy . . . 190-?," Oliver Wendell Holmes Mss. and Documents, CHM. It is unlikely that this account was written in the 1900s, though. The reminiscence appears to be the typed original of an article that later appeared in *Scribner's*. Dwight, "Reminiscences of Dr. Holmes"; *Catalogue of the Officers and Students of Harvard College*, 67.

31. Holmes, *Introductory Lecture*, 32-34. First quote on 32. Second quote on 33.

32. Holmes, *Introductory Lecture*, 33; Berkowitz, *Charles Bell*, 49-60.

33. Vol. 1: notes 1850-1851, HLA; Pickering, *Races of Man*, 4-5, 187.

34. HLA.

35. The syllabus only gives a taste of what Cabell might have covered in class, as these are "the mere heads of the topics which are to be fully expounded in the oral discourses of the teacher." Cabell, *Syllabus*, iii, 58-59. First quote on 58-59, second quote on iii.

36. *Annual Announcement of the Trustees and Faculty*, 4, 7, 11. First quote on 7. Second quote on 4. Stanton, *Leopard's Spots*, 53.

37. For more on Heth, see chapter 4.

38. Bogdan, *Freak Show*, 128. For more on popular anatomy, see Sappol, *Traffic of Dead Bodies*, 168-211. For more on Maximo and Bartola in the context of the greater fetishizing of the history of pre-Columbian American civilizations in this period, see Evans, *Romancing the Maya*, 84-87.

39. Warren, "Two Remarkable Indian Dwarfs," 285. First and second quotes on 285. D. T. Brown to J. Mason Warren, December 26, 1850; and D. T. Brown to J. Mason Warren, February 5, 1851, John Collins Warren Papers, Massachusetts Historical Society, Boston. Third quote from the December 26 letter.

40. Warren, "Two Remarkable Indian Dwarfs," 285-90.

41. Warren, "Two Remarkable Indian Dwarfs," 285-91; D. T. Brown to J. Mason Warren, February 5, 1851, John Collins Warren Papers, Massachusetts Historical Society, Boston.

42. For more on Barnum, see Reiss, *Showman and the Slave*.

43. Berry, *Price for Their Pound of Flesh*, 101-7; Deetz, "Finding the Bones of Nat Turner."

44. Johnson, *River of Dark Dreams*, 21-22; Brown, *Reaper's Garden*, 135-37.

45. Kenny, "Medical Museums in the Antebellum American South," 34-38.

46. *Catalogue of Anatomical Preparations*, 135, 150, 167, 183, 188, 190-92, 194, 196. The Hunterian catalog does not give dates, so these objects represent the collection as of 1840, but anecdotal evidence proves earlier racial collecting. Winthrop Jordan discusses John Hunter's interest in racial classification of skulls. Charles White is quoted in Jordan, *White Over Black*, 498-501. White, *Account of the Regular Gradation in Man*, 61.

47. Berkowitz, *Charles Bell*, 54. Ponce, "They Increase in Beauty and Elegance," 347-49.

48. Berkowitz, *Charles Bell*, 49; John Collins Warren to J. B. S. Jackson, October 6, 1849, Records of the Warren Anatomical Museum, 1828-1892, CHM.

49. Before unpacking the record's complexity, it is worth noting that Warren Anatomical Museum curator Dominic Hall was indispensable to conducting this

research. His work at organizing the museum and its records has been phenomenal. Dominic's aid made this research possible.

Discerning how the skulls were arranged at the Warren Anatomical Museum was both an incredibly complex and simple task. On the one hand, their organization fit within contemporary racial ideas. However, a lack of clear visual or written evidence from the antebellum period made this project notably difficult. First, while antebellum handwritten catalogs of the museum exist, these were living documents created or annotated by multiple professors, including, and at least, John Collins Warren and J. B. S. Jackson. John Collins Warren had his own numbering system for the initial donation of the museum, and Jackson renumbered the objects upon their contribution in 1847, and then again in 1870 for the published catalog. The last changes were made to reconcile the addition of the artifacts from the Boston Phrenological Society and the Boston Society for Medical Improvement. This is the system still used to number items in the museum. Second, many of these catalogs are undated or have multiple dates attributed to their composition.

Third, the Warren Collection comprises at least three collections that began converging in 1847. In practice, though, the Boston Society for Medical Improvement's collections were not consolidated into the Warren Museum until the decade after their official donation in 1871, even as the Warren and phrenological collections were consolidated in the late 1840s. However, beginning in 1847, Jackson was technically curating all three collections, as he was the curator for the Warren Museum and the Boston Society for Medical Improvement's museum, which was at a separate location.

Fourth, until 2011, the Warren Anatomical Museum's records existed somewhat in a state of disorder. In 2011, archivists officially processed the collection for the Center for the History of Medicine. While they continue to refine and add to the finding aid, their work has made writing this and other histories of the museum much easier. The documents' numerous authors and unclear organization make most conclusions about the antebellum era inherently guarded. Finally, the oldest available written description of where the objects were physically placed in the museum is from 1871 (See "Designation of the Place of Each Specimen, 1871" below).

Despite these difficulties, we can have a great deal of confidence that my description of the racial skulls' organization is broadly accurate. First, from the antebellum to the progressive eras, catalogs always grouped the racial skulls together. Second, prior to their combination, all three initial museums arranged the skulls together racially. These were never random skulls used to illustrate gross anatomy. Third, the earliest and latest descriptions of the museum's spatial organization grouped the racial skulls together, further signaling their continuity as a coherent collection. The image of the Grove Street location that spanned the antebellum and postbellum period and images of a later location in Building A of the Longwood Campus also depicted the skulls together, or at least the phrenological casts in the case of Grove Street. Finally, logic dictates that a collection of skulls whose purpose was to depict racial difference would be organized in an overtly racial manner.

Here is a list of the core sources used to create this map. Because it required a cross listing of many sources that can be found on the collection's finding aid, I have tried to be as explicit and detailed as possible in describing the records that I consulted. I should thank Dominic Hall again for reading and giving feedback on this note. Any failings in the note or research are, of course, my own. Folder 7, "Catalogue of the Museum Index"; Folder 8, "Catalogue of Preparations Belonging to the Anatomical Cabinet of the Massachusetts Medical College"; "Folder 9: Catalog of the Cabinet, undated"; Folder 11, "Descriptive Catalogue of the Cabinet, Volume II, Wyman Collection, ca. 1837–1847"; Folder 12, "Descriptive Catalogue of the Cabinet, Volume 3, Wyman Collection, ca. 1847–1877"; and Folder 13, "Designation of the Place of Each Specimen, 1871," Box 10; John Collins Warren, "Catalogue of Preparations Deposited in the Massachusetts Medical College November 1st, 1847," Box 17, Collection Registration Records; "Descriptive Catalogue of the Museum of the Mass. Medical College, August 1850," Box 17; Catalog of unknown origin; "Second Catalogue," 1861; "Descriptive Catalogue of the Museum of the Mass. Medical College. 2nd Volume. January 1866"; and "WAM Volume 15 #07001–08683," all in WAMR; *Catalogue of Phrenological Specimens*; Jackson, *Descriptive Catalogue of the Anatomical Museum of the Boston Society*; Jackson, *Descriptive Catalogue of the Warren Anatomical Museum*; Warren, "Collection of the Boston Phrenological Society," 1–11.

50. Nearly any page in either catalog would uphold this practice. For example, the entry immediately following "vulva of a Black infant" was "viscera of pelvis in female infant, minutely injected." Horner, *Catalogue of the Wistar*, 11.

51. Jackson, *Descriptive Catalogue of the Warren Anatomical Museum*, 74.

52. Horner, *Catalogue of the Wistar*, 11, 33, 38.

53. Forwood, "Negro—a Distinct Species," 228–31; Jordan, *White Over Black*, 458–60.

54. The diverse provenance of these human remains will be covered in greater depth in the next chapter. Horner, *Catalogue of the Wistar*, 57.

55. Horner, *United States Dissector*, 19–25, 26–30, 31–33. First quote on 31. Second quote on 32. The first edition was published in 1823. Italics for emphasis added. Jackson, *Descriptive Catalogue of the Warren Anatomical Museum*, viii. Sappol, *Traffic of Dead Bodies*, 93–94; Berkowitz, *Charles Bell*, 61.

56. While it is no longer available, Eastman's 1854 thesis was titled "Some of the Differences between the Saxon and Negro." J. H. F. Milton to Joseph Leidy, June 29, 1860; and T. J. Eastman to Joseph Leidy, January 21, 1863, Leidy Family Papers, College of Physicians of Philadelphia; *Catalogue of the Alumni*, 51, 125.

57. Sappol, *Traffic of Dead Bodies*, 274–80; Kenny, "Medical Museums in the Antebellum American South," 38; Berkowitz, *Charles Bell*, 49.

58. McDow, "Essay on the Negro," no page number, MDUPST.

59. McDow, "Essay on the Negro," no page number.

60. McDow, "Essay on the Negro," no page number.

61. Hogarth, *Medicalizing Blackness*, 2–3. Berkowitz, *Charles Bell*, 75.

62. Newton C. Miller, "Inaugural Dissertation on the Diversity of the Human Species," 17–21, Erskind Biomedical Library, Vanderbilt University, Nashville, Tenn.

63. Westmoreland, "Inaugural Dissertation on the Anatomical and Physiological Difference," 12–16, Erskind Biomedical Library, Vanderbilt University, Nashville, Tenn. MDUP student George C. Harlan also explained, "In the negro, the iris has its share of the general excess of pigment and its hue is so dark as to be scarcely indistinguishable from that of the pupil." Harlan, "Essay on Iris," 6, MDUPST.

64. Myers, "Essay on the Human Family," 19, MDUPST.

65. Westmoreland, "Inaugural Dissertation on the Anatomical and Physiological," 13–14; Miller, "Inaugural Dissertation on the Diversity of the Human Species."

66. Gibson, "Essay on Plurality," 13, MDUPST.

67. Italics for emphasis in original. Myers, "Essay on the Human Family," 16–19, MDUPST. First quote on 16. Second quote on 17. Third, fourth, fifth, and sixth quotes on 18.

68. Myers, "Essay on the Human Family," 24–27, MDUPST. First quote on 26, Second and third quotes on 24, and fourth quote on 25. Also worth noting, there appear to have been even more theses written on racial anatomy during this period at MDUP. A number of MDUP students whose theses are no longer extant also gave their works quite provocative titles: Francis B. Carter's "Some of the Physical Peculiarities and Diseases of Southern Negroes" (1838), Thomas J. Eastman's "Some of the Differences Observed between the Saxon and Negro" (1854), David Minis Jr.'s "Special Anatomy of the Negro" (1854), and Thomas Cooper Rogers's "The Negro—a Distinct Species" (1855). *Catalogue of the Alumni*, 51, 125, 155.

69. Ball, "The Origin of the Different Human Species," no page numbers, WHL. For more on Caldwell's racial science monograph, see chapter 1. For more on Caldwell's role in popularizing phrenology, see Poskett, *Materials of the Mind*.

70. Prichard, *Natural History of Man*, 1:115–17, 339; John Bachman, excerpt from *The Doctrine of the Unity of the Human Race*, in *John Bachman: Selected Writings*, 259–60.

71. Examination Book, 1838–1841, School of Medicine, Student Records, 1828–1952, University Archives and Records Center, University of Pennsylvania, Philadelphia; *Catalogue of the Alumni*, 28.

72. "A Singular Trial—Distinction between Indians and Negroes. From the Southern (S.C.) Patriot," *Sacramento (Calif.) Union*, November 28, 1854.

73. "Singular Trial." Gibbes's testimony was also discussed in a pro-polygenesis piece written a few years later by MDUP graduate William Stump Forwood. Forwood, "Negro—a Distinct Species," 229–31. Records of MCSC's purchase of the casts are contained in correspondence with Samuel Morton. S. G. Morton to J. C. Warren, April 13, 1849, John Collins Warren Papers, Massachusetts Historical Society, Boston.

CHAPTER 5

1. "Descriptive Catalogue of the Cabinet, Volume II, Wyman Collection, ca. 1837–1847," Folder 11, Box 10, Collection Registration Records, WAMR. While the catalog does not explicitly place this head as a part of the first Opium War, the date of its entrance into the society's collection and the reason for the smugglers' beheading make this circumstance highly likely.

2. For a good introduction to the history of empire and modernity, see Streets-Salter and Getz, *Empires and Colonies*.

3. "Descriptive Catalogue of the Cabinet, Volume II, Wyman Collection, ca. 1837–1847," 284–85.

4. Fabian, *Skull Collectors*, 2–6; Kenny, "Medical Museums in the Antebellum American South," 35. In her study of Samuel G. Morton's skulls, scholar Ann Fabian reveals the international and imperialist nature of his collection, which was opportunistically tied to the violence of capitalism and colonialism. Likewise, in his study of medical museums in the antebellum South, Stephen Kenny argues that museum

curators built their exhibitions with the remains of enslaved people. In their work, Fabian and Kenny reveal how the violence of imperialism and slavery were not just the context for the rise of the medical and scientific professions, but also integral influences on their material and intellectual cultures.

5. Beckert, *Empire of Cotton*, xi–xviii. Wilder, *Ebony & Ivy*, 70–77. This literature is growing at a rapid pace, but for other examples of the new history of slavery and capitalism, see also Rosenthal, *Accounting for Slavery*; Berry, *Price for Their Pound of Flesh*; Fett, *Recaptured Africans*; and Beckert and Rockman, *Slavery's Capitalism*.

6. Rana Hogarth has shown that in the antebellum South, allopathic physicians used their self-proclaimed expertise on race as an essential tool to enhance their prestige and market institutions such as slave hospitals, training hospitals, and medical schools. *Medicalizing Blackness*, 184–86.

7. By 1822, Warren was already publishing on cranial capacity and race, as can be seen in appendix H of his monograph on the comparative anatomy of the nervous system. Warren, *Sensorial and Nervous Systems*, 129–43; Warren, "Collection of the Boston Phrenological Society," 7–9; John Collins Warren, "Catalogue of Preparations Deposited in the Massachusetts Medical College, November 1st, 1847," 1–13, Box 17, Collection Registration Records, WAMR.

8. Beckert, *Empire of Cotton*, xv.

9. Karp, *This Vast Southern Empire*, 1–8. Strang, "Violence, Ethnicity, and Human Remains," 986.

10. Skotnes, "Introduction," 19–20. See also White, "Traffic in Heads," 325–38.

11. *Catalogue of Phrenological Specimens*, 29, 39. "Object 373a" is a handwritten addition to the text. "Object 747" and "Object 1300," in "Descriptive Catalogue of the Cabinet, Volume 3, Wyman Collection, ca. 1847–1877," Folder 12, Box 10, Collection Registration Records, WAMR. This catalog does not have traditional page numbers, but the Okinawan skull is "Object 1300" and located on the page marked "1300-4." The skull is referred to as being from the island of "lew-chew." "Descriptive Catalogue of the Museum of the Mass. Medical College, August 1850," Box 17, 232, WAMR.

12. For a detailed description of my method for recreating the organizational system of the Warren Museum, see chapter 4, note 49.

13. Jackson, *Descriptive Catalogue of the Anatomical Museum of the Boston Society for Medical Improvement*, 4–10; Jackson, *Descriptive Catalogue of the Warren Anatomical Museum*, 706–7.

14. Mussey, *Anatomical Cabinet, Belonging to R. D. Mussey*, 14.

15. Unsurprisingly, the politics of these names are very complicated, with the Khoe and the San representing two different language groups. I have elected to use Khoisan, as it is one of the least problematic terms adopted by historians. Holt, "Inquiry into Hereditary Predisposition," 8, WHL; Gaffney, "Dissertation on the Psychology of Man," 7, WHL.

16. Cooke, "Inaugural Dissertation," 31, MDUPST.

17. Here, I should note that it is unclear to what degree the people that I am researching would have wanted their stories told under the best of circumstances, much less when mediated through often-racist archival documents. Yet I still believe it is essential to tell their stories, as doing so draws attention to and humanizes the violence of many modern sciences. It is my hope that greater consideration and

humanization of those exploited by science might be a route to preventing future transgressions and rethinking contemporary scientists' global impacts.

18. Strang, "Violence, Ethnicity, and Human Remains," 979–83; Brown, *Reaper's Garden*, 218; Reis, *Death Is a Festival*, 67–69.

19. Through the concept of "soul values," historian Daina Ramey Berry explains the ability of subjugated peoples to construct alternative definitions of their worth, even as whites monetized and racialized their bodies. Berry defines soul value as "an intangible marker that often defied monetization yet spoke to the spirit and soul of who they [enslaved individuals] were as human beings. It represented the self-worth of the enslaved." Berry, *Price for their Pound of Flesh*, 6.

20. These stories provide another opportunity for the "holistic retrieval of owned" people's lives in the history of medicine, as described by historian Deirdre Cooper Owens. Building on the work of Cooper Owens, as well as scholars Marisa J. Fuentes and Elise A. Mitchell, this narrative applies a similar method to the records of Harvard's racial skull collection, reincorporating back into the history of the anatomy museum the stories of a few individuals whose bodies were stolen. Fuentes, *Dispossessed Lives*, 4–7; Cooper Owens, *Medical Bondage*, 3; Mitchell, "Unbelievable Suffering." In *Materials of the Mind*, historian James Poskett at times also works to center the stories of those described by phrenologists, and in *Maladies of Empire*, Jim Downs makes a similar move, highlighting the hidden roles of enslaved and colonized people in creating the field of epidemiology.

21. Clarence, *Aborigines of South Africa*, 6–8, 23–24; Crais and Scully, *Sara Baartman and the Hottentot Venus*, 138–41. It is worth noting that Sturmann was called many variations of this name in the U.S. and South African press, and he sometimes was referred to with variations of the last name Jantjes. I have elected to call him Sturmann, because the name was common in Little Namaqualand, although typically spelled "Stuurman." Likewise, Sturmann was the name used by Walter Clarence in the exhibit promotional pamphlet. Clarence's pamphlet is the backbone of my account, and it would appear that Clarence spoke directly to Sturmann to prepare this document. Worth noting, Matthew Smith Miller, a Harvard undergraduate, wrote a fantastic bachelors thesis on the entire exhibit in 2011. Miller, "Surely His Mother Mourns." For more on the name Stuurman, see Penn, "Note on the Name Stuurman." Nigel Penn was nice enough to share this unpublished essay with me, for which I am grateful.

22. Clarence, *Aborigines of South Africa*, 6–8, 23–24. I should also thank Clifton Crais. While at Emory, I shared the account of Sturmann with him, and he set me on the path to reconstructing some of the basic facts of Sturmann's life in southern Africa. Any flaws in this account are, of course, my own fault.

23. As historian of the Khoisan in Little Namaqualand Nigel Penn explains,

Such words are also not timeless ahistorical categories but historical categories and social constructions. "Khoisan," which has become the convenient generic name for both the Khoikhoi and San peoples, implies that there is a relationship between them. The term means one thing when used in the precolonial context and another in the colonial context. In the former, the processes the word implies relate to the transition of societies or individuals from a predominantly hunting and gathering mode of existence to a predominantly pastoralist mode, and vice versa. (According to this model, if a Khoikhoi fell on hard times and lost his livestock he could revert to hunting and gathering, while a hunter-gatherer could attain the status of pastoralist by acquiring livestock.) However, the arrival of the Europeans fundamentally changed the cycle itself. It was no longer possible for either Khoikhoi or San to experience upward mobility, and the relationship between Khoikhoi and San itself was changed. The realities behind the word "Khoisan" are therefore very different in the eighteenth and in the sixteenth century. The historical records of the eighteenth century suggest that there were indeed real differences between Khoikhoi and San. . . .

The approach of this book is a pragmatic one. "Khoisan" is used when the identity of the indigenous societies is uncertain or when it is clear that both Khoikhoi and San are involved together. But that there were distinct hunter-gatherer societies, distinct from pastoralist ones, is taken as given. This is not to say that the colonists did not exaggerate San difference (or equate hostile Khoikhoi with the San) when it suited them to do so (Penn, *Forgotten Frontier*, 8–9).

24. Clarence, *Aborigines of South Africa*, 7.

25. Quoted in Skotnes, "Introduction," 17.

26. Clarence, *Aborigines of South Africa*, 7–8.

27. Clarence, *Aborigines of South Africa*, 8; "Five Native Africans," *Congregationalist* (Boston) January 15, 1861.

28. For more on Heth's case, see Reiss, *Showman and the Slave* and chapter 3 of this book.

29. "Five Native Africans."

30. "Boston Aquarial and Zoological Gardens," *Boston Evening Transcript*, October 3, 1860. The men's names were given in an earlier article by the *Transcript*. "An Extraordinary Importation from South Africa," *Boston Evening Transcript*, September 28, 1860.

31. "Suicide of a Hottentot at the Aquarial Gardens," *Boston Traveler*, April 29, 1861; "Suicide at the Aquarial Gardens," *Boston Evening Transcript*, April 29, 1861; Clarence, *Aborigines of South Africa*, 9.

32. Historical records of Khoisan religions are scant, but I am continuing to search for scholarship on Khoe beliefs about what follows death. It is also possible that Sturmann was a Christian. Penn, *Forgotten Frontier*, 5. While I caution against lumping all Khoisan beliefs together or putting too much confidence in attributing modern Khoisan beliefs to historical figures like Sturmann, anthropologist Alan Barnard asserts of contemporary Khoisan beliefs about the afterlife, "All Khoisan peoples claim belief in a high god. Some peoples attribute to him both good and evil characteristics, and others separate these characteristics, and attribute them to two beings. Some, notably the pre-Christian Damara, the !Kung, and the Khoe Bushman of the central Kalahari, say that he lives in the sky and the souls of the dead travel to his village after death and burial." Barnard, *Hunters and Herders of Southern Africa*, 252.

33. I do not bring up Central and West African beliefs on suicide to say that the Khoisan peoples shared cosmologies with these groups. Rather, these views on suicide among some Central and West Africans should caution scholars against assuming that all people shared Euro-Christian beliefs about suicide. This was clearly not the case among some African groups. Snyder, *Power to Die*, 9. Discussing suicide in the Middle Passage, historian Sowande' M. Mustakeem explains, "Fully aware of and intentional about their impending death, bondspeople willingly sought to sever the ties of slavery, end their physical existence in bondage, and gain permanent freedom." Mustakeem, *Slavery at Sea*, 107. For more on suicide in Africa, see Bohannan, *African Homicide and Suicide*.

34. "Descriptive Catalog of the Museum of the Mass. Medical College, August 1850," Box 17, 1–13, 444, WAMR.

35. Wyman, "Skeleton of a Hottentot," 330–35. Quote on 330. I also consulted a pamphlet version of this source, held at the Countway Library, but it lacks clear publication information.

36. "Descriptive Catalog of the Museum of the Mass. Medical College, August 1850," Box 17, 1–13, 444 (quote on 444), WAMR.

37. This skull was originally apart of the society's collection before merging with the Warren Museum. To avoid confusion, I often refer to the skull as being at Harvard in the text. Jackson, *Descriptive Catalogue of the Anatomical Museum of the Boston Society for Medical Improvement*, 7; "Descriptive Catalogue of the Cabinet, Volume II, Wyman Collection, ca. 1837–1847," 264, Folder 11, Box 10, Collection Registration Records, WAMR.

38. Jackson, *Descriptive Catalogue of the Anatomical Museum of the Boston Society for Medical Improvement*, 7.

39. Reis, *Slave Rebellion in Brazil*, 5–7, 94–111; Reis, *Death Is a Festival*, 25.

40. Reis, *Slave Rebellion in Brazil*, 112–19.

41. Reis, *Slave Rebellion in Brazil*, 73–92, 114–15. Quote on 114.

42. Reis, *Slave Rebellion in Brazil*, 5–7, 94–111, 118–19.

43. Jackson, *Descriptive Catalogue of the Warren Anatomical Museum*, 702; "Designation of the Place of Each Specimen, 1871," 127–30, Box 10, Folder 13, WAM.

CHAPTER 6

1. McDow, "Essay on the Negro," no page numbers, MDUPST.

2. McDow, "Essay on the Negro," no page numbers.

3. Stepan, *Picturing Tropical Nature*, 16–17.

4. Cartwright, "Extract of a Letter to the Editor," 73; Samuel Morton, Journal, 1833–ca. 1837, SGMP; Pickering, *Races of Man*.

5. Italics for emphasis in original. Jeffries Wyman to Elizabeth A. Wyman, November 9, 1844, and October 12, 1844, JWP.

6. Jeffries Wyman to Elizabeth A. Wyman, December 24, 1844, JWP.

7. Jeffries Wyman to Elizabeth A. Wyman, November 18, 1847, JWP. For an annotated transcription of this letter focused on Saamaka history and other excerpts from Wyman's writings about his trip among the Saamaka, See Price and Willoughby, "Harvard Physician's Reports."

8. Diary entries from April 5, 11, and 14, 1857 (quote from April 14), vol. 1, JWP.

9. Jeffries Wyman to Morrill Wyman, April 15, 1857, JWP.

10. Diary entry, April 5, 1857, vol. 2, JWP.

11. Diary entry, March 3, 1857, vol. 2, JWP; Jeffries Wyman to Morrill Wyman, April 15, 1857, JWP.

12. Diary entries, April 14 and 22, 1857, vol. 2, JWP; diary entry, April 27, 1857, vol. 2, JWP.

13. Diary entry, April 27 and May 1, 1857, vol. 2, JWP.

14. Jeffries Wyman to Elizabeth A. Wyman, May 19, 1857, JWP. While Wyman did not describe the Maroon community as Saamaka, they, among other related groups, were certainly the people he was visiting. He named the "great captain" as Joannis Arabbi, who might have been a descendant of Johannis Arabie mentioned by Richard Price. Likewise, Price shows that Saamaka villages were along the Suriname River, where Wyman traveled. Price, *Alabi's World*, xiii, 229.

15. Jeffries Wyman to Elizabeth A. Wyman, May 19, 1857, JWP.

CHAPTER 7

1. Henry, "Essay on Bilious Fever," 16–17, MDUPST; Daughtry, "Essay on Febris Remittens," 3, MDUPST; Smith, "Essay on Bilious Remittent Fever," no page numbers, MDUPST. Parts of this chapter were originally printed as an article in the *Journal of the History of Medicine and Allied Sciences*. See Willoughby, "'His Native, Hot Country,'" 328–51.

2. Fett, *Recaptured Africans*, 31; Sinha, *Counterrevolution of Slavery*, 125–27; Horne, *Deepest South*, 107–10; Karp, *This Vast Southern Empire*.

3. Attempting to compete with perceptions of Black people's natural resistance to tropical diseases, some whites even attempted to contract tropical ailments. They believed doing so would acclimate them to the local environment, and some white doctors even encouraged such practices, hoping to increase and whiten local labor markets. Olivarius, "Immunity, Capital, and Power."

4. For Rush's theory of Blackness as a form of leprosy, see Elijah Griffiths, Notes from Dr. Rush's Lectures, 1797–1798 Session, vol. 2, College of Physicians of Philadelphia; Rush, "Black Color (as It Is Called) of the Negroes," 289–97; and Warner, *Therapeutic Perspective*, 58–59.

5. Historian Melissa Stein argues that this was true through the history of racial science in the nineteenth and twentieth centuries, asserting, "The sciences of race, from ethnology to eugenics, were fundamentally applied sciences." Stein, *Measuring Manhood*, 262.

6. Valenčius, *Health of the Country*, 236.

7. Rush, "Black Color (as It Is Called) of the Negroes," 297.

8. Rush, *Medical Inquiries and Observations*, 2:428. In 1809 MDUP student Thomas Harris explained, "Hence I would Infer that the difference of colour in the human species is entirely dependent on the climate in which they live, and not to any specific difference in the original stamina. Negro children, those considerably white at birth, become Black when exposed to the solar rays, and I am inclined to believe they would continue so, even if practicable for them to live without being exposed to the light."

Harris, "Stimulating and Nutritive Effects of Light," no page numbers, MDUPST. One student in the 1820s pushed a similar narrative of racial formation, explaining, "The cause of a change in man, is his mode of life, climate, diet, dress, and all the variety which enter into the means of man's support." Holt, "Inquiry into the Hereditary Predisposition," no page numbers, WHL. Rush, "Black Color (as It Is Called) of the Negroes," 296–97. Conevery Valenčius argues that by the antebellum era, monogenists and polygenists viewed race and environment in largely similar ways, explaining, "And no matter how they posited racial origins or environmental causality, few in the white majority questioned the main conclusion that human peoples intrinsically belonged to the locales for which they were suited." Valenčius, *Health of the Country*, 236.

9. Rush divided stimuli on the body into "external" and "internal forces." He explained, "The external are light, sound, odours, air, heat, exercise, and the pleasures of the senses. The internal stimuli are food, drinks, chyle, the blood, a certain tension of the glands, which contain secreted liquors, and the exercise of the faculties of the mind." Rush, *Medical Inquiries and Observations*, 2:378–83. Quote in note on 378, first quote in text on 378, and second quote in text on 382.

10. Rush, *Medical Inquiries*, 2:395–96.

11. William E. Horner, Lecture Notes, 1813, 27 (first quote), 309 (second quote), College of Physicians of Philadelphia.

12. Cartwright, "Slavery in the Light of Ethnology," 722–24. Rush was also an important figure in the Philadelphia Abolition Society, helping write its constitution in 1787 and freeing his only enslaved laborer in 1788. Nash, *Forging Freedom*.

13. Altschuler, "From Blood Vessels to Global Networks of Exchange," 216. Discussing Jamaica, historian Sasha Turner highlights how many British abolitionists understood ending the slave trade as a part of larger imperial schemes to civilize non-whites. *Contested Bodies*, 20, 28–37.

14. Finger, *Contagious City*, 129; Nash, *Forging Freedom*, 122.

15. Bryant, "Inaugural Dissertation on Tetanus," 1–2, MDUPST; Hugh Holmes McGuire echoed Bryant's position on tetanus in his 1822 thesis, McGuire, "Tetanus," no page numbers, MDUPST. See also Boyd, "Dissertation on Typhus Fever," MDUPST; Cook, "Sketch of the Autumnal Fever," MDUPST; Ashmead, "Tetanus," MDUPST; Heston, "Inaugural Essay on Tetanus," MDUPST; Milligan, "Inaugural Dissertation on Tetanus," WHL.

16. Heston, "Inaugural Essay on Tetanus."

17. Waring, "Inaugural Dissertation on Typhus Gravior," no page numbers, WHL; Toole, "Dissertation on Typhoid Fever," 24, WHL; Fishburne, "Inaugural Dissertation on Enteric Fever," 13–14, WHL.

18. Dickson, *Essays on Life, Sleep, Pain, Etc.*, 236. For Dickson on racial science and slavery, see his *Remarks on Certain Topic*.

19. Boyd, "Inaugural Dissertation on Hydrops," no page numbers, WHL (first quote); Warner, *Therapeutic Perspective*, 58–59; Dickson, *Elements of Medicine*, 24 (second quote).

20. Warner, *Therapeutic Perspective*, 69–75.

21. Warner, *Against the Spirit of System*, 180–82, 282–83.

22. Karp, *This Vast Southern Empire*, 6–7.

23. Lewis, "Essay on Difficulties," 5–9, MDUPST. Quote on 5.

24. Radbill, *Samuel Henry Dickson*, 282–86; S. H. Dickson Memoranda Book, 1824–1860, WHL.

25. Dickson, *Syllabus*, 51.

26. See Dickson's *Essays on Life, Sleep, Pain, Etc.* as described on the preceding page and his *Remarks on Certain Topics*.

27. Dickson, *Syllabus*, 88. For more on the environment, slavery, yellow fever, and malaria during this period, see Willoughby, *Yellow Fever, Race, and Ecology*, and McCandless, *Slavery, Disease, and Suffering*.

28. Dickson, *On Dengue*, 12–13; Osgood, "Remarks on the Dengue," 562.

29. Dickson, *Syllabus*, 98.

30. Drake, *Letters on Slavery to Dr. John C. Warren*, 65 (first quote), 66 (second quote). For more on Lugenbeel, see Clegg, *Price of Liberty*, 176–79.

31. Stein, *Measuring Manhood*, 41–42. Notably, two scholars have broken this mold in their treatment of Nott, depicting him as a complicated scientist whose views were deeply rooted in contemporary culture. See Keel, "Religion, Polygenism, and the Early Science of Human Origins," 3–32; and Horsman, *Josiah Nott of Mobile*. Nott and Gliddon, *Indigenous Races of the Earth*, 354.

32. Nott and Gliddon, *Indigenous Races of the Earth*, 356–66. Quote on 356.

33. Nott and Gliddon, *Indigenous Races of the Earth*, 356–66. First and second quotes on 366. James E. Nott to John Collins Warren, April 27, 1845, John Collins Warren Papers, Massachusetts Historical Society, Boston. In discussing physicians in British India during this period, historian Mark Harrison reveals a similar trend. There, physicians viewed local observations as in conversation with a transnational discourse on natural history, and they embraced a polygenesis-inspired version of environmental determinism. Harrison, *Climates and Constitutions*, 220–25.

34. Italics for emphasis in original. Nott and Gliddon, *Indigenous Races of the Earth*, 368.

35. Quoted in Nott and Gliddon, *Indigenous Races of the Earth*, 380. For more on disease, medicine, and slavery in West Africa and the slave trade, see Barcia, *Yellow Demon of Fever*.

36. For more on race and health in the age of empire, see Espinosa, *Epidemic Invasions*; Sutter, "Nature's Agents or Agents of Empire?"; Anderson, *Colonial Pathologies*; Downs, *Maladies of Empire*; Harrison, *Climates and Constitutions*; and Savitt, *Medicine and Slavery*.

37. Nott and Gliddon, *Indigenous Races of the Earth*, 357–58, 366, 371–372.

38. Nott and Gliddon, *Indigenous Races of the Earth*, 374–76.

39. Johnson, *River of Dark Dreams*, 14–15. Nancy Stepan makes a similar claim, stating, "From the 1830s on, Latin America was considered part of the 'manifest destiny' of the United States." Stepan, *Picturing Tropical Nature*, 92.

40. Nott and Gliddon, *Indigenous Races of the Earth*, 374.

41. Nott and Gliddon, *Indigenous Races of the Earth*, 393.

42. Nott and Gliddon, *Indigenous Races of the Earth*, 379.

43. Nott and Gliddon, *Indigenous Races of the Earth*, 371–72.

44. Kvach, *"De Bow's Review,"* 42–44.

45. Nott and Gliddon, *Indigenous Races of the Earth*, 399.

46. Italics for emphasis in original. Nott and Gliddon, *Indigenous Races of the Earth*, 400.

47. Nott and Gliddon, *Indigenous Races of the Earth*, 401.

48. Knox, *Races of Men*, 210.

49. Dunn, "Inaugural Essay on Tetanus," no page numbers, MDUPST; Wood, *Treatise on the Practice of Medicine*, 2:789.

50. Bull, "Thesis on Tetanus," no page numbers, WHL. Bull, however, was slightly more confident in the cause of the disproportionate number of cases of tetanus among Black people. Most students agreed that Black people contracted the ailment more often than whites, and unlike Bull or earlier students, they largely avoided providing a causational narrative for this disparity. Lassiter, "Thesis on Tetanus," 18, WHL; Hoof, "Essay on Tetanus," 18, MDUPST; Pope, "Tetanus," 20, WHL; Fleming, "Essay on Tetanus," 11–12, MDUPST; Miller, "Essay on Tetanus," 15, MDUPST.

51. Historian Melissa Stein explores the concept of the "social doctor" in her discussion of turn-of-the-twentieth-century sexologists who were "optimistic about science's potential to reform society." Stein, *Measuring Manhood*, 237.

52. Nott and Gliddon, *Indigenous Races of the Earth*, 363–64.

53. Quoted in Nott and Gliddon, *Indigenous Races of the Earth*, 380.

54. Smith, "Essay on Bilious Remittent Fever," no page numbers, MDUPST.

55. The figures are based on a spreadsheet that I compiled from reading all of the antebellum manuscript medical theses from MCSC and MDUP, totaling more than 4,000 individual essays. To give a bit more information on the scope of these collections and how race is depicted in them, MDUP's collection contains 2,244 theses (1807–61), and MCSC has 1,900 theses (1825–60). Race is most often discussed in theses about specific ailments (also the most common type of thesis in general), the top six being malaria / bilious fever, typhoid/ typhus fever, pneumonia, yellow fever, intermittent fever, and tetanus. MDUPST; Medical College of South Carolina Student Theses, WHL.

56. Bonner, "Malaria," 15–16, MDUPST; Horn, "Inaugural Dissertation on the Subject Is Yellow Fever Contagious," no page numbers, WHL.

57. Fishburne, "Inaugural Dissertation on Enteric Fever," 13, WHL. Many students commenting on typhoid fever shared this measured approach; Fladger, "Inaugural Dissertation on Typhoid Fever," 1, WHL; Dade, "Inaugural Dissertation on Typhus Fever," 8–9, WHL; Cunningham, "Dissertation on Typhoid Fever," 9, WHL.

58. Dawson, "Essay on the Theory of Cholera," no page numbers, MDUPST; Unknown Author, "Epidemic Cholera—Cholera Asphyxia," no page numbers, WHL; Cuckow, "Essay on Cholera," 9, WHL.

59. Theses on dysentery that are skeptical or undecided about the cause of these differing rates of contracting the illness include Weston, "Dissertation on Epidemic Dysentery," 4–5, WHL; Cowell, "Essay on Acute Dysentery," 14, MDUPST; and Galphin, "Inaugural Dissertation on Dysentery," no page numbers, WHL.

60. Snow, "Inaugural Dissertation on Menstruation," 2–3, WHL; Weathersbee, "Treatise on Menstruation," 4, WHL.

61. Schwartz, *Birthing a Slave*, 75–81. For more students on race and menstruation, see Brabham, "Inaugural Dissertation on Menstruation," WHL; and Murchison, "Inaugural Dissertation on Amenorrhoea," WHL.

62. Paxson, "Inaugural Dissertation on Pneumonia Typhodes," no page numbers, MDUPST. Du Bose, "Inaugural Dissertation on Pneumonia Propria," 3, WHL.

63. Mellichamp, "On the Causes of Insanity," no page numbers, WHL. For more on the history of theories of slavery and mental health, see Myers, "'Drapetomania'"; Fett, *Working Cures*; and McCandless, *Moonlight, Magnolias, & Madness*.

64. Mellichamp, "On the Causes of Insanity."

65. Miller, "Remarks on Insanity," no page numbers, WHL.

66. Mellichamp, "On the Causes of Insanity."

67. O'Sullivan, "Dyspepsia," 1, MDUPST.

68. Furse, "Inaugural Dissertation on Dyspepsia," 7–8, WHL.

69. Nott and Gliddon, *Indigenous Races of the Earth*, 368.

70. Nott and Gliddon, *Indigenous Races of the Earth*, 369; Savitt, *Medicine and Slavery*, 12–14.

71. McCloud, "Hints on the Medical Treatment of Negroes," 21, WHL.

72. Carter, "Essay on Empresma Pulmonitis," no page numbers, WHL.

73. Westmoreland, "Inaugural Dissertation on the Anatomical and Physiological," 26, Erskind Biomedical Library, Vanderbilt University, Nashville, Tenn.; McCloud, "Medical Treatment of Negroes," 17; Carter, "Empresma Pulmonitis"; Jerman, "Essay on Pneumonia," 17, WHL; Fuller, "Treatise on Pneumonia," 13, WHL; Freeman, "Thesis on Pneumonia," 32–33, WHL; Brickell, "Essay on Typhoid Pneumonia," 45, MDUPST; Huger, "Dissertation on the Medical Topography," no page numbers, WHL; Smith, "Inaugural Thesis on Climacterical Influences," 33, WHL; and McPheeters, "Essay on Pneumonia," 18, MDUPST.

74. McCloud, "Medical Treatment of Negroes," 3, 10; G. H. Wikoff, "Copy of a *Course of Medical Lectures Delivered by Nathaniel Chapman*," 2 vols., 1843, 1:53, College of Physicians of Philadelphia. It is unclear whether Wikoff was the actual writer of the quote, although he certainly made the original copy of Chapman's lectures. Wikoff did attend MDUP, but numerous students seem to have possessed these notes at various points.

75. Smith, "Inaugural Thesis on Climacterical Influences," 27–28.

76. Cheves, "Some Remarks upon Hereditary Tendencies," no page numbers, WHL; McDow, "Essay on the Negro," no page numbers, MDUPST.

77. Cheves, "Some Remarks upon Hereditary Tendencies," no page numbers.

78. Cheves, "Some Remarks upon Hereditary Tendencies," no page numbers.

EPILOGUE

1. Charles R. Pryor to Joseph Leidy, March 12, 1861, JLP; "Thomas Jefferson on Secession," *Dallas Herald*, March 13, 1861.

2. Francis S. Holmes to Joseph Leidy, January 7, 1861; and William A. B. Norcom to Joseph Leidy, April 30, 1866, JLC.

3. Josiah Nott to Ephraim G. Squier, May 3, 1861, E. G. Squier Papers (Microfilm), Library of Congress, Washington, D.C.; William Stump Forwood to Samuel Cartwright, May 13, 1861, WSFP.

4. J. Edwards Holbrook to Joseph Leidy, February 24, 1861, JLC.

5. Francis S. Holmes to Joseph Leidy, December 9, 1865, JLC.

6. Josiah Nott to Joseph Leidy, September 19, 1866, JLC.

7. Horsman, *Josiah Nott of Mobile*, 310–21.

8. James L. Cabell to Jeffries Wyman, March 2, 1868, JWP.

9. For an effective synthesis of this history of medical experimentation on Black people, see Washington, *Medical Apartheid*. Likewise, Terence Keel has illustrated the enduring effects of polygenesis on medical thought after the Darwinian revolution. Keel, "Charles V. Roman and the Spectre of Polygenism," 742–66.

10. For more on the history of craniometry and skull collecting after the Civil War, see Redman, *Bone Rooms*.

11. Charles Darwin to Joseph Leidy, March 4, 1860, JLC; Warren, *Joseph Leidy*, 272n5.

12. Hollingsworth Neill, "Some Anatomical Peculiarities of the Negro" (M.D. thesis, University of Pennsylvania, 1874), 10–15, MDUPST.

13. Neill, "Some Anatomical Peculiarities," 17.

14. Neill, "Some Anatomical Peculiarities," 24.

15. Humphreys, *Marrow of Tragedy*, 6–8. See also Devine, *Learning from the Wounded*. Humphreys and Devine do a great deal to complicate the history of the Civil War as medical progress, but both accounts ultimately depict the period as in many ways a great break with the previous era of medical practice. Likewise, Humphreys and Jim Downs have both shown that inferior medical practice on Black people was often a characteristic of the war. Humphreys, *Intensely Human*, 7–11. Downs, *Sick from Freedom*, 4.

16. Worth noting, records of Holmes's lectures do not exist for every term. The 1871–72 and 1875–76 sessions are the only postbellum ones where Holmes kept lecture notes and did not mention racial science. Holmes Lectures on Anatomy, 1850–1882, HLA; "WAM Volume 15 #07001–08683," WAMR.

17. Redman, *Bone Rooms*, 18; Schwalm, "Black Bodies, Medical Science, and the Age of Emancipation."

18. "WAM Volume 15 #07001–08683."

19. Delany, *Principia of Ethnology*, ix–1.

20. Bay, *White Image in the Black Mind*, 96–97; Du Bois, *Health and Physique of the Negro American*.

21. For more on race, science, and medicine in the twentieth century, see Stein, *Measuring Manhood*; Yudell, *Race Unmasked*; Reverby, *Examining Tuskegee*; Dorr, *Segregation's Science*; Washington, *Medical Apartheid*; Anderson, *Colonial Pathologies*; Wailoo, *Dying in the City of Blues*; and Jones, *Bad Blood*.

22. Polk, *Contagions of Empire*, 13–76. See also Espinosa, *Epidemic Invasions*.

23. Anderson, *Colonial Pathologies*, 1–12. See also Kramer, *Blood of Government*.

24. Willoughby, *Yellow Fever, Race, and Ecology*, 157–60.

25. Shah, *Body Hunters*.

26. Hoffman et al., "Racial Bias in Pain Assessment and Treatment Recommendations," 4296–4301. Quote on 4298. According to the article's informetric (accessed November 1, 2020), the study had been "picked up by 274 news outlets," https://www.pnas.org/content/early/2016/03/30/1516047113/tab-article-info.

27. Hoffman et al., "Racial Bias in Pain Assessment and Treatment Recommendations," 4296–4301. First quote on 4299 and second quote on 4300.

BIBLIOGRAPHY

ARCHIVAL SOURCES
Boston, Mass.
  Center for the History of Medicine, Francis A. Countway Library of
        Medicine, Harvard Medical School
    Benjamin Waterhouse Papers
    Holmes Lectures on Anatomy, 1850–1882
    Jeffries Wyman Papers
    Oliver Wendell Holmes Mss. and Documents
    Petitions and Correspondence, Re Admission of Colored Students
    Records of the Warren Anatomical Museum, 1828–1892
    Warren Anatomical Museum Records, 1835–2010
  Massachusetts Historical Society
    John Collins Warren Papers
Cambridge, Mass.
  University Archives, Harvard University
    Wyman Family Papers
Chapel Hill, N.C.
  Southern Historical Collection, Louis Round Wilson Library, University of North
        Carolina at Chapel Hill
    William Stump Forwood Papers
Charleston, S.C.
  Waring Historical Library, Medical University of South Carolina
    Medical College of South Carolina Theses
      Ball, Dyer. "The Origin of the Different Human Species." M.D. thesis,
        Medical College of South Carolina, 1837.
      Boyd, William D. "An Inaugural Dissertation on Hydrops." M.D. thesis,
        Medical College of South Carolina, 1830.
      Brabham, S. J. "An Inaugural Dissertation on Menstruation." M.D. thesis,
        Medical College of South Carolina, 1856.
      Bull, W. J., Jr. "A Thesis on Tetanus." M.D. thesis, Medical College of South
        Carolina, 1860.
      Caffey, John. "A Thesis on Calomel in Southern Fevers." M.D. thesis,
        Medical College of South Carolina, 1839.
      Carter, Benjamin F. "An Essay on Empresma Pulmonitis." M.D. thesis,
        Medical College of South Carolina, 1852.
      Cheves, R. N. "Some Remarks upon Hereditary Tendencies." M.D. thesis,
        Medical College of South Carolina, 1852.
      Cleckley, James D. "A Dissertation on the Modus Operandi of Emetics."
        M.D. thesis, Medical College of South Carolina, 1854.

Compton, W. P., "An Inaugural Treatise on Iodine." M.D. thesis, Medical College of South Carolina, 1844.

Cuckow, William K. "An Essay on Cholera." M.D. thesis, Medical College of South Carolina, 1826.

Cunningham, William Augustus. "A Dissertation on Typhoid Fever." M.D. thesis, Medical College of South Carolina, 1856.

Dade, Robert F. "An Inaugural Dissertation on Typhus Fever." M.D. thesis, Medical College of South Carolina, 1842.

Du Bose, McNeely. "An Inaugural Dissertation on Pneumonia Propria." M.D. thesis, Medical College of South Carolina, 1854.

Fishburne, Benjamin C. "An Inaugural Dissertation on Enteric Fever." M.D. thesis, Medical College of South Carolina, 1856.

Fladger, R. B. "An Inaugural Dissertation on Typhoid Fever." M.D. thesis, Medical College of South Carolina, 1853.

Freeman, W. C. "A Thesis on Pneumonia." M.D. thesis, Medical College of South Carolina, 1856.

Fuller, William. "A Treatise on Pneumonia." M.D. thesis, Medical College of South Carolina, 1857.

Furse, George C. "An Inaugural Dissertation on Dyspepsia." M.D. thesis, Medical College of South Carolina, 1842.

Gaffney, Joseph G. "A Dissertation on the Psychology of Man." M.D. thesis, Medical College of South Carolina, 1836.

Galphin, George. "An Inaugural Dissertation on Dysentery." M.D. thesis, Medical College of South Carolina, 1831.

Higgins, C. Caldwell. "An Inaugural Dissertation on Cutaneous Absorption." M.D. thesis, Medical College of South Carolina, 1846.

Holt, Samuel D. "An Inquiry into Hereditary Predisposition of Mind and Body." M.D. thesis, Medical College of South Carolina, 1827.

Horn, Peter L. "An Inaugural Dissertation on the Subject Is Yellow Fever Contagious." M.D. thesis, Medical College of South Carolina, 1860.

Huger, William Harleston. "A Dissertation on the Medical Topography of St. John's Berkley." M.D. thesis, Medical College of South Carolina, 1849.

Jerman, J. P. "An Essay on Pneumonia." M.D. thesis, Medical College of South Carolina, 1849.

Lassiter, Craven. "A Thesis on Tetanus." M.D. thesis, Medical College of South Carolina, 1853.

Leak, Jeremiah F. "A Thesis on the Modus Operandi of Medicines." M.D. thesis, Medical College of South Carolina, 1851.

McCloud, Moses. "Hints on the Medical Treatment of Negroes." M.D. thesis, Medical College of South Carolina, 1850.

Mellichamp, Joseph Hinson. "On the Causes of Insanity in the United States." M.D. thesis, Medical College of South Carolina, 1852.

Miller, William C. "Remarks on Insanity." M.D. thesis, Medical College of South Carolina, 1845.

Milligan, Joseph. "An Inaugural Dissertation on Tetanus." M.D. thesis, Medical College of South Carolina, 1826.

Murchison, A. A. "An Inaugural Dissertation on Amenorrhoea." M.D. thesis, Medical College of South Carolina, 1860.

Phillips, Josiah. "An Inaugural Dissertation on the Modus Operandi of Opium." M.D. thesis, Medical College of South Carolina, 1843.

Pope, Daniel T. "Tetanus." M.D. thesis, Medical College of South Carolina, 1860.

Raysor, William A. "Inaugural Dissertation on the Modus Operandi of Cathartics and Their Therapeutical Application to Diseases." M.D. thesis, Medical College of South Carolina, 1852.

Smith, J. Calvin. "An Inaugural Thesis on Climacterical Influences." M.D. thesis, Medical College of South Carolina, 1848.

Snow, Lewellyn E. "An Inaugural Dissertation on Menstruation." M.D. thesis, Medical College of South Carolina, 1857.

Thornton, John Hancock. "An Inaugural Dissertation upon Iodine." M.D. thesis, Medical College of South Carolina, 1847.

Toole, E. G. "A Dissertation on Typhoid Fever." M.D. thesis, Medical College of South Carolina, 1855.

Unknown author. "Epidemic Cholera—Cholera Asphyxia." M.D. thesis, Medical College of South Carolina, 1832.

Waring, Morton, Jr. "An Inaugural Dissertation on Typhus Gravior." M.D. thesis, Medical College of South Carolina, 1830.

Weathersbee, W. "A Treatise on Menstruation." M.D. thesis, Medical College of South Carolina, 1855.

Weston, A. G. "A Dissertation on Epidemic Dysentery as It Existed in South Alabama in 1851-2." M.D. thesis, Medical College of South Carolina, 1853.

Minutes of the Medical Society of South Carolina

Lexington, Ky.

Special Collections Department, J. Douglas Gay Jr. / Francis Carrick Thomas Library, Transylvania University

Addams, Abraham. "An Inaugural Dissertation on the Internal Changes Produced by the Operation of the Remote Causes of Fever." M.D. thesis, Medical Department of Transylvania University, 1828.

Louisville, Ky.

History Collections, Kornhauser Health Sciences Library, University of Louisville

David Pusey Papers

Nashville, Tenn.

Erskind Biomedical Library, Vanderbilt University

Miller, Newton C. "An Inaugural Dissertation on the Diversity of the Human Species." M.D. thesis, University of Nashville, 185[?].

Westmoreland, Theophilis. "An Inaugural Dissertation on the Anatomical and Physiological Differences in the Ethiopian and White Man." M.D. thesis, University of Nashville, 1855.

New York, N.Y.

Archives and Special Collections, August C. Long Health Sciences Library,
Columbia University

Drake, Charles. Notes on Smith's Anatomy Lectures, 1812–1813.

Taulman, John. Lecture Notes, 1812–1813 Session.

New York Historical Society

Titus Munson Coan Papers

Philadelphia, Pa.

Academy of Natural Sciences of Drexel University

Joseph Leidy Memorial Albums

Joseph Leidy Papers

P. A. Browne Hair Albums

American Philosophical Society

Samuel George Morton Letters (Microfilm)

Samuel George Morton Papers

College of Physicians of Philadelphia

Barton, Benjamin Smith. "Notes from Dr. Barton's Lectures on Natural
History, or Zoology, 1809–1810."

Carson, Joseph. History of the Medical Department of the University of
Pennsylvania Scrapbooks.

Griffiths, Elijah. Notes from Dr. Rush's Lectures, 1797–1798 Session.

Horner, William E. Lecture Notes, 1813.

Joseph Leidy Papers

Leidy Family Papers

Leidy, Joseph. Notes to his Courses on Anatomy at the University of
Pennsylvania.

Wikoff, G. H. "A Copy of a *Course of Medical Lectures Delivered by Nathaniel
Chapman*." 2 vols.

Kislak Center for Special Collections, Rare Books and Manuscripts, Van Pelt
Library, University of Pennsylvania

Medical Department of the University of Pennsylvania Theses

Ashmead, Theodore. "Tetanus." M.D. thesis, University of Pennsylvania,
1822.

Bettner, George S. "An Inaugural Essay on Ulceration of the Intestines."
M.D. thesis, University of Pennsylvania, 1828.

Bonner, J. P. "Malaria." M.D. thesis, University of Pennsylvania, 1850.

Boyd, John C. "A Dissertation on Typhus Fever." M.D. thesis, University of
Pennsylvania, 1820.

Brickell, William Edwin. "An Essay on Typhoid Pneumonia." M.D. thesis,
University of Pennsylvania, 1853.

Bryant, Thomas. "An Inaugural Dissertation on Tetanus." M.D. thesis,
University of Pennsylvania, 1807.

Carrington, William W. "An Inaugural Essay on Hydrophobia." M.D.
thesis, University of Pennsylvania, 1828.

Caruthers, John W. "An Essay on Emetics and Their Mode of Action." M.D.
thesis, University of Pennsylvania, 1857.

Cook, James. "A Sketch of the Autumnal Fever, as It Prevailed in the Town of Fredericksburg, Virginia, 1821." M.D. thesis, University of Pennsylvania, 1822.

Cooke, Singleton Jones. "An Inaugural Dissertation on the Mechanism and Physiology of the Human Head." M.D. thesis, University of Pennsylvania, 1829.

Cowell, William H. "An Essay on Acute Dysentery." M.D. thesis, University of Pennsylvania, 1855.

Daughtry, William Henry. "An Essay on Febris Remittens." M.D. thesis, University of Pennsylvania, 1855.

Dawson, John. "An Essay on the Theory of Cholera Asiatic Epidemics." M.D. thesis, University of Pennsylvania, 1848.

Dunn, Theophilus C. "An Inaugural Essay on Tetanus." M.D. thesis, University of Pennsylvania, 1821.

Fleming, Albert Wayne. "An Essay on Tetanus." M.D. thesis, University of Pennsylvania, 1860.

Gambel, William. "An Essay on Organic Forms or Species." M.D. thesis, University of Pennsylvania, 1848.

Gibson, Tully S. "An Essay on Plurality of Origin of the Races." M.D. thesis, University of Pennsylvania, 1855.

Gwathmey, William. "Cholera Infantum, an Essay." M.D. thesis, University of Pennsylvania, 1819.

Harlan, George C. "An Essay on Iris." M.D. thesis, University of Pennsylvania, 1858.

Harris, Thomas. "Stimulating and Nutritive Effects of Light." M.D. thesis, University of Pennsylvania, 1809.

Hayley, L. B. "An Essay on Thesis." M.D. thesis, University of Pennsylvania, 1860.

Henry, T. G. "An Essay on Bilious Fever." M.D. thesis, University of Pennsylvania, 1851.

Heston, Gilbert. "An Inaugural Essay on Tetanus." M.D. thesis, University of Pennsylvania, 1825.

Hoof, James H. "An Essay on Tetanus." M.D. thesis, University of Pennsylvania, 1859.

Lewis, Joel B. "An Essay on Difficulties Attending the Practice of Medicine in the Country at the South." M.D. thesis, University of Pennsylvania, 1860.

McDow, John Ramsay. "An Essay on the Negro and the White Man." M.D. thesis, University of Pennsylvania, 1855.

McGuire, Hugh Holmes. "Tetanus." M.D. thesis, University of Pennsylvania, 1822.

McPheeters, William A. "An Essay on Pneumonia." M.D. thesis, University of Pennsylvania, 1855.

Miller, George W. "An Essay on Tetanus." M.D. thesis, University of Pennsylvania, 1860.

Morrill, Henry Edwin. "An Essay on the Formation of Medical Character." M.D. thesis, University of Pennsylvania, 1840.

Myers, Arthur B. "An Essay on the Human Family—Diversities and Causes of Those Diversities." M.D. thesis, University of Pennsylvania, 1857.

Neill, Hollingsworth. "Some Anatomical Peculiarities of the Negro." M.D. thesis, University of Pennsylvania, 1874.

O'Sullivan, John J. "Dyspepsia." M.D. thesis, University of Pennsylvania, 1827.

Paxson, William A. "An Inaugural Dissertation on Pneumonia Typhodes." M.D. thesis, University of Pennsylvania, 1817.

Schaffer, Charles. "An Essay on Experiments on the Heart's Action." M.D. thesis, University of Pennsylvania, 1859.

Smith, Elliott. "An Essay on Bilious Remittent Fever." M.D. thesis, University of Pennsylvania, 1857.

University Archives and Records Center, University of Pennsylvania
    School of Medicine, Student Records, 1828–1952
    William Edmonds Horner Papers
Washington, D.C.
    Library of Congress
        E. G. Squier Papers (Microfilm)

NEWSPAPERS

Boston Daily Atlas
Boston Evening Transcript
Boston Investigator
Boston Traveler
Congregationalist (Boston)
Daily Advertiser (New York, N.Y.)
Daily National Intelligencer (Washington, D.C.)
Daily National Journal (Washington, D.C.)
Dallas Herald
Evening Post (New York, N.Y.)
Herald (New York, N.Y.)
Liberator (Boston)
Louisiana Advertiser
Newport (R.I.) Mercury
New York Tribune
Pennsylvania Chronicle, and Universal Advertiser
Raleigh Register, and North-Carolina State Gazette
Sacramento (Calif.) Union
Southern Patriot (Charleston, S.C.)
United States Telegraph (Washington, D.C.)
Virginia Free Press

PRINTED PRIMARY SOURCES

Annual Announcement of the Trustees and Faculty of the Medical College of the State of South Carolina for the Session of 1840–41. Charleston, S.C.: Burges & James, 1840.

Annual Circular of the Medical Department of the University of Louisiana. Session of 1859-60. New Orleans: Picayune Print, 1859.

Bachman, John. *The Doctrine of the Unity of the Human Race Examined on the Principles of Science.* Charleston, S.C.: C. Canning, 1850.

———. *John Bachman: Selected Writings on Science, Race, and Religion.* Edited by Gene Waddell. Athens: University of Georgia Press, 2011.

———. "A Reply to the Letter of Samuel George Morton, M.D., on the Question of Hybridity in Animals Considered in Reference to the Unity of the Human Species." *Charleston Medical Journal and Review* 5, no. 4 (July 1850): 466–508

———. "Second Letter to Samuel G. Morton, M.D., on the Question of Hybridity in Animals, Considered in Reference to the Unity of the Human Species." *Charleston Medical Journal and Review* 5, no. 5 (September 1850): 621–60.

Baldwin, H. R. "Unity of the Human Race." *Medical & Surgical Reporter* 11 (1858): 141–51.

Bartlett, Elisha. *An Essay on the Philosophy of Medical Science.* Philadelphia: Lea & Blanchard, 1844.

Barton, Benjamin Smith. "Account of Henry Moss, a White Negro." *Philadelphia Medical and Physical Journal* 2, no. 2 (September 1806): 3–18.

Beaumont, William. *Experiments and Observations on the Gastric Juice, and the Physiology of Digestion.* Edinburgh ed. Edinburgh: MacLachlan & Stewart, 1838.

Brown, John. *Slave Life in Georgia: A Narrative of the Life, Sufferings, and Escape of John Brown, a Fugitive Slave, Now in England.* Edited by L. A. Chamerovzow. London: L. A. Chamerovzow, 1855.

Browne, P. A. *The Classification of Mankind, by the Hair and Wool of their Head.* Philadelphia: A. Hart, 1850.

Bunyavanich, Supinda, Chantal Grant, and Alfin Vicencio. "Racial/Ethnic Variation in Nasal Gene Expression of Transmembrane Serine Protease 2 (TMPRSS2)." *Journal of the American Medical Association* 324, no. 15 (September 10, 2020): 1567–68. https://jamanetwork.com/journals/jama/fullarticle/2770682. Accessed September 12, 2020.

Cabell, J. L. *Syllabus of the Lectures on Physiology and Histology: Including the Outlines of Comparative Anatomy Delivered at the University of Virginia.* Charlottesville, Va.: McKennie & Son, 1853.

———. *The Testimony of Modern Science to the Unity of Mankind.* New York: Carter & Brothers, 1859.

Caldwell, Charles. *Autobiography of Charles Caldwell, M.D. with a Preface, Notes, and Appendix by Harriot W. Warner.* Philadelphia: Lippincott, Grambo, 1855.

———. *Thoughts on the Original Unity of the Race.* New York: E. Bliss, 1830.

Carroll, Charles. *"The Negro a Beast"; or, "In the Image of God"; the Reasoner of the Age, the Revelator of the Century! The Bible as It Is! The Negro and His Relation to the Human Family!* St. Louis, Mo.: American Book and Bible House, 1900.

Carson, Joseph. *A History of the Medical Department of the University of Pennsylvania from its Foundation in 1765.* Philadelphia: Lindsay & Blakiston, 1869.

Cartwright, Samuel A. "Extract of a Letter to the Editor, on the Art of Acquiring Knowledge." *Western and Southern Medical Recorder* 1, no. 1 (November 1841): 71–73.

———. "Report on the Diseases and Physical Peculiarities of the Negro Race (Continued)." *New Orleans Medical and Surgical Journal* 8 (1852): 187–94.

———. "Report on the Diseases and Physical Peculiarities of the Negro Race." *New Orleans Medical and Surgical Journal* 7 (1851): 691–715.

———. "Slavery in the Light of Ethnology." In *Cotton is King, and Pro-slavery Arguments*, edited by E. N. Elliot, 691–728. Augusta, Ga.: Pritchard, Abbot, & Loomis, 1860.

Catalogue of Anatomical Preparations in the Hunterian Museum, University of Glasgow. Glasgow: George Richardson, 1840.

A Catalogue of Phrenological Specimens, Belonging to the Boston Phrenological Society. Boston: Printed by John Ford, 1835.

Catalogue of the Alumni of the Medical Department of the University of Pennsylvania, 1765–1877. Philadelphia: Collins, 1877.

A Catalogue of the Officers and Students of Harvard College, for the Academical Year 1850–51. Cambridge, Mass.: Metcalf, 1850.

Catlin, A. "Another Ethiopian Turning to a White Man." *Medical Repository* (1802): 83–84.

"Census of the Blockley Alms House and Philadelphia Hospital, January 10, 1844." *Medical Examiner and Record of Medical Science* 7, no. 6 (March 1844): 61.

Clarence, Walter. *The Aborigines of South Africa, Now on the Exhibition at the New Boston Aquarial and Zoölogical Gardens*. Boston: J. P. Plumer, 1860.

Code of Ethics of the American Medical Association Adopted May 1847. Philadelphia: T. K. & P. G. Collins, 1848.

Coles, Abraham. "The Unity of the Origin of Mankind, Supported by Scripture, by Reason, and by the Investigations of Science." *Medical and Surgical Reporter* 10, no. 12 (December 1857): 582–99.

Colman, Benjamin. *Some Observations on the New Method of Receiving the Small-Pox by Ingrafting or Inoculating*. Boston: B. Green, 1721.

Comings, B. N. *Class-Book of Physiology: for the Use of Schools and Families; Comprising the Structure and Functions of the Organs of Man, Illustrated by Comparative Reference to Those of Inferior Animals*. 2nd ed. New York: D. Appleton, 1854.

"The Commissioners of the Alms-House vs. Alexander Whistelo, a Black Man"; Being a Remarkable Case of Bastardy, Tried and Adjudged by the Mayor, Recorder, and Several Aldermen of the City of New York. New York: David Longworth, 1808.

"A Declaration of the Immediate Causes Which Induce and Justify the Secession of the State of Mississippi from the Federal Union." 1861. The Avalon Project: Documents in Law, History, and Diplomacy. Yale University. https://avalon .law.yale.edu/19th_century/csa_missec.asp. Accessed August 11, 2015.

Delany, Martin R. *Principia of Ethnology: The Origin of Races and Color, with an Archaeological Compendium of Ethiopian and Egyptian Civilization from Years of Careful Examination and Inquiry*. 2nd and rev. ed. Philadelphia: Harper & Brother, 1880.

Dickson, S. Henry. *Elements of Medicine: A Compendious View of Pathology and Therapeutics; or the History and Treatment of Diseases*. Philadelphia: Blanchard & Lea, 1855.

——. *Essays on Life, Sleep, Pain, Etc.* Philadelphia: Blanchard & Lea, 1852.

——. *On Dengue: Its Theory, Pathology, and Treatment.* Philadelphia: Haswell, Barrington, & Haswell, 1839.

——. *Remarks on Certain Topics Connected with the General Subject of Slavery.* Charleston, S.C.: Observer Office Press, 1845.

——. *Syllabus of Part of the Course of Lectures of S. Henry Dickson, M.D.: Professor of the Institutes and Practices of Medicine in the Medical College of South-Carolina.* Charleston, S.C.: James S. Burges, 1830.

Douglass, Frederick. *The Claims of the Negro, Ethnologically Considered.* Rochester, N.Y.: Lee, Mann, Daily American Office, 1854.

Drake, Daniel. *Dr. Daniel Drake's Letters on Slavery to Dr. John C. Warren, of Boston: Reprinted from "The National Intelligencer" Washington, April 3, 5 and 7, 1851 with an Introduction by Emmet Field Horine, M.D. of Louisville, Kentucky.* New York: Schuman, 1940.

Du Bois, W. E. B. *The Health and Physique of the Negro American.* Atlanta: Atlanta University Press, 1906.

Dwight, Thomas. "Reminiscences of Dr. Holmes as Professor of Anatomy." *Scribner's* 17, no. 1 (January 1895): 121–28.

Ewcorstart, John K. "The Negro Not a Distinct Species." *Medical and Surgical Reporter* 10, no. 12 (December 1857): 577–82.

Forwood, William Stump. "Ethnological Papers." *Maryland and Virginia Medical Journal* 15, no. 2 (August 1860): 114–30.

——. "The Negro—a Distinct Species." *Medical and Surgical Reporter* 10, no. 5 (May 1857): 225–34.

Gibson, William. *Rambles in Europe in 1839.* Philadelphia: Lea & Blanchard, 1841.

Gobineau, Comte de. *The Moral and Intellectual Diversity of Races, with Particular Reference to Their Respective Influence in the Civil and Political History of Mankind. From the French of Count A De Gobineau: With an Analytical Introduction and Copious Historical Notes. By H. Hotz. To Which Is Added an Appendix Containing a Summary of the Latest Scientific Facts Bearing upon the Question of Unity or Plurality of Species. By J. C. Nott, M.D.* Translated by Henry Hotz. Philadelphia: J. B. Lippincott, 1856.

Gorham, John. "Cases in Morbid Anatomy." *New England Journal of Medicine and Surgery, and Collateral Branches of Science* 12, no. 4 (October 1823): 344–50.

——. "Collections in Morbid Anatomy: No. III, Organic Disease of the Heart, with Dissection." *New England Journal of Medicine and Surgery, and Collateral Branches of Science* 3, no. 1 (January 1814): 34–36.

Gross, S. D. *History of American Medical Literature, from 1776 to the Present Time.* Philadelphia: Collins, 1876.

Heck, J. G. *Iconographic Encyclopædia of Science, Literature, and Art.* Translated by Spencer F. Baird. 4 vols. New York: Rudolph Garrigue, 1851.

Holmes, Oliver Wendell. *An Introductory Lecture, Delivered at the Massachusetts Medical College, November 3, 1847.* Boston: William D. Ticknor, 1847.

Home, Everard. *Lectures on Comparative Anatomy: In Which Are Explained the Preparations in the Hunterian Collection.* 6 vols. London: Longman, Hurst, Rees, Orme & Brown, 1823.

Home, Henry. *Six Sketches on the History of Man. Containing, the Progress of Men as Individuals.* Philadelphia: R. Bell & R. Aitken, 1776.

Hood, E. C. "Another White African." *Southern Medical & Surgical Journal* 9 (1853): 461.

Horner, William E. *Catalogue of the Wistar, or Anatomical Museum of the University of Pennsylvania.* Philadelphia: L. R. Bailey, 1850.

———. *A Treatise on Special and General Anatomy.* 2nd ed. 2 vols. Philadelphia: Carey & Lea, 1830.

———. *The United States Dissector, or Lessons in Practical Anatomy.* Edited by Henry H. Smith. 4th ed. Philadelphia: Lea & Blanchard, 1846.

Hutchison, Joseph C. "A Remarkable Case of Change of Complexion with Loss of the Sense of Smell." *American Journal of Medical Science* 23, no. 1 (January 1852): 146–48.

Jackson, J. B. S. *A Descriptive Catalogue of the Anatomical Museum of the Boston Society for Medical Improvement.* Boston: Ticknor, 1847.

———. *A Descriptive Catalogue of the Warren Anatomical Museum.* Boston: A. Williams, 1870.

Jefferson, Thomas. *Notes on the State of Virginia.* Philadelphia: Prichard & Hall, 1788.

Knox, Robert. *A Manual of Artistic Anatomy, for the Use of Sculptors, Painters, and Amateurs.* London: Henry Renshaw, 1852.

———. *Races of Men: A Fragment.* Philadelphia: Lea & Blanchard, 1850.

Lee, Charles A. *Human Physiology for the Use of Elementary Schools.* Philadelphia: Lippincott, Grambo, 1854.

Lehlbach, Charles F. J. "Is the Negro a Distinct Species?—a Reply to 'Senex,' and an Anti-Criticism to Dr. Cole's Criticism of Nott and Gliddon's Works." *Medical and Surgical Reporter* 10, no. 11 (November 1857): 532–41.

Leidy, Joseph. *An Elementary Treatise on Human Anatomy.* Philadelphia: J. B. Lippincott, 1861.

Linnaeus, Carolus. *A General System of Nature.* Translated by William Turton. English ed. 7 vols. London: Lackington, Allen, 1802.

Louis, P. Ch. A. *An Essay on Clinical Instruction.* Translated by Peter Martin. London: S. Highley, 1834.

McKnight, W. J. *A Pioneer Outline of Northwestern Pennsylvania.* Philadelphia: J. B. Lippincott, 1905.

Morton, Samuel George. *Catalogue of Skulls of Man and the Inferior Animals in the Collection of Samuel George Morton.* 3rd ed. Philadelphia: Merrihew & Thompson, 1849.

———. *Crania Aegyptiaca; or, Observations on Egyptian Ethnography, Derived from Anatomy, History and the Monuments.* Philadelphia: John Penington, 1844.

———. *Crania Americana; or, a Comparative View of the Skulls of Various Aboriginal Nations of North and South America.* Philadelphia: J. Dobson, 1839.

———. *An Illustrated System of Human Anatomy, Special, General and Microscopic.* Philadelphia: Grigg, Elliot and Co., 1849.

Mussey, R. D. *Anatomical Cabinet, Belonging to R. D. Mussey, M.D., Professor of Surgery in the Medical College of Ohio.* Cincinnati [?], 1837.

Nott, Josiah, and George R. Gliddon. *Indigenous Races of the Earth*. Philadelphia: J. B. Lippincott, 1857.

———. *Types of Mankind: or, Ethnological Researches*. Philadelphia: Lippincott, Grambo, 1854.

Osgood, David. "Remarks on the Dengue." *Boston Medical and Surgical Journal* 1, no. 36 (October 1828): 561–63.

Parsons, Usher. *The Importance of the Sciences of Anatomy and Physiology as a Branch of General Education: Being an Introduction to the Upper Classes in Brown University*. Cambridge, Mass.: Hilliard & Metcalf, 1826.

Pickering, Charles. *The Races of Man: And Their Geographical Distribution*. New ed. London: H. G. Bohn, 1854.

Prichard, James Cowles. *The Natural History of Man: Comprising Inquiries into the Modifying Influences of Physical and Moral Agencies on the Different Tribes of the Human Family*. Edited by Edwin Norris. 4th ed. 2 vols. New York: H. Baillière, 1855.

"Review of Cartwright *On the Diseases and Physical Peculiarities of the Negro Race*." *Charleston Medical Journal & Review* 7 (1852): 89–98.

Richardson, T. G. *Elements of Human Anatomy: General, Descriptive, and Practical*. Philadelphia: Lippincott, Grambo, 1854.

Richerand, Anthelme. *Elements of Physiology*. Translated by G. J. M. De Lys and John D. Godman. Edited by Nathaniel Chapman. 5th ed. Philadelphia: James E. Moore, 1823.

Rollin, Francis A. *Life and Public Services of Martin R. Delany*. Boston: Lee & Shepard, 1883.

Rush, Benjamin. *Medical Inquiries and Observations*. 4 vols. Philadelphia: J. Conead, 1805.

———. "Observations Intended to Favour the Supposition That the Black Color (as It Is Called) of the Negroes Is Derived from the Leprosy." *Transactions of the American Philosophical Society* 4 (1799): 289–97.

———. *A Syllabus of a Course of Lectures on the Institutes and Practices of Medicine*. Philadelphia: Thomas & Samuel F. Bradford, 1798.

Senex. "Is the Negro a Distinct Species? Answered in the Negative, Being a Continuation of the Discussion from the June Number of the Reporter." *Medical and Surgical Reporter* 10, no. 8 (August 1857): 375–86.

———. "The Negro Not a Distinct Species." *Medical and Surgical Reporter* 10, no. 6 (June 1857): 288–301.

Smith, Henry H. *Anatomical Atlas, Illustrative of the Structure of the Human Body, under the Supervision of William E. Horner*. Philadelphia: Blanchard & Lea, 1854.

Thornton, S. C. "The Ethnological Question." *Medical and Surgical Reporter* 10, no. 11 (November 1857): 541–46.

Todd, Robert Bentley. *The Descriptive and Physiological Anatomy of the Brain, Spinal Cord, and Ganglions, and of Their Coverings. Adapted for the Use of Students*. London: Sherwood, Gilbert, & Piper, 1845.

Warren, J. Mason. "An Account of Two Remarkable Indian Dwarfs Exhibited in Boston under the Name Aztec Children." *American Journal of the Medical Sciences* 21, no. 42 (April 1851): 285–97.

Warren, John Collins. *A Comparative View of the Sensorial and Nervous Systems in Men and Animals*. Boston: Joseph W. Ingraham, 1822.

Warren, John Collins, Jr. "The Collection of the Boston Phrenological Society—a Retrospect." *Annals of Medical History* 3, no. 1 (1921): 1–11.

Webster, James. *Facts Concerning Anatomical Instruction in Philadelphia*. Philadelphia, 1832.

White, Charles. *An Account of the Regular Gradation in Man, and in Different Animals and Vegetables*. London: C. Dilly, 1799.

Wistar, Caspar. *A System of Human Anatomy for the Use of Students*. 2 vols. Philadelphia: Thomas Dobson, 1811.

Wood, George B. *A Treatise on the Practice of Medicine*. 5th ed. 2 vols. Philadelphia: J. B. Lippincott, 1858.

Wyman, Jeffries. "Observations on the Skeleton of a Hottentot." *Anthropological Review* 3, no. 11 (October 1865): 330–35.

SECONDARY SOURCES

Ackerknecht, Erwin. *Medicine at the Paris Hospital, 1794–1848*. Baltimore: Johns Hopkins University Press, 1967.

Altschuler, Sari. "From Blood Vessels to Global Networks of Exchange: The Physiology of Benjamin Rush's Early Republic." *Journal of the Early Republic* 32, no. 2 (Summer 2012): 207–31.

———. *The Medical Imagination: Literature and Health in the Early United States*. Philadelphia: University of Pennsylvania Press, 2018.

Anderson, Warwick. *Colonial Pathologies: American Tropical Medicine, Race, and Hygiene in the Philippines*. Durham, N.C.: Duke University Press, 2006.

Augstein, H. F. *James Cowles Prichard's Anthropology: Remaking the Science of Man in Early Nineteenth Century Britain*. Atlanta: Rodopi B. V., 1999.

Bankole-Medina, Katherine. *Slavery and Medicine: Enslavement and Medical Practices in Antebellum Louisiana*. New York: Garland Publishing, 1998.

Barcia, Manuel. *The Yellow Demon of Fever: Fighting Disease in the Nineteenth-Century Transatlantic Slave Trade*. New Haven, Conn.: Yale University Press, 2020.

Barnard, Alan. *Hunters and Herders of Southern Africa: A Comparative Ethnography of the Khoisan Peoples*. New York: Cambridge University Press, 1992.

Bates, A. W. *The Anatomy of Robert Knox: Murder, Mad Science and Medical Regulation in Nineteenth-Century Edinburgh*. Portland, Ore.: Sussex Academic, 2010.

Bay, Mia. *The White Image in the Black Mind: African-American Ideas about White People, 1830–1925*. New York: Oxford University Press, 2000.

Beckert, Sven. *Empire of Cotton: A Global History*. New York: Alfred A. Knopf, 2014.

Beckert, Sven, and Seth Rockman, eds. *Slavery's Capitalism: A New History of American Economic Development*. Philadelphia: University of Pennsylvania Press, 2016.

Berkowitz, Carin. *Charles Bell and the Anatomy of Reform*. Chicago: University of Chicago Press, 2015.

Berry, Daina Ramey. *The Price for Their Pound of Flesh: The Value of the Enslaved from Womb to Grave, in the Building of a Nation*. Boston: Beacon, 2017.

Blackett, R. J. M. *The Captive's Quest for Freedom: Fugitive Slaves, Fugitive Slave Law, and the Politics of Freedom*. New York: Cambridge University Press, 2018.

Bogdan, Robert. *Freak Show: Presenting Human Oddities for Amusement and Profit*. Chicago: University of Chicago Press, 1988.

Bohannan, Paul, ed. *African Homicide and Suicide*. Princeton, N.J.: Princeton University Press, 1960.

Braude, Benjamin. "The Sons of Noah and the Construction of Ethnic and Geographical Identities in the Medieval and Early Modern Periods." *William and Mary Quarterly* 54, no. 1 (January 1997): 103–42.

Breeden, James O. "Body Snatchers and Anatomy Professors: Medical Education in Nineteenth-Century Virginia." *Virginia Magazine of History and Biography* 83, no. 3 (July 1975): 321–45.

Brophy, Alfred L. *University, Court, & Slave: Pro-slavery Thought in Southern Colleges & Courts & the Coming of the Civil War*. New York: Oxford University Press, 2016.

Brown, Vincent. *The Reaper's Garden: Death and Power in the World of Atlantic Slavery*. Cambridge, Mass.: Harvard University Press, 2008.

Browne, Randy M. *Surviving Slavery in the British Caribbean*. Philadelphia: University of Pennsylvania Press, 2017.

Bylebyl, Jerome J. "William Beaumont, Robley Dunglison, and the 'Philadelphia Physiologists.'" *Journal of the History of Medicine and Allied Sciences* 25, no. 1 (January 1970): 3–21.

Cash, Phillip. "Pride, Prejudice, and Politics." *Harvard Medical Alumni Gazette* 54 (December 1980): 20–25.

Cassedy, James H. *American Medicine and Statistical Thinking, 1800–1860*. Cambridge, Mass.: Harvard University Press, 1984.

———. "The Flourishing Character of Early American Medical Journalism, 1797–1860." *Journal of the History of Medicine and Allied Sciences* 38, no. 2 (April 1983): 135–50.

———. *Medicine and American Growth, 1800–1860*. Madison: University of Wisconsin Press, 1986.

Chaplin, Joyce. *Subject Matter: Technology, the Body, and Science on the Anglo-American Frontier, 1500–1676*. Cambridge, Mass.: Harvard University Press, 2001.

Clegg, Claude A., III. *The Price of Liberty: African Americans and the Making of Liberia*. Chapel Hill: University of North Carolina Press, 2004.

Cooper Owens, Deirdre. "Manifesting Power through the Degraded Body: Enslaved and Irish-Immigrant Women and Antebellum-Era Modern American Gynecology." In *Power in History: From the Medieval to the Post-modern World*, edited by Anthony McElligott, Liam Chambers, Ciara Breathnach, and Catherine Lawless, 167–84. Dublin: Irish Academic, 2011.

———. *Medical Bondage: Race, Gender, and the Origins of American Gynecology*. Athens: University of Georgia Press, 2017.

Corgan, James X. "Some Medical Dissertations: Written by Tennesseans before 1846." *Tennessee Historical Quarterly* 63, no. 2 (Summer 2004): 71–85.

Crais, Clifton, and Pamela Scully. *Sara Baartman and the Hottentot Venus: A Ghost Story and a Biography*. Princeton, N.J.: Princeton University Press, 2009.

Curran, Andrew S. *The Anatomy of Blackness: Science & Slavery in an Age of Enlightenment*. Baltimore: Johns Hopkins University Press, 2011.

Curtin, Phillip D. *The Atlantic Slave Trade: A Census*. Madison: University of Wisconsin Press, 1969.

Dain, Bruce. *A Hideous Monster of the Mind: American Race Theory in the Early Republic*. Cambridge, Mass.: Harvard University Press, 2002.

Deetz, Kelley Fanto. "Finding the Bones of Nat Turner, American Rebel." *National Geographic*, November 4, 2019. https://www.nationalgeographic.com/history /history-magazine/article/nat-turner-slave-rebellion-southampton-virginia. Accessed June 1, 2020.

DeLancey, Dayle B. "Vaccinating Freedom: Smallpox Prevention and the Discourses of African American Citizenship in Antebellum Philadelphia." *Journal of African American History* 95 (July 2010): 296–321.

Desmond, Adrian. *The Politics of Evolution: Morphology, Medicine, and Reform in Radical London*. Chicago: University of Chicago Press, 1989.

Devine, Shauna. *Learning from the Wounded: The Civil War and the Rise of American Medical Science*. Chapel Hill: University of North Carolina Press, 2014.

DiPiero, Thomas. "Missing Links: Whiteness and the Color of Reason in the Eighteenth Century." *Eighteenth Century* 40, no. 2 (Summer 1999): 155–74.

Dorr, Gregory Michael. *Segregation's Science: Eugenics and Society in Virginia*. Charlottesville: University of Virginia Press, 2008.

Downs, Jim. *Maladies of Empire: How Colonialism, Slavery, and War Transformed Medicine*. Cambridge, Ma.: Belknap Press of Harvard University Press, 2021.

———. *Sick from Freedom: African-American Illness and Suffering during the Civil War and Reconstruction*. New York: Oxford University Press, 2012.

Dracobly, Alex. "Ethics and Experimentation on Human Subjects in Mid-nineteenth-century France: The Story of the 1859 Syphilis Experiments." *Bulletin of the History of Medicine* 77, no. 2 (Summer 2003): 332–66.

Duffy, John. *The Tulane University Medical Center: One Hundred and Fifty Years of Medical Education*. Baton Rouge: Louisiana State University Press, 1984.

Duster, Troy. *Backdoor to Eugenics*. 2nd ed. New York: Routledge, 2003.

Espinosa, Mariola. *Epidemic Invasions: Yellow Fever and the Limits of Cuban Independence, 1878–1930*. Chicago: University of Chicago Press, 2009.

Evans, R. Tripp. *Romancing the Maya: Mexican Antiquity in the American Imagination, 1820–1915*. Austin: University of Texas Press, 2004.

Fabian, Ann. *The Skull Collectors: Race, Science, and America's Unburied Dead*. Chicago: University of Chicago Press, 2010.

Fett, Sharla M. *Recaptured Africans: Surviving Slave Ships, Detention, and Dislocation in the Final Years of the Slave Trade*. Chapel Hill: University of North Carolina Press, 2017.

———. *Working Cures: Healing, Health, and Power on Southern Slave Plantations*. Chapel Hill: University of North Carolina Press, 2002.

Fields, Karen E., and Barbara J. Fields. *Racecraft: The Soul of Inequality in American Life*. New York: Verso, 2012.

Finger, Simon. *The Contagious City: The Politics of Public Health in Early Philadelphia*. Ithaca, N.Y.: Cornell University Press, 2012.

Force, Pierre, and Susan Dick Hoffius. "Negotiating Race and Status in Senegal, Saint-Domingue, and South Carolina: Marie-Adélaïde Rossingal and Her Descendants." *Early American Studies* 16, no. 1 (Winter 2018): 124–50.

Ford, Lacy K. *Deliver Us from Evil: The Slavery Question in the Old South*. New York: Oxford University Press, 2009.

Forrest, John N., Jr. "Introduction: The Medical Student Thesis at Yale." *Yale Journal of Biology and Medicine* 62 (1989): 291–92.

Foucault, Michel. *The Birth of the Clinic: An Archaeology of Medical Perception*. Translated by A. M. Sheridan Smith. New York: Vintage Books, 1994. Original French ed., 1963.

Fredrickson, George M. *The Black Image in the White Mind: The Debate over Afro-American Character and Destiny, 1817–1914*. Middleton: Wesleyan University Press, 1987.

———. *Racism: A Short History*. Princeton, N.J.: Princeton University Press, 2002.

Freehling, William W. *The Road to Disunion*. Vol. 1, *Secessionists at Bay, 1776–1854*. New York: Oxford University Press, 1990.

———. *The Road to Disunion*. Vol. 2, *Secessionists Triumphant, 1854–1861*. New York: Oxford University Press, 2007.

Fuentes, Marisa J. *Dispossessed Lives: Enslaved Women, Violence, and the Archive*. Philadelphia: University of Pennsylvania Press, 2016.

Fye, W. Bruce. *The Development of American Physiology: Scientific Medicine in the Nineteenth Century*. Baltimore: Johns Hopkins University Press, 1987.

Goldberg, David Theo. *Racist Culture: Philosophy and the Politics of Meaning*. Oxford, U.K.: Blackwell, 1993.

Gómez, Pablo. *The Experiential Caribbean: Creating Knowledge and Healing in the Early Modern Atlantic*. Chapel Hill: University of North Carolina Press, 2017.

Gonaver, Wendy. *The Peculiar Institution and the Making of Modern Psychiatry, 1840–1880*. Chapel Hill: University of North Carolina Press, 2018.

Gossett, Thomas. *Race: The History of an Idea in America*. Dallas: Southern Methodist University Press, 1963.

Greenberg, Kenneth S. "Introduction, *The Confessions of Nat Turner*: Text and Context." In *The Confessions of Nat Turner and Related Documents*, edited by Kenneth S. Greenberg, 1–35. Boston: Bedford / St. Martin's, 1996.

Gross, Ariela J. *Double Character: Slavery and Mastery in the Antebellum Southern Courtroom*. Princeton, N.J.: Princeton University Press, 2000.

Hahn, Stephen. *A Nation under Our Feet: Black Political Struggles in the Rural South from Slavery to the Great Migration*. Cambridge, Mass.: Belknap Press of Harvard University Press, 2003.

Haller, John S. "The Negro and the Southern Physician: A Study of Medical and Racial Attitudes, 1800–1860." *Medical History* 16, no. 3 (July 1972): 238–53.

Hannaford, Ivan. *Race: The History of an Idea in the West*. Baltimore: Johns Hopkins University Press, 1996.

Harris, Leslie M., James T. Campbell, and Alfred L. Brophy, eds. *Slavery and the University: Histories and Legacies*. Athens: University of Georgia Press, 2019.

Harrison, Mark. *Climates and Constitutions: Health, Race, Environment and British Imperialism in India, 1600-1850*. Oxford: Oxford University Press, 1999.

Headrick, Daniel R. *The Tools of Empire: Technology and European Imperialism in the Nineteenth Century*. New York: Oxford University Press, 1981.

Hoffman, Kelly M., Sophie Trawalter, Jordan R. Axt, and M. Norman Oliver. "Racial Bias in Pain Assessment and Treatment Recommendations, and False Beliefs about Biological Differences between Blacks and Whites." *Proceedings of the National Academy of Sciences of the United States of America* 113, no. 16 (April 2016): 4296-301.

Hogarth, Rana A. "Charity and Terror in Eighteenth-Century Jamaica: The Kingston Hospital and Asylum for Deserted 'Negroes.'" *African and Black Diaspora: An International Journal* 10, no. 3 (March 2016): 1-18.

———. "Comparing Anatomies, Constructing Races: Medicine and Slavery in the Atlantic World, 1787-1838." PhD diss., Yale University, 2012.

———. *Medicalizing Blackness: Making Racial Difference in the Atlantic World, 1780-1840*. Chapel Hill: University of North Carolina Press, 2017.

Horne, Gerald. *The Deepest South: The United States, Brazil, and the African Slave Trade*. New York: New York University Press, 2007.

Horsman, Reginald. *Josiah Nott of Mobile: Southerner, Physician, and Racial Theorist*. Baton Rouge: Louisiana State University Press, 1987.

———. *Race and Manifest Destiny: The Origins of American Racial Anglo Saxonism*. Cambridge, Mass.: Harvard University Press, 1981.

Humphrey, David C. "Dissection and Discrimination: The Social Origins of Cadavers in America, 1760-1915." *Bulletin of the New York Academy of Medicine* 49 (1973): 819-27.

Humphreys, Margaret. *Intensely Human: The Health of the Black Soldier in the American Civil War*. Baltimore: Johns Hopkins University Press, 2008.

———. *Marrow of Tragedy: The Health Crisis of the American Civil War*. Baltimore: Johns Hopkins University Press, 2013.

Hunt-Kennedy, Stefanie. *Between Fitness and Death: Disability and Slavery in the Caribbean*. Urbana: University of Illinois Press, 2020.

Jensen, Niklas Thode. *For the Health of the Enslaved: Slaves, Medicine and Power in the Danish West Indies, 1803-1848*. Copenhagen, Denmark: Museum Tusculanum Press, 2012.

Johnson, Walter. *River of Dark Dreams: Slavery and Empire in the Cotton Kingdom*. Cambridge, Mass.: Belknap Press of Harvard University Press, 2013.

———. *Soul by Soul: Life inside the Antebellum Slave Market*. Cambridge, Mass.: Harvard University Press, 1999.

Jones, David S. *Rationalizing Epidemics: Meanings and Uses of American Indian Mortality since 1600*. Cambridge, Mass.: Harvard University Press, 2004.

Jones, James H. *Bad Blood: The Tuskegee Syphilis Experiment*. New York: Free Press, 1981.

Jordan, Winthrop D. *White Over Black: American Attitudes toward the Negro, 1550-1812*. Chapel Hill: University of North Carolina Press & the Institute for Early American History & Culture, 1968.

Karp, Matthew. *This Vast Southern Empire: Slaveholders at the Helm of American Foreign Policy*. Cambridge, Mass.: Harvard University Press, 2016.

Keel, Terence D. "Charles V. Roman and the Spectre of Polygenism in Progressive Era Public Health Research." *Social History of Medicine* 28, no. 4 (2015): 742–66.

———. *Divine Variations: How Christian Thought Became Racial Science*. Stanford, Calif.: Stanford University Press, 2019.

———. "Religion, Polygenism, and the Early Science of Human Origins." *History of the Human Sciences* 26, no. 2 (April 2013): 3–32.

Kelton, Paul. *Cherokee Medicine, Colonial Germs: An Indigenous Nation's Fight against Smallpox, 1518–1824*. Norman: University of Oklahoma Press, 2018.

———. *Epidemics and Enslavement: Biological Catastrophe in the Native Southeast, 1492–1715*. Lincoln: University of Nebraska Press, 2007.

Kenny, Stephen C. "The Development of Medical Museums in the Antebellum American South: Slave Bodies in Networks of Anatomical Exchange." *Bulletin of the History of Medicine* 87, no. 1 (Spring 2013): 32–62.

———. "'A Dictate of Both Interest and Mercy'?: Slave Hospitals in the Antebellum South." *Journal of the History of Medicine and Allied Sciences* 65, no. 1 (January 2010): 1–47.

———. "Power, Opportunism, Racism: Human Experiments under American Slavery." *Endeavour* 39, no. 1 (2015): 10–20.

Kidd, Colin. *The Forging of Races: Race and Scripture in the Protestant Atlantic World, 1600–2000*. Cambridge: Cambridge University Press, 2006.

Kilbride, Daniel. *An American Aristocracy: Southern Planters in Antebellum Philadelphia*. Columbia: University of South Carolina Press, 2006.

Kiple, Kenneth F. *The Caribbean Slave: A Biological History of Black People*. Cambridge: Cambridge University Press, 1984.

Kramer, Paul A. *The Blood of Government: Race, Empire, the United States, and the Philippines*. Chapel Hill: University of North Carolina Press, 2006.

Kvach, John F. *"De Bow's Review": The Antebellum Vision of a New South*. Lexington: University Press of Kentucky, 2013.

Lederer, Susan. *Subjected to Science: Human Experimentation in America before the Second World War*. Baltimore: Johns Hopkins University Press, 1995.

Lesch, John E. *Science and Medicine in France: The Emergence of Experimental Physiology, 1790–1855*. Cambridge, Mass.: Harvard University Press, 1984.

Lindquist, Wendi A. "Stealing from the Dead: Scientists, Settlers, and Indian Burial Sites in Early-Nineteenth-Century Oregon." *Oregon Historical Quarterly* 115, no. 3 (Fall 2014): 324–43.

Livingstone, David N. *Adam's Ancestors: Race, Religion, and the Politics of Human Origins*. Baltimore: Johns Hopkins University Press, 2008.

Long, Gretchen. *Doctoring Freedom: The Politics of African American Medical Care in Slavery and Emancipation*. Chapel Hill: University of North Carolina Press, 2012.

MacDonald, Helen. *Human Remains: Dissection and Its Histories*. New Haven, Conn.: Yale University Press, 2005.

McCandless, Peter. *Moonlight, Magnolias, & Madness: Insanity in South Carolina from the Colonial Period to the Progressive Era*. Chapel Hill: University of North Carolina Press, 1996.

———. "The Political Evolution of John Bachman: From New York Yankee to South Carolina Secessionist." *South Carolina Historical Magazine* 108, no. 1 (January 2007): 6–31.

———. *Slavery, Disease, and Suffering in the Southern Lowcountry.* Cambridge: Cambridge University Press, 2011.

McGregor, Deborah Kuhn. *From Midwives to Medicine: The Birth of American Gynecology.* New Brunswick, N.J.: Rutgers University Press, 1998.

Medford, Edna Greene, Emilyn L. Brown, Selwyn H. H. Carrington, Linda Heywood, and John Thornton. "'By the Visitations of God': Death, Burial, and the Affirmation of Humanity." In *Historical Perspectives of the African Burial Ground: New York Blacks and the Diaspora,* edited by Edna Greene Medford, 85–90. Washington, D.C.: Howard University Press, 2009.

Miller, Matthew Smith. "Surely His Mother Mourns for Him: Africans on Exhibition in Boston and New York, 1860–1861." BA thesis, Harvard University, 2011.

Mintz, Sidney. *Sweetness and Power: The Place of Sugar in Modern History.* New York: Viking, 1985.

Mitchell, Elise A. "Unbelievable Suffering: Rethinking Feigned Illness in Slavery and the Slave Trade." In *Medicine and Healing in the Age of Slavery,* edited by Sean Morey Smith and Christopher D. E. Willoughby, 99–120. Baton Rouge: Louisiana State University Press, 2021.

Morgan, Jennifer. *Laboring Women: Reproduction and Gender in New World Slavery.* Philadelphia: University of Pennsylvania Press, 2004.

Murray, Robert. "Bodies in Motion: Liberian Settlers, Medicine, and Mobility in the Atlantic World." *Journal of the Early Republic* 39, no. 4 (Winter 2019): 615–46.

Mustakeem, Sowande' M. *Slavery at Sea: Terror, Sex, and Sickness in the Middle Passage.* Urbana: University of Illinois Press, 2016.

Myers, Bob Eberly, II. "'Drapetomania': Rebellion, Defiance and Free Black Insanity in the Antebellum United States." PhD diss., University of California, Los Angeles, 2014.

Naramore, Sarah. "I Sing the Body Republic: How Benjamin Rush Created American Medicine." PhD diss., Notre Dame University, 2018.

Nash, Gary B. *Forging Freedom: The Formation of Philadelphia's Black Community, 1720–1840.* Cambridge, Mass.: Harvard University Press, 1988.

Numbers, Ronald L., and William J. Orr Jr. "William Beaumont's Reception at Home and Abroad." *Isis* 72, no. 4 (December 1981): 590–612.

Oast, Jennifer. *Institutional Slavery: Slaveholding Churches, Schools, Colleges, and Businesses in Virginia, 1680–1860.* Cambridge: Cambridge University Press, 2015.

Olivarius, Kathryn. "Immunity, Capital, and Power in Antebellum New Orleans." *American Historical Review* 124, no. 2 (April 2019): 425–55.

Paugh, Katherine. *The Politics of Reproduction: Race, Medicine, and Fertility in the Age of Abolition.* New York: Oxford University Press, 2017.

Peabody, Sue. *"There Are No Slaves in France": The Political Culture of Race and Slavery in the Ancien Régime.* New York: Oxford University Press, 1996.

Penn, Nigel. *The Forgotten Frontier: Colonist and Khoisan on the Cape's Northern Frontier in the 18th Century.* Athens: Ohio University Press, 2005.

———. "Note on the Name Stuurman." Unpublished essay shared with the author by Nigel Penn in January 2022.

Perry, Warren R., Jean Howson, and Barbara A. Bianco. *The Archaeology of the African Burial Ground.* 3 vols. Washington, D.C.: Howard University Press, 2009.

Pitcock, Cynthia DeHaven. "William Beaumont, M.D. and Malpractice: The Mary Dugan Case, 1844." *Journal of the History of Medicine and Allied Sciences* 47, no. 2 (April 1992): 153–62.

Polk, Khary Oronde. *Contagions of Empire: Scientific Racism, Sexuality, and Black Military Workers Abroad, 1898–1948.* Chapel Hill: University of North Carolina Press, 2020.

Ponce, Rachel N. "'They Increase in Beauty and Elegance': Transforming Cadavers and the Epistemology of Dissection in Early Nineteenth-Century American Medical Education." *Journal of the History of Medicine and Allied Sciences* 68, no. 3 (July 2013): 331–76.

Poskett, James. *Materials of the Mind: Phrenology, Race, and the Global History of Science.* Chicago: University of Chicago Press, 2019.

Price, Richard. *Alabi's World.* Baltimore: Johns Hopkins University Press, 1990.

Price, Richard, and Christopher D. E. Willoughby. "A Harvard Physician's Reports on an 1857 Visit to the Saamaka." *New West Indian Guide* 93, nos. 3–4 (2019): 259–78.

Radbill, Samuel X. *Samuel Henry Dickson: Pioneer Southern Medical Educator.* New York: Paul B. Hoeber, 1942.

Redman, Samuel. *Bone Rooms: From Scientific Racism to Human Prehistory in Museums.* Cambridge, Mass.: Harvard University Press, 2016.

Reis, João José. *Death Is a Festival: Funeral Rights and Rebellion in Nineteenth-Century Brazil.* Translated by H. Sabrina Gledhill. Chapel Hill: University of North Carolina Press, 2003.

———. *Slave Rebellion in Brazil: The Muslim Uprising of 1835 in Bahia.* Translated by Arthur Brakel. Baltimore: Johns Hopkins University Press, 1993.

Reiss, Benjamin. *The Showman and the Slave: Race, Death, and Memory in Barnum's America.* Cambridge, Mass.: Harvard University Press, 2001.

Reverby, Susan M. *Examining Tuskegee: The Infamous Syphilis Study and Its Legacy.* Chapel Hill: University of North Carolina Press, 2009.

Richardson, Ruth. *Death, Dissection, and the Destitute.* 2nd ed. Chicago: University of Chicago Press, 2000.

Roberts, Dorothy. *Fatal Invention: How Science, Politics, and Big Business Re-create Race in the Twenty-First Century.* New York: New Press, 2011.

Rosenthal, Caitlin. *Accounting for Slavery: Masters and Management.* Cambridge, Mass.: Harvard University Press, 2018.

———. "Slavery's Scientific Management: Masters and Managers." In *Slavery's Capitalism: A New History of American Economic Development*, edited by Sven Beckert and Seth Rockman, 62–86. Philadelphia: University of Pennsylvania Press, 2016.

Rothstein, William G. *American Medical Schools and the Practice of Medicine: A History.* New York: Oxford University Press, 1987.

———. *American Physicians in the 19th Century: From Sects to Science*. Baltimore: Johns Hopkins University Press, 1985.

Sappol, Michael. *A Traffic of Dead Bodies: Anatomy and Embodied Social Identity in Nineteenth-Century America*. Princeton, N.J.: Princeton University Press, 2002.

Savitt, Todd L. *Medicine and Slavery: The Diseases and Health Care of Blacks in Antebellum Virginia*. Urbana: University of Illinois Press, 1978.

———. "The Use of Blacks for Medical Experimentation and Demonstration in the Old South." *Journal of Southern History* 48, no. 3 (August 1982): 331–48.

Schiebinger, Londa. "The Anatomy of Difference: Race and Sex in Eighteenth-Century Science." *Eighteenth-Century Studies* 23, no. 4 (Summer, 1990): 387–405.

———. "Medical Experimentation and Race in the Eighteenth-Century Atlantic World." *Social History of Medicine* 26, no. 3 (2013): 364–82.

———. *Secret Cures of Slaves: People, Plants, and Medicine in the Eighteenth-Century Atlantic World*. Stanford: Stanford University Press, 2017.

Schwalm, Leslie A. "Black Bodies, Medical Science, and the Age of Emancipation." In *Medicine and Healing in the Age of Slavery*, edited by Sean Morey Smith and Christopher D. E. Willoughby, 182–97. Baton Rouge: Louisiana State University Press, 2021.

Schwartz, Marie Jenkins. *Birthing a Slave: Motherhood and Medicine in the Antebellum South*. Cambridge, Mass.: Harvard University Press, 2006.

Sera-Shriar, Efram. "Ethnology in the Metropole: Robert Knox, Robert Gordon Latham and Local Sites of Observational Training." *Studies in the History and Philosophy of Biological and Biomedical Sciences* 42, no. 4 (December 2011): 486–96.

Seth, Suman. *Difference and Disease: Medicine, Race, and the Eighteenth-Century British Empire*. Cambridge: Cambridge University Press, 2018.

Shah, Sonia. *The Body Hunters: Testing New Drugs on the World's Poorest Patients*. New York: New Press, 2006.

Sheridan, Richard. *Doctors and Slaves: A Medical and Demographic History of Slavery in the British West Indies, 1680–1834*. Cambridge: Cambridge University Press, 1985.

Sinha, Manisha. *The Counterrevolution of Slavery: Politics and Ideology in Antebellum South Carolina*. Chapel Hill: University of North Carolina Press, 2000.

Skotnes, Pippa. "Introduction." In *Miscast: Negotiating the Presence of the Bushmen*, edited by Pippa Skotnes, 15–23. Cape Town, South Africa: University of Cape Town Press, 1996.

Skotnes, Pippa, ed. *Miscast: Negotiating the Presence of the Bushmen*. Cape Town, South Africa: University of Cape Town Press, 1996.

Smedley, Audrey. *Race in North America: Origin and Evolution of a Worldview*. Boulder, Co.: Westview, 1993.

Smith, Mark M. *How Race Is Made: Slavery, Segregation, and the Senses*. Chapel Hill: University of North Carolina Press, 2006.

———. "Transcending, Othering, Detecting: Smell, Premodernity, Modernity." *Postmedieval: A Journal of Medieval Cultural Studies* 3 (2012): 380–90.

Smith, Sean Morey, and Christopher D. E. Willoughby, eds. *Medicine and Healing in the Age of Slavery*. Baton Rouge: Louisiana State University Press, 2021.

Snyder, Terri L. *The Power to Die: Slavery and Suicide in British North America*. Chicago: University of Chicago Press, 2015.

Stanton, William. *The Leopard's Spots: Scientific Attitudes toward Race in America, 1815-59*. Chicago: University of Chicago Press, 1960.

Stein, Melissa N. *Measuring Manhood: Race and the Science of Masculinity, 1830-1934*. Minneapolis: University of Minnesota Press, 2015.

Stepan, Nancy. *The Idea of Race in Science: Great Britain, 1800-1960*. London: MacMillan, 1982.

———. *Picturing Tropical Nature*. London: Reaktion Books, 2001.

Stephens, Lester D. *Science, Race, and Religion in the American South: John Bachman and the Charleston Circle of Naturalists, 1815-1895*. Chapel Hill: University of North Carolina Press, 2000.

Stowe, Stephen M. *Doctoring the South: Southern Physicians and Everyday Medicine in the Mid-Nineteenth Century*. Chapel Hill: University of North Carolina Press, 2004.

Strang, Cameron B. *Frontiers of Science: Imperialism and Natural Knowledge in the Gulf South Borderlands*. Williamsburg, Va.: Omohundro Institute of Early American History and Culture & the University of North Carolina Press, 2018.

———. "Violence, Ethnicity, and Human Remains during the Second Seminole War." *Journal of American History* 100, no. 4 (March 2014): 973-94.

Streets-Salter, Heather, and Trevor R. Getz. *Empires and Colonies in the Modern World*. 2nd ed. New York: Oxford University Press, 2016.

Sutter, Paul S. "Nature's Agents or Agents of Empire? Entomological Workers and Environmental Change during the Construction of the Panama Canal." *Isis* 98, no. 4 (December 2007): 724-54.

Swan, Robert J. "Prelude and Aftermath of the Doctors' Riot of 1788: A Religious Interpretation of White and Black Reaction to Grave Robbing." *New York History* 81, no. 4 (October 2000): 417-56.

Sweet, James H. *Domingos Álvares, African Healing, and the Intellectual History of the Atlantic World*. Chapel Hill: University of North Carolina Press, 2011.

———. "The Iberian Roots of American Racist Thought." *William and Mary Quarterly* 54, no. 1 (January 1997): 143-66.

Sweet, John Wood. *Bodies Politic: Navigating Race in the American North, 1730-1830*. Philadelphia: University of Pennsylvania Press, 2003.

Thompson, Courtney E. *An Organ of Murder: Crime, Violence, and Phrenology in Nineteenth-Century America*. New Brunswick, N.J.: Rutgers University Press, 2021.

Thornton, John. *Africa and Africans in the Making of the Atlantic World, 1400-1800*. 2nd ed. Cambridge: Cambridge University Press, 1998. 1st ed, 1992.

Troutman, Phillip. "Grapevine in the Slave Market: African American Geopolitical Literacy and the 1841 *Creole* Revolt." In *The Chattel Principle: Internal Slave Trades in the Americas*, edited by Walter Johnson, 203-33. New Haven, Conn.: Yale University Press, 2004.

Turner, Sasha. *Contested Bodies: Pregnancy, Childrearing, and Slavery in Jamaica.* Philadelphia: University of Pennsylvania Press, 2017.

Valenčius, Conevery Bolton. *The Health of the Country: How American Settlers Understood Themselves and Their Land.* New York: Basic Books, 2002.

Wailoo, Keith. *Dying in the City of Blues: Sickle Cell Anemia and the Politics of Race and Health.* Chapel Hill: University of North Carolina Press, 2001.

Warner, John Harley. *Against the Spirit of System: The French Impulse in Nineteenth-Century American Medicine.* Baltimore: Johns Hopkins University Press, 1998.

———. *The Therapeutic Perspective: Medical Practice, Knowledge, and Identity in America, 1820–1885.* Cambridge, Mass.: Harvard University Press, 1986.

Warner, John Harley, and James M. Edmonson. *Dissection: Photographs of a Rite of Passage in American Medicine, 1880–1930.* New York: Blast Books, 2009.

Warner, Sam Bass. *The Private City: Philadelphia in Three Periods of Its Growth.* Rev. ed. Philadelphia: University of Pennsylvania Press, 1987.

Warren, Leonard. *Joseph Leidy: The Last Man Who Knew Everything.* New Haven, Conn.: Yale University Press, 1998.

Washington, Harriett. *Medical Apartheid: The Dark History of Medical Experimentation on Black Americans from Colonial Times to the Present.* New York: Harlem Moon, 2006.

Weaver, Karol K. *Medical Revolutionaries: The Enslaved Healers of Eighteenth-Century Saint Domingue.* Urbana: University of Illinois Press, 2006.

White, Luis. "The Traffic in Heads: Bodies, Borders and the Articulation of Regional Histories." *Journal of Southern African Studies* 23, no. 2 (June 1997): 325–38.

Wilder, Craig Steven. *Ebony & Ivy: Race, Slavery, and the Troubled History of America's Universities.* New York: Bloomsbury, 2013.

Wilf, Steven Robert. "Anatomy and Punishment in Late Eighteenth-Century New York." *Journal of Social History* 22, no. 3 (Spring 1989): 507–30.

Wilkinson, Doris Y. "The 1850 Harvard Medical School Dispute and the Admission of African American Students." *Harvard Library Bulletin* 3, no. 3 (Fall 1992): 13–27.

Williams, Eric. *Capitalism & Slavery.* 2nd ed. Chapel Hill: University of North Carolina Press, 1994. 1st ed., 1944.

Willoughby, Christopher D. E. "'His Native, Hot Country': Racial Science and Environment in Antebellum American Medical Thought." *Journal of the History of Medicine and Allied Sciences* 72, no. 3 (July 2017): 328–51.

———. "Running Away from Drapetomania: Samuel Cartwright, Medicine, and Race in the Antebellum South." *Journal of Southern History* 84, no. 3 (August 2018): 579–614.

Willoughby, Urmi Engineer. *Yellow Fever, Race, and Ecology in Nineteenth-Century New Orleans.* Baton Rouge: Louisiana State University Press, 2017.

Worboys, Michael. "Medical Perspectives on Health and Disease." *A Cultural History of the Human Body.* 6 vols. Edited by Michael Sappol and Stephen P. Rice. Vol. 5, *In the Age of Empire.* New York: Berg, 2010.

Yudell, Michael. *Race Unmasked: Biology and Race in the 20th Century.* New York: Columbia University Press, 2014.

INDEX

Page numbers in italics refer to illustrations.

anatomical objects. *See* anatomical models; casts of human remains; human remains; skulls

anatomy, 5-6, 14, 71-72, 76-77, 93-122; in popular culture, 71-72, 76-77, 101, 107-8, 134; and racial science, 5-6, 14, 93-122

anatomy riots, 70, 77, 79, 82-83, 211n26

anesthesia, 84, 86

Anglo-Saxon. *See* whiteness

Anthing, Louis, 133

anthropology, 54, 136, 144-45, 185-86

apes: comparisons with Black people, 34, 36, 43, 71-72, 130-31, 136-37, 186; dissection of, 71-72; racial science myths about reproduction with Black people, 35-36

apprenticeships, 15, 20, 26-27, 78, 209n44

Arabbi, Joannis, 225n14

Arkansas, 120

Army Medical Museum (United States), 187

Ashanti people, 136

Atlantic slave trade, 5, 22-23, 131, 134, 138, 152-53, 156-57, 165

Atlantic World, 5, 8, 10, 13, 22-25, 36-38, 49-50, 53-56, 68, 82, 116, 140, 144, 156-57, 163-65

Audubon, John James, 38

autopsy, 50-52, 56, 71, 75-77

Aztec children (Maximo and Bartola) 100-101, 107-8

Baartman, Sara, 132, 136

Bachman, John, 36-42, 46; on fertility of mixed-race people, 38; proslavery beliefs of, 37-38; support for monogenesis, 36-38, 40-42; support for South Carolina's secession, 37-38

Baird, Spencer F., 54

Ball, Dyer, 43-44, 118-19

Baltimore, 70-71, 74, 80, 184, 211n21

Bankole-Medina, Katherine, 201n18

Barbados, 55

Barnard, Alan, 223n32

Barnum, P. T., 76-77, 108, 134

Bartlett, Elisha, 51

Barton, Benjamin Smith, 4, 19-20, 30, 32, 97

Batavia, 168

Bay, Mia, 188

Bayle, Gaspard Laurent, 50-51

Beaumont, William, 86-88

Beckert, Sven, 12, 128

Benin, 138

Berkowitz, Carin, 94-95

Bernard, Claude, 84-85, 88

Berry, Daina Ramey, 11, 69, 211n21, 222n19

Bettner, George S., 75, 212n28

Bichat, Xavier, 50, 215n16

Black people. *See* African descendants

"Bleeding Kansas," 3, 98

Blockley Almshouse, 211n27

bloodletting, 33, 49, 50, 52-53, 83, 176-77

Blumenbach, Johann Friedrich, 36

body snatching, 67-83; from Black cemeteries, 77-78, 80; Black people's resistance to, 77-78; governmental complicity with, 79-80; legality of, 68, 70, 76-77, 81-82; at northern medical schools, 69-80, 211n26; from public graveyards, 79-80; riots in response to, 70, 77, 79, 82-83, 211n26; at southern medical schools, 81-83

Boerhaave, Herman, 208n18

Boers, 133-34

Bogdan, Robert, 216n26

Bonner, J. P., 172

Boston, 16, 39, 60, 75-76, 80, 101, 107-8, 125-26, 132-38, 145

Boston Aquarial and Zoölogical Gardens, 132-33

Boston Phrenological Society, 128, 217-19n49

Boston Society for Medical Improvement, 72, 125-26, 128-29, 137, 187, 217-19n49

Boston Society of Natural History, 136

Boudin, Jean Christian Marc, 165

Bowen, Francis, 74, 211n21

M.D. theses, 1, 8, 12–13, 26, 36, 43–45, 60–61, 67–68, 75, 85, 87–91, 94–96, 115–19, 130–31, 142–43, 151, 157, 170–90, 206–7n102, 213n72, 220n68, 226n15, 228n55, 228n59; experiments on enslaved people discussed in, 87–91; faculty assessment of, 119; racial, supposed, anatomical differences listed in, 115–19, 130–31, 186; about racial science and medicine, 36, 43–44, 60–61, 115–19, 130–31, 142–43, 157, 170–79, 186, 188, 220n68

MDUP. *See* University of Pennsylvania

measles, 69, 88–90, 172

Medical and Surgical Reporter, 1–2, 30, 216n28

Medical Association of Louisiana, 42

Medical College of Alabama, 35, 39–40, 43, 184

Medical College of Ohio, 43, 130, 162

Medical College of South Carolina (MCSC): enslaved cadavers dissected at, 81; medical museum of, 107; pedagogical approach to race at, 35, 43, 107, 118–20, 130, 158–60, 170, 172–78, 182, 215n10, 216n28; student theses from, 1, 12–13, 51–52, 88–91, 118–19, 130, 170, 172–78, 213n72, 228n55

medical journals, 1, 20–21, 28–30, 45, 183; proliferation of, 30, 45; racial science published in, 1–2, 42–43, 45, 202n10

medical licensing, 28–29

medical museums: donation of objects by students and alumni for, 113–14; enslaved people's remains displayed in, 7–8, 11, 13, 109, 137–40, 220–21n4; in Europe, 110–11; medical students use of, 63, 94–95, 101–2, 106, 108–11, 114–15, 121, 185; methods of preparing anatomical objects for, 114; racialized objects in, 7–8, 13, 16, 61, 72, 95, 101, 106, 109–10, 113–15, 119, 125–41, 185; reliance on theft of human remains for, 7–8, 11, 113–14, 125–41; reproductive organs in, 72, 110, 113,

187; skull collections in, 7–8, 13, 95, 101, 109–11, 113, 125–41, 185–87, 217–19n49, 224n37; in the United States, 7–8, 11, 13, 16, 47, 61, 72, 94–95, 101–2, 106–11, 113–15, 119, 121, 125–41, 185–88, 217–19n49, 220–21n4, 224n37

medical profession (United States), 1–3, 5–6, 11–13, 16, 20–21, 26–33, 37, 45–46, 49, 52, 63, 72, 75–76, 79–84, 91–92, 94, 109, 114, 126, 144, 150, 153–54, 159–60, 164, 172, 179, 181–85, 187–88, 191–92, 209n42, 212n50, 220–21n4

medical record books, 52–53

medical regionalism, 159–61, 163, 169, 179–80

medical schools: admittance and exclusion of Black students from, 27–29, 80, 100–101, 130, 183, 185, 187–88; competition among, 25–26; effects of U.S. Civil War on, 16, 27, 105–6, 181–90; exclusion of female students from, 27; founded by Black people, 27, 183; number of graduates from, 27–28; proliferation of, 27–28; requirements to obtain a degree from, 26–27; typical courses offered in, 26

Medical Society of South Carolina, 28–29

medical students: as body snatchers, 67–83; donation of human remains by, 113–14; racial science and medicine theses by, 36, 43–44, 60–61, 115–19, 130–31, 142–43, 157, 170–79, 186, 188, 220n68

medical textbooks: anatomy textbooks, 16, 60–61, 67, 76, 94–101, 114, 215n10, 216n27; craniometry in, 60, 96–100, 118–19; phrenology in, 97; racial discussion of disease in, 4; racial discussion of intelligence in, 98–100; racial discussion of skin in, 97, 215n11

medicine, professionalization of, 2, 11, 31, 60

Meigs, James Aitken, 206n87

Mellichamp, Joseph Hinson, 1, 174–75

Mendizabel, J., 168

menstruation, 173–74

mental illness, 173–75, 179, 229n63

Mexico, 168

microscope, 61

Miller, Newton C., 116–17

Milton, J. H. F., 114

Mississippi, 44–45, 117, 207n105

Mississippi River, 14

Mitchell, Samuel L., 31–33

Mitchell, Silas Weir, 85

Mobile (Alabama), 39–40, 47, 62, 163

monogenesis, 4, 6, 21, 34–38, 43, 116–19, 153, 155–59, 185, 206n98; Christianity's influence on, 6, 21, 117–18; craniometry's influence on, 34–37, 116–19, 185; in M.D. theses, 36, 116–19; relationship to abolitionism, 36–38, 155–57

monogenists. *See* craniometry; monogenesis; Morton, Samuel G.; Nott, Josiah; polygenesis; racial science; skull collectors

Montreal, 211n21

Moreau de Jonnès, Alexandre, 165–67

Morgan, John, 5, 26

Morrill, Henry Edwin, 67–68

Morris (human trafficker), 107

Morton, Samuel G.: anatomical textbook of, 96–97, 99–100, 215n9, 215n10; curated casts of skulls of, 111, 113–14, 120, 220n73; devices for measuring crania of, 58–60, *58, 59,* 63; influence on medical students of, 44, 60–61, 116, 178, 209n44; medical career of, 35, 38, 49–50, 63, 96–97, 145, 206n84, 215n9, 215n10, 216n26; study of Egyptology, 39–40, 178; study of human crania, 39–40, 53–54, 57–62, 111, 113–14, 126–28, 205n81, 220n4; support for polygenesis, 15, 34–36, 38–40, 46; views of Black people, 13–14, 39–40, 96, 205n81; views of Native Americans, 13–14, 57, 96; views on slavery, 55–56, 205n77, 208n28

Morton, William T. G., 86

Moss, Henry, 19–20, 30, 32–33, 142

Moultrie, James, 107

Mount Hope Cemetery, 75–76

Muslim uprising, 8, 137–40; history of, 138–40; human remains stolen from, 137–38; role of Islam in, 138–39

Mussey, Reuben, 80, 130

Mustakeem, Sowande' M., 224n33

Myers, Arthur B., 117–18

Nagô people, 137–39

Namibia, 132

National Medical Association, 183

Native Americans: displacement of, 14–15; genocide of, 14–15, 22–23, 128; healers, 28; racial scientists' fascination with cranial manipulation of, 57, 60, 97; racial theories about, 13–15, 22–25, 120, 128, 175; and virgin soil epidemics, 22–23

naturalists. *See* craniometry; monogenesis; Morton, Samuel G.; Nott, Josiah; polygenesis; racial science; skull collectors

natural history. *See* racial science

natural selection, theory of, 3, 186. *See also* Darwin, Charles

Nazi Germany, 92

Neill, Hollingsworth, 186, 188

Newark (New Jersey), 62

New England Journal of Medicine & Surgery, 75

New Hampshire, 130

New Orleans, 16, 29, 42, 45, 109

newspapers, 29, 40–41, 70, 76, 81, 134–35, 181; body snatching discussed in, 70, 81; racial science discussed in, 40–41; slavery discussed in, 152–53

New York (state), 170, 210n10

New York Alms-House, 31–33

New York City, 25, 31–33, 38, 69–71, 75–78, 80, 164, 182, 184, 211n21, 211n26

New York College of Physicians and Surgeons, 25–26, 31, 73, 76

New York University Medical College, 35, 43, 158
New Zealand, 61
nicotine, 69
Nigeria, 138
Norcom, William A. B., 182
North Carolina, 20
Nott, James E., 164
Nott, Josiah: criticism of, 39–41, 187; discussions of craniometry's limits, 62, 209n50; early life of, 47–48; education at the University of Pennsylvania, 29, 48, 97, 176–77; education in Paris, 47–53; founding of the Medical College of Alabama, 35; medical career of, 15, 29, 35, 61, 150, 182, 184, 206n84, 227n31; opposition to imperialism, 167–70, 179; proslavery politics of, 54–55, 200n14; slave ownership of, 54–55; studies of race and hat size by, 62; support for polygenesis, 34, 39–41, 46–49, 62–63, 127, 163–72; views on race and disease, 163–72, 174–76
numerical method, 50–53, 60, 62–63, 129–30, 136–37, 140–41; in Parisian medicine, 50–53; popularity among U.S. physicians of, 51–52; shortcoming of, 53; use of by racial scientists, 53, 60, 62–63, 129–30, 136–37, 140–41

Okinawa, 129, 221n11
Opium Wars, 8, 125, 140, 220n1
orangutans. *See* apes
Orisha, 138
Osgood, David, 162
Otis, J. H., 129
Ottoman Empire, 57
Owen, Richard, 102
Oxford University, 128–29

Pacific World, 187
Paris, 15, 29, 47–53, 62–63, 85, 87–89, 91, 132, 136, 159; American medical students in, 47–53, 63, 159; and

clinical medicine, 47–53, 62–63, 85; as home to racial scientists, 15, 48–49; hospitals in, 50–51, 87–89, 91; medical museum objects sold in, 47, 49
pathology, 51, 53, 97, 116, 142
Paxson, William, 174
Peabody Museum of Archaeology and Anthropology, 136
Peale's museum, 71–72
Pearl River, 125–26
Penn, Nigel, 222n21, 222–23n23
Pennsylvania, 27, 30, 41, 70, 78–79; abolition of slavery in, 27, 70
Pennsylvania Medical College, 38, 43, 96
Pepick (Winnebago chief), 129
Peru, 24, 60, 111, 127–29; skulls of Native Americans stolen from, 60, 111, 127–29
Perry, Matthew, 129
Phelps, Edward E., 80
Philadelphia, 1, 5, 13, 19–20, 29, 38–39, 41, 45, 61, 69, 75, 79–80, 85, 96, 111, 117, 164, 176, 181, 183, 186, 204n46; as center of U.S. medical education, 1, 5, 13, 29, 38, 45, 69, 96, 117, 181, 183, 204n46; as center of U.S. racial science, 38–39, 41, 61, 111
Philadelphia Abolition Society, 226n12
Philadelphia Almshouse, 75, 176
Philippines, 189
Phrenological Association, 39
phrenology, 39, 60, 97, 107, 119, 128, 186, 200n10, 217–19n49, 220n69, 222n20
phthisis, 13, 75, 171
physicians, allopathic: as racial experts in courts, 31–33, 93–94, 119–20; in slave markets, 54
physiognomy, 6, 19, 178
physiology, 24, 43, 48, 53, 84–91, 95, 97, 107, 117, 162, 173–74, 180; and experimentation on live subjects, 84–91; and racial science, 24, 43, 48, 89–90, 97, 107, 117, 162, 173–74, 180
Pickering, Charles, 100–101, 145; *The Races of Man*, 104-6, *106*

Tulloch (British major), 167

Turner, Nat, 81, 98, 109

Turner, Sasha, 226n13

Tuskegee syphilis experiments, 92, 188

Types of Mankind (Nott and Gliddon), 40–41, 62, 206n84, 206n87; national appeal of, 41; in popular culture, 41

typhoid fever, 51, 157–58, 172–73, 228n55, 228n57

typhus fever, 162, 228n55

United Fruit Company, 189–90

United States Exploring Expedition, 104–5, 145

universities (non-medical), 11–12, 20, 126, 190

University of Alabama at Birmingham. *See* Medical College of Alabama

University of Edinburgh, 36–38, 155–56, 208n18

University of Göttingen, 36

University of Leiden, 208n18

University of Louisiana, 35, 39–40, 43, 100, 216n23

University of Louisville, 35, 43, 100

University of Nashville, 13, 116–17, 177

University of Pennsylvania (MDUP), 1–6, 13, 19–20, 25–27, 29–30, 33, 35, 37–38, 40, 43–45, 47–48, 60, 67, 70, 72, 75–76, 79, 83, 85, 93–94, 96–98, 101, 104, 113–15, 117, 119, 128, 130, 142, 152, 170–72, 174, 177, 181–82, 186, 216n27, 216n28, 219n63, 220n68, 225–26n8, 228n55; Black cadavers used at, 67, 70, 72, 75–76; class sizes of medical department, 1, 6; geographic origins of student body, 2, 20–21, 45; pedagogical approach to race in the medical department at, 2, 4–5, 19, 33, 44, 67, 93–94, 96, 98, 101,113, 115, 117, 119, 128, 130, 142, 152, 157, 161, 165, 170–72, 174, 177, 184, 215n10, 216n27, 216n28, 219n63, 220n68, 225–26n8, 228n55

University of Vermont, 80

University of Virginia (UVA), 13, 43, 106–7, 181, 184–85, 190–91; after the Civil War, 184–85; in the present, 190–91; racial pedagogy at, 13, 43, 106–7

UVA. *See* University of Virginia

Valenčius, Conevery, 225–26n8

variolation, 88–89

vesicovaginal fistula, 213n65

Virginia, 19, 30, 39, 43, 69, 81, 90, 109, 130–31, 144–46, 148, 174, 177, 181, 184

Virginia and Maryland Medical and Surgical Reporter, 30

vitiligo, 142–43

vivisection, 85

Voltaire, 24

Wake Forest University, 74

Walker, Joseph, 128

Ward, H. A., 129

Warren, John Collins, 49, 51, 57, 60, 107, 111, 120, 127–28, 162–64, 211n21, 217–19n49, 221n7

Warren, Jonathan Mason, 107–8

Warren Anatomical Museum, 8, 61, 102, *110*, 110–11, 113, 125–42, 186, 217–19n49; national skulls in, 111, 113, 125–42, 186, 217–19n49

Washington, D.C., 146

Washington, Harriet, 12, 230n9

Waterhouse, Benjamin, 34

Weathersbee, W., 173

Webster, James, 79–80

Western Reserve College, 40

West Indies, 32, 55, 145, 165, 167–68

Westmoreland, Theophilus, 116–17

Whistelo, Alexander, 31–32

White, Charles, 34–35, 111

whiteness, 27, 31, 34–35, 54, 93, 165

white supremacy, 2, 20, 48, 94, 95–97, 102, 105–6, 108–11, 113, 116–17, 120, 127, 131, 137, 141, 156, 173, 179, 185

Wilder, Craig Steven, 11–12

Williams, Lucy, 31–32

Wisconsin, 114

Wistar, Caspar, 96–98, 100, 215n10, 215n11

Wood, George Bacon, 4, 170

Worboys, Michael, 209n42

World War II, 86

Wyman, Jeffries, 16, 35, 39, 49, 62–63, 72, 74, 136–37, 142–51, 184–85, 211n21, 224n7, 225n14; description of Sturmann's remains, 136–37; expedition to Suriname, 144–50, 225n14; experience at Hampden-Sydney College, 39, 81, 143–46; observations of enslaved people, 16, 145–49; racial science of, 63, 72, 136–37; views on slavery, 16, 74

yellow fever, 5, 25, 88–90, 153–54, 162, 165, 168, 171–73, 175, 177–79, 189–90, 228n5; relationship to climate, 5, 89–90, 154, 168, 171, 175, 179, 189–90; supposed resistance of Black people to, 25, 89–90, 153–54, 162, 165, 168, 171–73, 175, 177–79, 189, 228n5

Yorubaland, 138

Yoruba people, 136

Zemurray, Samuel, 189–90

Printed in the USA
CPSIA information can be obtained
at www.ICGtesting.com
CBHW031344020424
6250CB00002B/63

9 781469 672120